HQ
764
S
2000
2009

SERIES EDITOR

K. Warner Schaie
Evan Pugh Professor of Human Development and Psychology
College of Health and Human Development
The Pennsylvania State University
University Park, PA

Affiliate Professor of Psychiatry and Behavioral Science
University of Washington
Seattle, WA

2008 Social Structures and Aging Individuals: Continuing Challenges
K. Warner Schaie and Ronald P. Abeles, Editors

2007 Social Structures: Demographic Changes and the Well-Being of
Older Persons
K. Warner Schaie and Peter Uhlenberg, Editors

2006 Social Structures, Aging, and Self-Regulation in the Elderly
K. Warner Schaie and Laura L. Carstensen, Editors

2005 Historical Influences on Lives and Aging
K. Warner Schaie and Glen H. Elder, Jr., Editors

2004 Religious Influences on Health and Well-Being in the Elderly
K. Warner Schaie, Neal Krause, and Alan Booth, Editors

2003 Impact of Technology on Successful Aging
Neil Charness and K. Warner Schaie, Editors

2002 Personal Control in Social and Life Course Contexts
Steven H. Zarit, Leonard I. Pearlin, and K. Warner Schaie, Editors

2002 Effective Health Behavior in Older Adults
K. Warner Schaie, Howard Leventhal, and Sherry L. Willis, Editors

2000 The Evolution of the Aging Self: The Societal Impact on the
Aging Process
K. Warner Schaie and Jon Hendricks, Editors

2000 Mobility and Transportation in the Elderly
K. Warner Schaie and Martin Pietrucha, Editors

1998 Impact of Work on Older Adults
K. Warner Schaie and Carmi Schooler, Editors

1997 Societal Mechanisms for Maintaining Competence in Old Age
Sherry L. Willis, K. Warner Schaie, and Mark Hayward, Editors

1996 Older Adults' Decision-Making and the Law
Michael Smyer, K. Warner Schaie, and Marshall B. Kapp, Editors

Social Structures and Aging Individuals

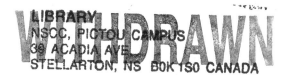

K. Warner Schaie, PhD, is the Evan Pugh Professor of Human Development and Psychology at the Pennsylvania State University. He also holds an appointment as affiliate professor of psychiatry and behavioral science at the University of Washington. He received his PhD in psychology from the University of Washington, an honorary DrPhil from the Friedrich-Schiller University of Jena, Germany, and an honorary ScD degree from West Virginia University. He received the Kleemeier Award for Distinguished Research Contributions from the Gerontological Society of America, the MENSA Lifetime Career Award, and the Distinguished Scientific Contributions Award from the American Psychological Association. He is author or editor of 54 books, including the textbook *Adult Development and Aging* (5th ed., with S. L. Willis, 2002) and the *Handbook of the Psychology of Aging* (6th ed., with J. E. Birren, 2006). He has directed the Seattle Longitudinal Study of cognitive aging since 1956 and is the author of more than 325 journal articles and chapters on the psychology of aging. His current research interests are the life course of adult intelligence, its antecedents and modifiability, the early detection of risk for dementia, and methodological issues in the developmental sciences.

Ronald P. Abeles, PhD, is a special assistant to the director of the Office of Behavioral and Social Sciences Research in the Office of the Director at the National Institutes of Health (NIH). From 1994 to 1998, he served as the associate director for behavioral and social research at the National Institute on Aging (BSR/NIA). Previously, he served at BSR/NIA as the deputy associate director (1980–1991) and acting associate director (1991–1994). He received the NIH Award of Merit twice for "leadership and contributions to the advancement of behavioral and social research on aging within the Federal Government and nationally" (1993) and for "exceptional leadership in advancing a program of research to understand and apply knowledge about the relationship between psychosocial factors and health" (2002).

Dr. Abeles has been instrumental in fostering behavioral and social research throughout the NIH. From 1980 to 1993, he served as the executive secretary and acting chair of the ad hoc NIH Working Group on Health and Behavior. From 1993 to the present, he was first the vice chair and then the chair of the NIH Health and Behavior Coordinating Committee and then of its successor, the NIH Behavioral and Social Sciences Research Coordinating Committee. The committee facilitates behavioral and social research across the NIH and is an advisory group to the director of the Office of Behavioral and Social Sciences Research. For these activities, he received the NIH Director's Award in 1990.

From June 1992 to October 1994, he served as the executive secretary for the congressionally mandated Task Force on Aging Research, which prepared recommendations on aging-related research by federal agencies for submission to the secretary, the U.S. Department of Health and Human Services, and Congress. He is a founding member (1985–2001) of the Advisory Panel on Behavioral and Social Sciences and the Humanities for the Brookdale National Fellowship Program in Gerontology, a founding member (1996) of and senior consultant (1997–) to the Board of Trustees (Kuratorium) of the German Center for Aging Research (Deutsches Zentrum für Alternsforschung, Heidelberg), and was cochair of the German–American Academic Council's project on Gerontological Research in Germany and the U.S.: Towards Intensified Cooperation and Future Strategies.

Dr. Abeles has held elected offices in the aging sections of the American Psychological Association (APA) and the American Sociological Association (ASA). He was the chair (1999–2000) and newsletter editor (1988–2002) of the ASA's Section on Aging and the Life Course. He was twice the program chair of the APA's Division (20) on Adult Development and Aging (1990 and 2000) and was its president (2001–2002). He is a Fellow of the APA, the American Psychological Society, the Society of Behavioral Medicine, and the Gerontological Society of America. In 2004, the APA presented him with its Meritorious Research Service Commendation, and APA Division 38 honored him with its Career Service to Health Psychology Award.

His 1971 doctoral degree in social psychology (with a minor in sociology) is from the Department of Social Relations, Harvard University. His experience as a staff associate at the Social Science Research Council (1974–1978) for the Committee on Work and Personality in the Middle Years and the Committee on Life Course Development stimulated his interest in life course issues. He has organized several symposia at the annual meetings of professional societies, published chapters, and edited books on various aspects of life course and aging research, most frequently in regard to sense of control and to the interface between social structure and behavior. He is the editor of *Life-span Perspectives and Social Psychology* (1987), the coeditor of *Aging, Health, and Behavior* (1993) and of *Aging and Quality of Life* (Springer, 1994), and an associate editor of three editions of *Handbook of the Psychology of Aging* (4th ed., 1996; 5th ed., 2001; 6th ed., 2006).

Social Structures and Aging Individuals

Continuing Challenges

K. WARNER SCHAIE, PhD

RONALD P. ABELES, PhD

Editors

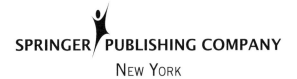

SPRINGER PUBLISHING COMPANY

NEW YORK

Springer Publishing Company, LLC
11 West 42nd Street
New York, NY 10036
www.springerpub.com

Acquisitions Editor: Sheri W. Sussman
Production Editor: Julia Rosen
Cover design: Joanne E. Honigman
Composition: Apex Publishing, LLC

07 08 09 10/ 5 4 3 2 1

Library of Congress Cataloging-in-Publication Data

Social structures and aging individuals : continuing challenges / K. Warner Schaie, Ronald P. Abeles, editors.

    p. cm.
  Includes bibliographical references and index.
  ISBN 978-0-8261-2408-1 (alk. paper)
  1. Aging—Social aspects—United States—Congresses.   2. Aging—Psychological aspects—Congresses.   3. Life cycle, Human—Social aspects—Congresses.   I. Schaie, K. Warner (Klaus Warner), 1928–
II. Abeles, Ronald P., 1944–
  HQ1064.U5S5982 2008

   305.260973—dc22   2008009537

Printed in the United States of America by Lightning Source.

Contents

Contributors

W. Andrew Achenbaum, PhD
Professor of History and Social Work
University of Houston
Houston, TX

David M. Almeida, PhD
Associate Professor
Gerontology Center
The Pennsylvania State University
University Park, PA

Vern L. Bengtson, PhD
AARP University Professor
of Gerontology
Professor of Sociology
Director, Division of Social and
Behavioral Services Research
Andrus Gerontology Center
University of Southern California
Los Angeles, CA

Fredda Blanchard-Fields, PhD
Professor of Psychology
Director, Adult Development
Laboratory
Georgia Institute of Technology
School of Psychology
Atlanta, GA

Michelle L. Bragg, PhD
Research Associate
Human Development and
Family Studies
The Pennsylvania State University
University Park, PA

Chalandra M. Bryant, PhD
Associate Professor
Human Development and
Family Studies
The Pennsylvania State University
University Park, PA

Leslie J. Caplan, PhD
Staff Scientist
National Institute of Mental Health
Division of Intramural Research
Programs
Section on Socio-Environmental
Studies
Bethesda, MD

Nathan Carlin, MS
Graduate Assistant
Department of Religious Studies
Rice University
Houston, TX

Laura L. Carstensen, PhD
Director, Stanford Center on
Longevity
Professor of Psychology
Stanford University
Stanford, CA

Susan Turk Charles, PhD
Associate Professor
Department of Psychology & Social
Behavior
University of California, Irvine
Irvine, CA

Neil Charness, PhD
William G. Chase Professor
of Psychology
Associate, Pepper Institute on
Aging and Public Policy
Florida State University
Tallahassee, FL

Thomas Cole, PhD
Professor and Director
Center for Health, Humanities, and
the Human Spirit
Houston School of Medicine
University of Texas
Houston, TX

Casey E. Copen
University of Southern California
Los Angeles, CA

Dale Dannefer, PhD
Selah Chamberlain Professor
of Sociology
Chair, Department of Sociology
Case Western Reserve University
Cleveland, OH

David J. Ekerdt, PhD
Professor of Sociology
Director, Gerontology Center
University of Kansas
Lawrence, KS

James L. Farr, PhD
Professor of Psychology
The Pennsylvania State University
University Park, PA

Christine L. Fry, PhD
Professor of Anthropology, Emerita
Loyola University of Chicago
Chicago, IL

Mark D. Hayward, PhD
Director, Population Research Center
and Department of Sociology

University of Texas at Austin
Austin, TX

Rukmalie Jayakody, PhD
Associate Professor
Department of Human Development
and Family Studies
Population Research Institute
The Pennsylvania State University
University Park, PA

Neal Krause, PhD
Professor of Health Behavior and
Health Education
School of Public Health and Senior
Research Scientist
Health Behavior and Health
Education
Survey Research Center
Institute of Gerontology
University of Michigan
Ann Arbor, MI

Elaine A. Leventhal, MD, PhD
Internal Medicine
Robert Wood Johnson University
Medical Group
School of Medicine
University of Medicine and Dentistry
of New Jersey
New Brunswick, NJ

Howard Leventhal, PhD
Board of Governors
Professor of Health Psychology
Institute for Health, Health Care
Policy and Aging Research
Rutgers, the State University
of New Jersey
New Brunswick, NJ

Casey Lindberg
Graduate Student
Department of Psychology
Stanford University
Stanford, CA

Sylvia Morelli
Graduate Student
University of California, Los Angeles
Los Angeles, CA

Tamara J. Musumeci, MS
Postdoctoral Fellow
Institute for Health, Health Care
Policy and Aging Research
Rutgers, the State University
of New Jersey
New Brunswick, NJ

Shevaun D. Neupert, PhD
Department of Psychology
North Carolina State University
Raleigh, NC

Norella M. Putney
College of Letters Arts and Sciences
University of Southern California
Los Angeles, CA

Nilam Ram, PhD
Assistant Professor

Human Development and
Family Studies
The Pennsylvania State University
University Park, PA

Carmi Schooler, PhD
Chief of Section on
Socioenvironmental Studies
Socio-Environmental Studies
Division of Intramural Research
Programs
National Institute of
Mental Health
Bethesda, MD

Alexander R. Schwall
Graduate Student, Psychology
The Pennsylvania State University
University Park, PA

Merril Silverstein, PhD
Leonard Davis School of
Gerontology
University of Southern California
Los Angeles, CA

Preface

This is the 20th and final volume in a series on the broad topic of the societal impact on aging. Lawrence Erlbaum Associates published the first five volumes of this series under the series title Social Structures and Aging. The present volume is the 15th published under the Springer Publishing Company imprint. It is the edited proceedings of a conference held at the Pennsylvania State University, October 9–10, 2006.

The series of Penn State Gerontology Center conferences originated from the deliberations of a subcommittee of the Committee on Life Course Perspectives of the Social Science Research Council, chaired by Matilda White Riley, in the early 1980s. That subcommittee was charged with developing an agenda and mechanisms that would serve to encourage communication between scientists who study societal structures that might affect the aging of individuals and those scientists who are concerned with the possible effects of contextual influences on individual aging. The committee proposed a series of conferences that would systematically explore the interfaces between social structures and behavior, and in particular, identify mechanisms through which society influences adult development. When the first editor was named director of the Penn State Gerontology Center in 1985, he was able to implement this conference program as one of the center's major activities. Matilda Riley attended the first few conferences in this series, and we are reprinting in this volume her preface to the first (1989) book emanating from it.

The previous 19 volumes in this series have dealt with the societal impact on aging in psychological processes (Schaie & Schooler, 1989); age structuring in comparative perspective (Kertzer & Schaie, 1989); self-directedness and efficacy over the life span (Rodin, Schooler, & Schaie, 1990); aging, health behaviors, and health outcomes (Schaie, Blazer, & House, 1992); caregiving in families (Zarit, Pearlin, & Schaie, 1993); aging in historical perspective (Schaie & Achenbaum, 1993); adult intergenerational relations (Bengtson, Schaie, & Burton, 1995); older adults' decision making and the law (Smyer, Schaie, & Kapp, 1996); the impact of social structures on decision making in the elderly (Willis, Schaie, & Hayward, 1997); the impact of the workplace on aging (Schaie & Schooler, 1998); mobility and transportation in the elderly (Schaie & Pietrucha, 2000); the evolution of the aging self (Schaie & Hendricks, 2000); societal impact on health behavior in the elderly (Schaie, Leventhal, & Willis, 2002); mastery and control in the elderly (Zarit, Pearlin, & Schaie, 2002); impact of technology on the elderly (Charness & Schaie, 2003); religious influences on health and well-being in the elderly (Schaie, Krause, & Booth, 2004); historical influences on lives and aging (Schaie & Elder, 2005); the impact of social structures on self-regulation in the elderly (Schaie & Carstensen, 2006); and demographic changes and the well-being of older persons (Schaie & Uhlenberg, 2007).

The strategy for each of these volumes has been to commission reviews on three major topics by established subject matter specialists who have credibility in aging research. We then invited two formal discussants for each chapter—usually, one drawn from the writer's discipline and one from a neighboring discipline. This format has provided a suitable antidote against the perpetuation of parochial orthodoxies and made certain that questions are raised in regard to the validity of iconoclastic departures in new directions.

To focus each conference, the organizers chose three aspects of the conference theme that were thought to be of broad interest to gerontologists. Social and behavioral scientists with a demonstrated track record were then selected and asked to interact with those interested in theory building within a multidisciplinary context.

The present volume reviews what has been learned as part of this series over the past two decades, but it also focuses on the continuing challenges for older persons in a rapidly changing society and tries to forecast what may be the next set of issues that may become important in the future at the intersection of social structures and the individual aging process. To do so, we invited a number of prominent scientists who have previously served as organizers and/or who have made significant contributions to the series. The resulting chapters in this volume therefore review both the accomplishments and omissions of our efforts, add some new timely topics, and provide guidelines for future research and theoretical explanations.

The volume begins with a conceptual and theoretical review of the theme that runs through the entire series (Dale Dannefer). We then organize the substantive material grouped by the themes of previous volumes into five broad topics. The first, addressed in volumes 4, 13, and 16, deals with the general topic of health and well-being, including the role of religion (Howard Leventhal, Tamara J. Musumeci, Elaine A. Leventhal, Neal Krause, David M. Almeida, Susan Turk Charles, and Shavaun D. Neupert). The second topic, addressed in volumes 1, 10, 11, and 15, reviews material on personality and cognition (Nilam Ram, Sylvia Morelli, Casey Lindberg, Laura L. Carstensen, Carmi Schooler, Leslie J. Caplan, and Fredda Blanchard-Fields). The third topic, addressed in volumes 2, 6, 17, and 19, deals with issues related to the impact of changes in technology and the workplace (Neil Charness, David J. Ekerdt, James L. Farr, and Alexander R. Schwall). The fourth topic deals with issues of sociocultural change and historical context (Thomas Cole, W. Andrew Achenbaum, Nathan Carlin, Christine L. Fry, and Rukmalie Jayakody). The fifth and final topic, addressed in volumes 5, 7, 8, and 9, provides examples of the family and societal context of aging (Vern L. Bengtson, Casey E. Copen, Norella M. Putney, Merril Silverstein, Mark D. Hayward, Chalandra M. Bryant, and Michelle L. Bragg).

We are grateful for the financial support of the conference that led to this volume, which was provided by conference grant R13 AG 09787 from the National Institute on Aging and by additional support from the College of Health and Human Development of the Pennsylvania State University. We are also grateful to Chriss Schultz for handling the conference logistics and to Jenifer Hoffman for coordinating the manuscript preparation.

K. Warner Schaie
January 2008

REFERENCES

Bengtson, V., Schaie, K. W., & Burton, L. K. (Eds.). (1995). *Adult intergenerational relations: Effects of societal change.* New York: Springer Publishing.

Charness, N., & Schaie, K. W. (Eds.). (2003). *Impact of technology on successful aging.* New York: Springer Publishing.

Kertzer, D., & Schaie, K. W. (Eds.). (1989). *Age structuring in comparative perspective.* Hillsdale, NJ: Erlbaum.

Rodin, J., Schooler, C., & Schaie, K. W. (Eds.). (1990). *Self-directedness and efficacy: Causes and effects throughout the life course.* Hillsdale, NJ: Erlbaum.

Schaie, K. W., & Achenbaum, W. A. (Eds.). (1993). *Societal impact on aging: Historical perspectives.* New York: Springer Publishing.

Schaie, K. W., Blazer D., & House, J. S. (Eds.). (1992). *Aging, health behaviors, and health outcomes.* Hillsdale, NJ: Erlbaum.

Schaie, K. W., & Carstensen, L. L. (Eds.). (2006). *Social structures, aging, and self-regulation in the elderly.* New York: Springer Publishing.

Schaie, K. W., & Elder, G. H., Jr. (Eds.). (2005). *Historical influences on lives and aging.* New York: Springer Publishing.

Schaie, K. W., & Hendricks, J. (Eds.). (2000). *The evolution of the aging self: The societal impact on the aging process.* New York: Springer Publishing.

Schaie, K. W., Krause, N., & Booth, A. (Eds.). (2004). *Religious influences on health and well-being in the elderly.* New York: Springer Publishing.

Schaie, K. W., Leventhal, H., & Willis, S. L. (Eds.). (2002). *Effective health behavior in older adults.* New York: Springer Publishing.

Schaie, K. W., & Pietrucha, M. (Eds.). (2000). *Mobility and transportation in the elderly.* New York: Springer Publishing.

Schaie, K. W., & Schooler, C. (Eds.). (1989). *Social structure and aging: Psychological processes.* Hillsdale, NJ: Erlbaum.

Schaie, K. W., & Schooler, C. (Eds.). (1998). *Impact of work on older adults.* New York: Springer Publishing.

Schaie, K. W., & Uhlenberg, P. (Eds.). (2007). *Social structures: Demographic changes and the well-being of older persons.* New York: Springer Publishing.

Smyer, M., Schaie, K. W., & Kapp, M. B. (Eds.). (1996). *Older adults' decision-making and the law.* New York: Springer Publishing.

Willis, S. L., Schaie, K. W., & Hayward, M. (Eds.). (1997). *Societal mechanisms for maintaining competence in old age.* New York: Springer Publishing.

Zarit, S. H., Pearlin, L., & Schaie, K. W. (Eds.). (1993). *Social structure and caregiving: Family and cross-national perspectives.* Hillsdale, NJ: Erlbaum.

Zarit, S. H., Pearlin, L. I., & Schaie, K. W. (Eds.). (2002). *Personal control in social and life course contexts.* New York: Springer Publishing.

Why This Book?

MATILDA WHITE RILEY
NATIONAL INSTITUTE ON AGING

A law enacted by Congress in mid-October 1986 symbolizes the changes of concern to us in this book. Congress voted that employers can no longer require workers to retire when they reach age 70 (with certain exceptions such as police officers and college professors). As Senator Heinz put it, this act does not end discrimination, but it does "guarantee freedom of choice, and sends strong messages to older workers that we do value their contributions" (Roberts, 1986, p. 33). In itself, of course, the act will affect only small numbers of people. But it may well portend a reversal of the century-long decline in labor force participation of men over 65.

Today we can look upon the act as a change in social structure made possible by psychological changes in attitudes of members of more recent cohorts. These changes precipitate ways in which some people will now spend their later years. The act illustrates the dialectical relationship implicit in the topic before us: social structure and the psychological aging processes.

On behalf of all participants in the conferences on social structures and aging, from which this book results, I want to express appreciation to Pennsylvania State University and to Warner Schaie in collaboration with Carmi Schooler for giving us the opportunity to discuss this topic. This book is the first in a series that will be adapted from conferences on biological as well as social and psychological aging. The conference grew out of several planning meetings of the Social Science Research Council. Those meetings were built on some 10 years of work done by the council's Committee on Life-Course Perspective (of which I was chairperson and with which Ronald Abeles and several of us at the conference were involved). Thus, we do not approach our topic de novo; rather, we are engaged in a scientific effort that has been and continues to be cumulative.

Our major objective within this series is to improve understanding of aging over the life course through

- Integrated conceptualizations that will bring together the relevant disciplines
- Research agenda that will lead to greater specification and clarification
- Improved methods that will be used for conducting the needed research
- Development of a knowledge base that will guide public policy and professional practice

In pursuit of this objective to enhance the scientific understanding of aging, our Social Science Research Council Planning Committee called for a series of conferences that would *view life-course development as interdependent with social structure and social change.* Three sets of interrelated variables were identified:

1. Processes of *aging* (or development), that is, aspects of the ways in which people grow older biologically, psychologically, and socially.
2. Age-related *social structures* and social changes, which include (a) *roles* (e.g., work roles, political roles) with their associated expectations, facilities, and rewards or punishments; (b) *values* that are built into these structures (i.e., standards of what is true, good, beautiful); and (c) *other people* who interact and are interrelated within these structures.
3. *Linkages,* that is, mechanisms that link aging processes with changing social structures. Such mechanism may be (a) psychological (e.g., coping, self-esteem, sense of personal control); (b) biological (e.g., changes in neural, sensorimotor, endocrine, immunological and other physiological systems that can impact directly on the aging process); (c) social (e.g., supportive or hostile relationships, opportunities or constraints affecting productive performance).

The planned series of books taken from these conferences thus focus on the nature of the interdependence among these three sets of variables.

For our deliberations here in this book—with our selected focus on the relationship between psychological aging processes and social structures—I see a twofold challenge: first, to *specify* these relationships and be done with abstract and global statements; second, to recognize the relationships as one of *dialectical interdependence,* that is, to recognize that social structure is both cause and consequence of psychological aging processes.

In regard to the first challenge, *specification* of the relationship, we all look forward to reports of current research work. Many scholars who have already made early contributions are with us today. For example, Warner Schaie and Sherry Willis have taught us a great deal about *what* psychological aging processes result in optimal performance in old age; Melvin Kohn and Carmi Schooler have shown *what* aspects of social structure lead to enhanced functioning; Alice Rossi has described *what* aspects of family structure relate to individual development; and so on. We need only read the table of contents to recognize the many contributions that relate to what aspects of psychological aging processes and the formulating testable hypotheses about the connecting *linkages.*

Even more exciting, I believe (although this is often overlooked), is my second challenge: to recognize and clarify the *dialectical interdependence* between social structure and psychological aging processes. This requires that we examine over time the interplay between aging individuals who are influenced *by* social structure and social structures that are *constructed,* as well as changed, by aging individuals. For example, the recent legislation abolishing mandatory retirement, a structural change, might be attributed to a shift in the predominate patterns of psychological aging, that is, a shift from a passive to an active orientation, from a widespread willingness for disengagement to a growing assertion of personal control. This and similar structural changes could markedly alter patterns of aging in the future. As one instance of such change, imagine what it would mean if older people were no longer stereotyped as universally incompetent (not a trivial suggestion)!

With these challenges in mind, the work resulting in this book constitutes an important beginning toward guiding future changes. This book, like those to follow, can help us formulate clearly specified hypotheses and examine them from the differing perspectives of multiple disciplines. I am proud to have participated in and opened the conference at Pennsylvania State University not only on behalf of the Social Science Research Council's Planning Committee but also for the National Institute on Aging, which supports such interdisciplinary work.

REFERENCE

Roberts, S. V. (1986). House votes to end mandatory retirement rules. *New York Times*, October 18, p. 33.

Introductory Overview

The Waters We Swim: Everyday Social Processes, Macrostructural Realities, and Human Aging

DALE DANNEFER

HUMAN NATURE AND HUMAN AGING: SOME FOUNDATIONAL PRINCIPLES

The project of understanding human development and human aging must be founded on a clear conception of human nature. The most central elements of this foundation concern the distinctive character of the human species and of human beings as living systems. The character of *Homo sapiens* involves sustained and profound interactions between individual and context, and a strong emphasis on context has been reflected in the Social Structure and Aging series over the past 20 years. I begin by sketching some of the key features of *Homo sapiens* that account for the exceptional importance of the role of context and the features of the organism that dictate particular modes of relating to context.

The Irreducible Sociality of *Homo Sapiens*

We are, of course, concerned primarily about aging, but human aging derives from the distinctive characteristics of the human species that are

Acknowledgments: I wish to thank Ron Abeles, Elaine Dannefer, Jonathan Micahel Dannefer, Susan Hinze, Robin Shura Patterson, Peter Uhlenberg, and Warner Schaie for suggestions and comments on an earlier version of this chapter.

present at the beginning and remain relevant throughout the life course. Thus, to understand the character of human aging, it will be useful also to consider how one becomes a young person. It does not just happen, and it clearly does not happen on one's own. It is trite to say the human being is a social product, yet the degree to which human individuals are shaped by experience, relationships, and cultural practices is something that is typically underestimated not only by the lay public, but also by social and behavioral scientists. We know this from many different kinds of evidence. Some of the most dramatic indicators of the depths to which human behavior relies on the internalization of social patterns come from those few and tragic cases of young human individuals who are truly on their own and deprived of human contact: feral children.

Consider Victor, the wild boy of Aveyron. More than two centuries after his capture in 1800, Victor still represents the best-documented and most influential case of a true feral child (Lane, 1976; Newton, 2003; Shattuck, 1994). Although he had a human body, Victor hardly seemed to be a human being when captured at about age 12 in the village of St. Sernin, in the French Pyrenees. Not just in manners and interests, but in perception, motor skills, and requirements for food and physical comfort, this child was extraordinary. Victor's posture and gait, his interests and daily rhythms, and his curious mix of physical abilities and limitations all made it clear that Victor had a unique perceptual apparatus and that his body had developed into a markedly different organism than that of a socialized human being. He was thought to be deaf because he paid no attention whatsoever to sounds to which humans would impute meaning, until it was discovered that he was highly attentive even to relatively faint sounds if they were relevant to his interests, such as nuts being cracked in another room. He had no interest in human comforts such as a warm bed on a cold winter night, preferring to crouch underneath in a thin nightshirt. Victor also liked to run naked in the snow, with no manifestation of being bothered by the cold. The differences extended to the musculoskeletal: his fingers would bend in every direction, providing exceptional dexterity and efficacy in such motor tasks as shucking peas and beans. On capture, Victor wanted only raw potatoes, roots, and nuts to eat, causing amazement among the doctors observing him and the capabilities of his digestive system. Victor was also observed to have an uncanny, eerily intense obsession with the moon and the wind (Lane, 1976).

Victor had apparently grown up for at least much, if not all, of his childhood in mountain forests, either all alone or with animals. This and other similar cases of feral children (Maclean, 1978; Newton, 2003) with remarkably similar behavioral patterns, including well-documented recent ones (Perry & Svalavitz, 2006) reveal the profound extent to which being human relies on the sustained immediacy of experience in a social context, and how the particular tastes and abilities one develops are provided by experience in the context.

The Flexibility of the Human Organism

Such cases are as close as the behavioral and social sciences can come to experimental conditions demonstrating the extraordinary flexibility of the human organism. At the beginning of the life course, flexibility is augmented by *exterogestation* (Montagu, 1989), a term referring to the fact that human birth occurs decidedly early compared to other species. If human neonates were as mature at birth as other species, gestation would last 21 months (Berger & Luckmann, 1967; Gould, 1977; Portmann, 1961). However, flexibility is not limited to the early years. It continues throughout the life course and is reflected in the distinctly human possibilities of lifelong learning, playfulness, and responsiveness that are reflected in the terms *neoteny* and *juvenescence* (Bromhall, 2003; Dannefer, 1999; Gould, 1977; Montagu, 1989), which refer to the childlike physical and developmental features of human adults. Age-related change in human beings thus always occurs in a social environment, and through the processes of socialization, human beings take on the particular character of their social environment.

It is thus crucially important to begin with a recognition that human beings are not hard-wired in the kind of deterministic sense that many other species are, and that provides the paradigmatic template of the organismic theory (Lerner & Walls, 2001; Reese & Overton, 1970). Humans are, instead, *hard-wired for flexibility*; we are "biologically cultural" (Rogoff, 2002, 2003, p. 63). As Berger and Luckmann (1967) emphasized earlier, this is one of the most central and distinctive aspects of human nature, and it is why others have suggested speaking of human *natures* rather than human nature (Ehrlich, 2000).

It is understandable that we are generally unaware of the profound dependency of human nature on social context or the degree to which patterns of physical and psychological as well as social aging are shaped by context. Individual human beings typically grow up in a local setting of taken-for-granted and largely unreflective routines. Processes of individual development and aging occur gradually over long sweeps of time and rarely are experienced directly as change. Reflecting on this circumstance brings to mind the assertion, often attributed to Marshall McLuhan, that "we don't know who discovered water, but we're certain it wasn't a fish." So it is with the force of social life in human development and aging. Everyday social relations are the invisible and unnoticed water we swim.

The water of social relationships and cultural practices that constitute our existence as human beings is not just a matter of childhood. Such practices govern most of daily life, organizing activity in the domains of work, family, and personal life; consumer and leisure activity, and so on. Indeed, these categories themselves reflect historically recent social arrangements: Work, family, and leisure were not experienced as segmented spheres of experience prior to the development of mercantilism and industrialization (Cott, 1997; Laslett, 2004). Of course, the regulation of individual activity by social expectations and practices extends to those most authentically felt by the individual, including culinary and other aesthetic preferences, sexual practices, religious beliefs and practices, and so on.

Thus human individuals continue to be shaped by social relations and by cultural practices throughout the life course, including through advanced old age. These effects clearly extend to the physical, as evidenced by cultural differences in health related to dietary and exercise practices. They also extend to age-related change in characteristics earlier assumed to be inevitable and universal concomitants of aging such as hypertension (Dressler, 1999; Fleming-Moran & Coimbra, 1990) and insulin resistance (Barzilai & Gupta, 1999; Ma et al., 2002; Rowe & Kahn, 1998).

The Force of the Individual: Organism and Actor

To emphasize the social organization of physical and mental aging does not mean that resilient features of the organism are unimportant, nor that there are no universal features of development (Dannefer & Perlmutter, 1990). For example, humans are born with a predisposition for language learning, and many researchers believe that the inability of feral children to acquire language reflects the importance of critical periods of brain growth and development for learning, and such organismically based physical changes occur throughout the life course.

Yet to focus on aspects of the universal or ontogenetic aspects of individual development as a way of preserving the individual against social determinism is to miss altogether the distinct significance and power of the individual human person, which is as a *world-constructing actor.* In acting in the world, the individual is doing more than "producing her own development" (Lerner & Walls, 1999); she is simultaneously co-constituting her own biography and social relationships, which form a central and proximate part of her environment (Berger & Luckmann, 1967; Dannefer, 1999; Mascolo, Fischer, & Neimeyer, 1999). With the potentials for learning and imagination provided by neoteny, this reconstitutive process also contains the potential for some degree of novelty and change. Thus, to emphasize the force of experience and context in shaping individual development is not to deny the agentic force of intentional action.

In sum, individual agency and social forces continuously shape each other in a reconstitutive, dialectical process. Although both are irreducibly important, they are not equal in their effects and potency. Each individual enters the world and human community helpless, and has her entire being shaped by the language and taken-for-granted practices of everyday life. The individual's actions, like those of the actors around her, largely conform to and thus reproduce those practices. Thus individuals are constituted and co-constituted in the context of preexisting social systems.

The Persistent Tendency Toward Reductionism in the Study of Human Aging

The importance of experience and context in influencing the way individuals develop and age has long been recognized, and it is an idea that received a transformative boost with the introduction of cohort analysis and the discovery of the radically different trajectories experienced by different cohorts (Schaie, 2005; Schaie & Baltes, 1996). Yet it has now been more than four decades since cohort analysis was introduced in 1965, and in many domains—including many psychological and psychosocial ones—researchers interested in age remain intellectually inclined to look for explanatory forces within the self-contained psychological and physical characteristics of the individual human being. There are indications that interest in cohort analysis itself has diminished even as the number of high-quality longitudinal data sets is increasing (Dannefer & Patterson, 2008). The relative lack of careful attention to cohort-related and other contextual factors in many recent analyses of age and development reveals a tendency toward reductionism.

Several factors contribute to the continued robustness of reductionist thinking. One that is frequently mentioned is the strong individualism of Western society that is deeply embedded in language, values, and social practices, including those of social and behavioral scientists. Westerners, and especially Americans, are said to be disinclined to be very skeptical and critical about individual-level explanations and about the unreflective use of age as an explanatory variable (Broughton, 1987; Dannefer, 1999; Morss, 1990).

Another reason that is more specific and potent, and yet much less recognized, has to do with the relationship between developing and aging individuals and social institutions. This is especially true for institutionalized social practices designed to take into account age and age-graded institutional forms, whether schools or geriatric institutions. Such institutions are deliberately designed with age-specific needs in mind. Yet when serving members of such a generative and responsive species as *Homo sapiens,* the dynamics involved are not so unidrectional and straightforward. Indeed, the interactive, responsive character of human development and human aging means that individual aging processes (both physical and psychological) occur in interaction with, and are to some extent shaped by, the institutional structures provided for them. Thus institutions create, to some degree, the very realities of human development and aging that they are also intended to accommodate.

The basic social processes by which institutional forces shape individual opportunity, individual activity, and self-definition are similar across age and across types of institutional setting. If older individuals begin to become frail and dependent, the dependency scripts that are part of nursing home practices further that dependence (Baltes & Wahl, 1992; Barkan, 2003; Thomas, 1996). Stroke patients who are unable to feed themselves but have a chance of recovering significant function are instead fed by nurse's aides and thus deprived of the opportunity to regain some independence (Dannefer & Daub, in press). Children who go to fabulous schools and excel are sorted into further enriched and stimulating educational environments that confirm earlier prediction of their potential and poise them for further affirmation of their brilliance, while children who attend poor schools that lack the resources to prepare them for advanced educational opportunities are declared to be slow learners and are excluded from such opportunities (Beyer & Apple, 1998; Kozol, 2005). Similar dynamics exist in the workplace, as demonstrated in the work of researchers such as Kohn and associates (e.g., Kohn & Slomczymski, 1990) and Marmot (2004). There is thus a kind of *surplus individualization* embedded in the very structure of institutions that have been designed to serve those who they actually are not just serving, but reconstituting (Baars, 1991; Dannefer, 1999). In this process, the individual is socially canalized further along trajectories either of further development and reward, or of increasing disability or disadvantage (Dannefer, 2003a). These dynamics thus may create a reification of organismic tendencies, even when they are tendencies that we would prefer to see minimized or ameliorated or that have the possibility of being reversed.

Constitutionalist Versus Accommodationist Views of Social Institutions

These considerations reveal the contrasting logics of two divergent views of institutional life, which may be called the *accommodationist* and *constitutionalist* perspectives on human institutions. The dynamics that I have just been describing relate to the constitutionalist view, which focuses on ways in which institutions, whether stratified educational systems or nursing homes, play an active role in creating the very conditions in individuals that require attention. From this perspective, institutions are viewed as actively contributing to the generation of problem conditions in the lives of the individuals they are intended to serve. Institutional processes sustain definitions of reality and legitimate differences between individuals and the distribution of opportunity among them. Thus they operate as subtle but powerful self-fulfilling prophecies, the effects of which are inscribed in the functional and performance-related outcomes of individuals.

In contrast, the accommodationist view is characterized by the assumption that the institutions we live in and are processed through—from preschools to retirement communities—are efficaciously designed to accommodate the needs and limitations of the individuals who are moving through them. School grades and tracks have been designed to accommodate differences in academic ability across age and among classmates, and vocational counseling and psychometric testing is claimed to help individuals learn where they fit in the occupational structure, like pegs in a pegboard. The progression of the nursing home career through stages of decline is justified on the basis that it provides an effective way of managing the needs of the aging residents. In sum, a presumption exists that human care organizations are functioning reasonably effectively and in line with their stated rationales, missions, and mandates.

Of course, neither of these views—accommodationist nor consti-tutionalist—is by itself entirely adequate. Constitutionalists can rightly say that to accommodationists, the active and constitutive force of social processes and social-structural constraints remains invisible because in-stitutions are creating as well as responding to human needs. Accom-modationists may reply that constitutionalists acknowledge neither the practical requirements of dealing with individual differences and needs, nor the value of presently existing institutions, despite their imperfec-tions. Clearly both perspectives are heuristically valuable as ideal types that capture the essential structural features of a particular perspective and point of view. Constitutionalists rightly emphasize the often adverse consequences of deliberately designed human care institutions based on the medical model. Nevertheless, they do not generally dispute the ne-cessity of such institutional structures, despite their destructive aspects. They are not institutional anarchists. On the other hand, few accom-modationists would deny that institutions can have adverse effects with long-term adverse consequences.

To acknowledge some validity to the social constitutionalist idea that institutions exacerbate or even create problems within the individuals who are processed through them is to acknowledge that to some de-gree, individual problems—including age-related problems—are part of an elaborate dynamic of self-fulfilling prophecy. This applies in all kinds of settings, both formal and informal; it can often be clearly seen in the more visible and predictable organization of everyday life that is imposed by age-graded human care institutions, whether elderhostels or K–12 schooling. With regard to schooling, for example, social science and related literatures contain innumerable, well-documented cases of high school students who act smart or not so smart based on what they are told by others about their abilities (e.g., Holstein & Gubrium, 1995; Jussim & Harber, 2005; Lucas & Good, 2001; Rist, 1979; Rosenthal, 1991). Equally apt examples can be drawn from studies approaching the end of the life course. As noted previously, the remaining skills and com-petencies of nursing home residents are removed by the regime of total dependency and powerlessness (Baltes & Wahl, 1992).

Such processes are unnoticed, continuous, seamless elements in the everyday lived experience of late modern society. Existing institutional arrangements and the social dynamics that derive from their organiza-tion are the waters we swim—taken for granted; accorded legitimacy by their very presence and power; always moving toward invisibility. These waters are so relentless and so seductive that they are difficult to discern even for critical observers such as behavioral and social scientists, who try to cultivate an analytical detachment and skepticism toward the social practices and institutional arrangements that organize our everyday lives and relationships.

INDIVIDUAL AGING, MACRO-LEVEL PROCESSES, AND THE MISSING MIDDLE: THE WATERS WE SWIM

This discussion has focused heavily on social structure and processes at the point of everyday life: the immediacy of microsocial interaction and the interface of experience with organizational dynamics, with little attention to the macrosocial. I begin with an emphasis on the micro- and mesolevels for two reasons: first, because it provides the basic foundation for studying distinctly human processes anchored in physical and developmental features of Homo sapiens, and second, because an understanding of the role of meso- and microdynamics that are proximate to the individual in everyday life in shaping aging is underdeveloped in the study of age. Because of this underdevelopment, the map of the social processes that shape individuals and that represent and reflect the impulses of broader social processes remains incomplete. For gerontological researchers, there has thus been a *missing middle* in the charting of social dynamics as they impact aging—a level that is critical to apprehending fully the relations between age and social structure. Examples of everyday interactional processes in which individuals' lives are constituted include a range of social relations and settings. They include the informal but habitualized patterns that characterize relationships in family life and among other consociates, and everyday experience that is organized by the reward structures and practices of formal organizational settings—in workplace, education, health care, and other contexts that involve assessment and gatekeeping of individuals. In addition to explicitly defined structures, an irreducible aspect of formal organizations is the concomitant existence of informal systems of social relations that can be centrally important to individual participants and to organizational life.

Across disciplines, the study of aging-in-context has tended to focus on understanding context through modes of social analysis several levels removed from everyday experience: through demographic analysis, through historical scholarship or cross-cultural comparisons, through examining macrostructural trends and policy initiatives, or through long-term longitudinal studies that track individual trajectories on repeated measures of snapshot characteristics. Such data are as invaluable as they are diverse, yet they share a common limitation: With such information, it is not possible to know in any detail the actual social processes of the everyday experiences that comprise the medium in which real-life individuals are constituted as living, developing, and aging beings. With demography and macrotrends at one level, and a focus on individual characteristics at the other, analysis of how the co-constitution of both actors and social relationships is accomplished and shaped in everyday interaction is typically undeveloped. As Diewald (2001) puts it, "psychological traits and functional capacities of individuals are mostly seen as being 'not social' and thus out of the realm of sociological explanations" (p. 228). This is a frequent assumption of both psychology and macrosociology, and it entails a remarkable omission in fields such as gerontology and the life course, where a central concern is to make connections between individual and social processes. These connections are required to understand human aging, and they require development of a middle level of social processes: the micro-meso-dynamics of informal social interaction and of the institutions that regulate it.

To point to this area of theoretical underdevelopment is not to detract from the value of the numerous traditions of research that have made seminal contributions to understanding the relation between age and social structure, whether long-term longitudinal studies of stability and change under varying conditions, or research demonstrating differential patterns of physical aging across time or across societies. Such discoveries have, in fact, provided some of the most compelling evidence requiring acknowledgment that human aging is something that can only be understood in context. Without cohort analysis and cross-cultural and historical research, and without population data and large-scale, representative studies, we would know much less about the power of social context to shape human development and aging. Yet that knowledge does not, in itself, provide an explicit conception of how development and aging actually occur.

Of course, it is not the task of historians or demographers, or even anthropologists, to articulate an explicit model of the person, even the person-in-context. Although these forms of analysis provide broad and comparative perspectives of change and difference in individual lives, they reveal little about the actual mechanisms through which changes in individual health, mental and physical functioning, aspirations, and values are produced. These are changes that happen to individuals and that are mediated in the proximate immediacy of everyday living, growing, and aging.

Notions of how these macro-level differences are linked to individual and micro-level realities often seem to be mystifying and the processes involved hidden in a black box. As so often happens, in such a situation, we tend to fall back, by default, on familiar, organismic conceptions of individual growth and aging. Almost by default, then, macro-level analyses have been wedded with quite traditional models of the individual that emphasize self-contained individual characteristics (e.g., coping style, temperament) that tend to be viewed either as stable or as changing in normative, age-graded, and implicitly organismically driven ways.

This tendency is evident in the resurgence of individual-level explanations, in the increasingly peripheral attention accorded to social context, and in the frequency with which cross-sectional data are employed to make inferences about age-related change, despite the dramatic expansion of quality longitudinal data. What remains to be developed, then, is a deliberate, systematic analysis of how individuals are actually constituted and change over time, processes which require, and in many respects take their character from, the waters we swim.

As noted previously, the work of some psychologists does bring us quite close to the dynamics of everyday life, as they study the personal consequences of conversational scripts (e.g., Baltes & Wahl, 1992) or of how modifying the context of everyday life can dramatically alter individual functioning (e.g., Grow & Ryan, 1999; Langer & Rodin, 1976). But these insights about the experiential and social contingency of individual change remain to be integrated both with sociological studies of interaction and with psychological studies of aging-in-context.

To make those connections in empirical research is not easy work, and it can be expensive. It requires at least some measure of labor-intensive data collection at the micro- and mesolevels of analysis. Consider Figure 1.1, depicting the cycle of induced incompetence, from Bengtson's (1973) early work (Kuypers & Bengtson, 1984). This diagram applies the principles of labeling theory to depict the sociogenic production of age-related incompetence. Beginning with a social definition of vulnerability, it traces how that definition can become a self-fulfilling prophecy—reified by others, and then internalized by the actor himself or herself. And the same applies to gaining competence and expertise. Neither competence nor incompetence is organismic; both are induced in the course of social interaction. This not something that happens just occasionally as a curious anomaly in social life; it depicts processes that are occurring constantly, for every human actor, all the time. Because we are swimming in it, it usually continues to go altogether unnoticed.

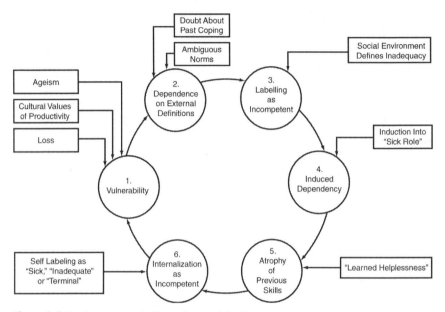

Figure 1.1 Sociogenic production of age-related incompetence.
From *The Social Psychology of Aging* by V. Bengtson, 1973, Indianapolis, IN: Bobbs-Merrill.

While this model is limited by a lack of structural connection, it is an exemplary effort to chart the interactive mechanisms of how individual identity and individual abilities are constituted in interaction.

The self-society dynamism has been a topic of this series (see, e.g., Gergen & Gergen, 1999; Gubrium, 1999), and research traditions relevant to social gerontology include some intriguing studies showing how individual abilities may be produced as outcomes of social processes (e.g., Diamond, 1995; Kanter, 1977; Holstein & Gubrium, 2000). These are relatively few in number, however, and seldom are efforts made to integrate them with systematic quantitative analyses of individual outcomes or of macro-level processes. Such studies also have the classic limitations of the ethnographic tradition, in their lack of representativeness, dearth of standardized concepts and measures, and so on. But there is much to recommend them. As symbolic interactionist pioneer Herbert Blumer (1969) challenged us, "the first task of a science is to respect its subject matter" (p. 41). If one accepts the premises of the social constitution and sustenance of the individual, and of humans being hard-wired for flexibility throughout the life course, the central necessity of detailing how the person is accomplished through the immediate processes of everyday life becomes clear.

LINKING AGE TO MACROSOCIAL FORCES: CONTINUING CHALLENGES

A widely recognized limitation of the classic interactionist tradition in sociology is its almost deliberate detachment of the processes it studies from larger structural realities and processes (e.g., Blumer, 1969). Such detachment is unnecessary and counterproductive because there are obvious connections between such levels. Consider, for example, the relation between kinds of treatment and diagnosis that occur in medical clinics and hospitals and their revenue streams. This is a relationship that is intricately informed by rules for Medicare, Medicaid, and insurance reimbursement, or by the models of human nature and human development contained in the curricula of nursing and medical schools. Yet the impact of macrostructural definitions of age is more pervasive still: Consider the images of aging that are reified by our entire culture—from social policy, to the educational system, to entertainment media, to advertising. Such macro-level forces organize and regulate the institutional practices and micro-level interactional processes that ethnographers study.

In modern bureaucratic states, the processes of everyday life and the organizational dynamics that so often define and direct the daily experiences of individuals are themselves organized, in substantial part, by macro-level processes of economic development. Since the advent of mass media, culture itself has become more centralized and homogenized, a macro-level force with great leverage over individual lives, as is evident by the resources individuals expend to achieve a properly informed and stylish presentation of self in matters ranging from music, media options, and books to designer clothing and trendy technology, whether handheld devices or SUVs.

The historian Stuart Ewen (1976) demonstrated how the force of advertising supplanted industrial development in shaping the consciousness of the population in the 20th century. More recently, the extraordinary deliberateness and effectiveness of efforts of marketers to extend the efforts that Ewen described to early childhood have been documented (e.g., Schor, 2004).

As historians of age have demonstrated, mass media (in entertainment programming, in advertising, and in authoritative public pronouncements from educational and medical experts) have played a central role in advancing particular forms of age consciousness (Chudacoff, 1989; Katz, 1994, 2006; see also Butsch, 2000). The images conveyed by media have produced an increasingly homogenized depiction of age across society, reflecting the increasingly standardized and normal life course patterns that reflect the institutionalization of the life course (Dannefer, 2003b; Kohli, 1986). As a result, the culturally pervasive images of age are now internalized by an entire society from early childhood onward—including, of course, gerontologists of every discipline.

Macro-level forces relevant to understanding aging thus include not only policies and programs, and not only populations and the broad-scale institutional configurations in which individuals live and age, but they also include the cultural definitions of age and old age that come to have their own power.

Because so many features of everyday life have implications for aging, the relevance of culture to age-related change is not at all limited to explicit references to age. Consider, for example, what is coming to be called the *pandemic of obesity*, which reflects a health issue that has major implications for the health and longevity of individuals as they age. For this, we can thank in part the combination of sedentariness and destructive diets, the latter aided by the fast-food industries. With utter predictability, the growing preoccupation with fat is spawning a host of antiobesity drugs, which are authoritatively announced as the answer in every form of advertising, including the Web. As one example, consider Lypozene, which claims that it enables the consumer to lose weight "without working hard at it," without changing lifestyle or diet, and while "eating what you want" (http://www.lipozene.com/).

In some cases, the targeting of key subpopulations has apparently been quite direct, as documented in Maxwell and Jacobson's (1989) investigative monograph *Marketing Disease to Hispanics.* While obesity may in some cases have a heritable component, a dramatic change in incidence or prevalence occurring within the span of a few decades cannot be genetic in origin. Obesity thus illustrates a problem in which (a) the long-term, age-related implications of everyday lifestyle practices and (b) macro-level dynamics (including corporate and other institutional interests) remain invisible and unacknowledged even as they continuously operate to organize people's daily routines. Aspects of these culturally organized routines are familiar and well publicized: minimal need or incentive to exercise, instant gratification and the sensitization of taste buds to junk food, the tendency to look to pharmaceuticals as a source of solutions. Thus the entire society is bathed in recommendations for culinary, lifestyle, and medical practices that are needed for profit margins of established product lines, while the role of products and the profits they provide as social forces that operate to constitute individual patterns and population processes of individual aging is unnoticed.

Of course, the fact that there is bad news here with respect to health and aging is irrelevant to the fundamental point that cultural knowledge and practices shape individual aging. Indeed, the news is not bad for everyone. Among elite subpopulations, there has now emerged a kind of counterculture that is obsessed with antiaging nutritional and lifestyle practices, and if such practices were to become universally practiced, it likely would have quite a profound effect on individual health and patterns of age-related health (Binstock, 2004). These practices, too, are socially generated and transmitted through information networks accessible to social and cultural elites. The effects of the stratification of such nutritional practices over extended periods of time are components in the ongoing process of cumulating dis/advantage in health (Crystal, 2006; Dannefer, 2003a; Douthit & Dannefer, 2007; Ferraro & Kelley-Moore, 2003). Thus the individual's location in networks of knowledge and opportunity may determine the extent to which the individual is at risk for obesity or good health (Christakis & Fowler, 2007). In sum, cultural practices, whether salutary or not, are an irrepressible, constant, and substantial element in the constitution of patterns of age-related change.

The linking of macro-level processes to age can be extended to the definitions of reality offered by the advertising and entertainment media that are key components of mass society. Often, such definitions have no obvious or inherent connection to age but nevertheless have profound implications for health. As long as individuals take them for granted as inevitable features of everyday life, the socially specific configuration of social forces that operate at every level—micro, meso, and macro—to produce age-related outcomes, those forces will remain the unacknowledged, unexplored water in which we all swim. The application of principles and insights in the behavioral and social sciences to the study of age has contributed a great deal to debunking the myths and fallacies of cohort-centrism (Riley, 1978) and ethnocentrism in the study of aging. Yet in deconstructing the power of social forces that shapes the reality of age and aging, an abundance of work remains to be done.

CONCLUSION: DISCOVERING THE WATERS WE SWIM

Immersion in the familiar, taken-for-granted, and relatively stable routines of everyday life obscures from view the necessity of social interaction as a precondition for becoming human and as a central regulator that sustains the socially specific practices and expectations that organize developmental and life course processes as individuals age.

The all-encompassing embrace of everyday social life calls to mind McLuhan's fish, who could not discover water since she was bathed in it as a continuous reality, without which she could not imagine existing, and indeed could not exist.

In the context of individualistically oriented societies, both the *lived experience* of aging in everyday life by the individual members of a society and *scientific inquiry about the experience of aging* tend to begin with an assumption of self-contained individual processes as strong determinants of age-related outcomes. Scholarship focused at both the individual level (e.g., psychological gerontology, lifespan development) and at the collective level (e.g., demography of age) has tended to rely on such assumptions and has thus omitted the crucial processes in between the individual level and the macro- and population levels. What has been thereby neglected are specific features both of individual human beings and of their interactions with each other and with the contexts in which they live, and through which they are constituted as developing and aging individuals, and which therefore must be made explicit to explain human aging.

These features include, at the individual level, the hard-wiring for flexibility of the human organism, and at the social level, the processes of social construction and social organization that regulate development and aging in a socially specific and culturally defined system of human relations.

In late modern societies, with centralized structures of knowledge and control, professional and "expert" knowledge about well-adjusted human behavior and normal aging and development gives legitimacy to the institutionalized life course and to mechanisms of stratification among age peers. Thus it serves as a powerful and established cultural force that defines and organizes the experience of individuals. Such institutionalized and professionalized declarations of age-graded normality are intended to accommodate the changing needs of individuals as they develop and age.

As social analysts are confronted simultaneously with a steady graying of the population and with increasing social inequality within age groups, the need to distinguish authentic age-related needs from the oppressive effects of surplus individualization and the invidious effects of mechanisms of stratification remains a centrally important yet undeveloped area of scholarship. By developing our understanding of these processes, scholarship will reveal the waters we swim, and suggest how they might be altered to enhance the possibilities of positive human development.

REFERENCES

Baars, J. (1991). The challenge of critical gerontology: The problem of social constitution. *Journal of Aging Studies, 5,* 219–243.

Baltes, M. M., & Wahl, H. (1992). The dependency-support script in institutions: Generalization to community settings. *Psychology of Aging, 7,* 409–418.

Barkan, B. (2003). The live oak regenerative community: Reconnecting culture within the long-term care environment. *Journal of Social Work in Long-Term Care, 2,* 197–221.

Barzilai, N., & Gupta, G. (1999). Interaction between aging and syndrome X: New insights on the pathophysiology of fat distribution. *Annals of the New York Academy of Science, 892,* 58–72.

Bengtson, V. (1973). *The social psychology of aging.* Indianapolis, IN: Bobbs-Merrill.

Berger, P., & Luckmann, L. (1967). *The social construction of reality: A treatise in the sociology of knowledge.* New York: Anchor.

Beyer, L. E., & Apple, M. W. (Eds.). (1998). *The curriculum: Problems, politics, and possibilities.* Albany, NY: SUNY Press.

Binstock, R. H. (2004). Anti-aging medicine and research: A realm of conflict and profound societal implications. *Journals of Gerontology, Ser. A, 59,* 523–533.

Blumer, H. (1969). *Symbolic interactionism: Perspective and method.* Englewood Cliffs, NJ: Prentice Hall.

Bromhall, C. (2003). *The eternal child: How evolution has made children of us all.* London: Ebury Press.

Broughton, J. (1987). *Critical theories of psychological development.* New York: Springer Publishing.

Butsch, R. (2000). *The making of American audiences: From stage to television, 1750–1990.* New York: Cambridge University Press.

Christakis, N., & Fowler, J. (2007). The spread of obesity in a large social network over 32 years. *New England Journal of Medicine, 9,* 357–370.

Chudacoff, H. (1989). *How old are you? Age consciousness in American culture.* Princeton, NJ: Princeton University Press.

Cott, N. (1997). *Bonds of womanhood: "Woman's sphere" in New England, 1780–1835.* New Haven, CT: Yale University Press.

Crystal, S. (2006). Dynamics of late-life inequality: Modeling the interplay of health disparities, economic resources, and public policies. In J. Baars, D. Dannefer, C. Phillipson, & A. Walker (Eds.), *Aging, globalization and inequality: The new critical gerontology* (pp. 205–214). Amityville, NY: Baywood.

Dannefer, D. (1999). Neoteny, naturalization and other constituents of human development. In C. Ryff & B. Marshall (Eds.), *Self and society of aging processes* (pp. 67–93). New York: Springer Publishing.

Dannefer, D. (2003a). Cumulative advantage and the life course: Cross-fertilizing age and social science knowledge. *Journals of Gerontology, Ser. B, 58,* S327–S337.

Dannefer, D. (2003b). Toward a global geography of the life course: Challenges of late modernity to the life course perspective. In J. T. Mortimer & M. Shanahan (Eds.), *Handbook of the life course* (pp. 647–659). New York: Kluwer.

Dannefer, D. & Daub, A. (in press). Extending the interrogation: Lifespan, Life course, and the subject matter of human aging. In T. Owens & A. de Ribaupierre (Eds.),

Linked lives and self-regulation: Lifespan—Life course, is it really the same? Advances in course research. Greenwich, CT: JAI Press.

Dannefer, D., & Patterson, R. S. (2008). The missing person: Some limitations in the contemporary study of cognitive aging. In S. Hofer & D. Alwin (Eds.), *Handbook of cognitive aging.* Thousand Oaks, CA: Sage.

Dannefer, D., & Perlmutter, M. (1990). Development as a multidimensional process: Individual and social constituents. *Human Development, 33,* 108–137.

Diamond, T. (1995). *Making gray gold: Narrative of nursing home care.* Chicago: University of Chicago Press.

Diewald, M. (2001). Unitary social science for causal understanding: Experiences and prospects for life course research. *Canadian Studies in Population, 28,* 219–248.

Douthit, K., & Dannefer, D. (2007). Social forces, life course consequences: Cumulative disadvantage and "getting Alzheimer's." In J. M. Wilmoth & K. F. Ferraro (Eds.), *Gerontology: Perspectives and issues* (pp. 223–243). New York: Springer Publishing.

Dressler, W. W. (1999). Modernization, stress, and blood pressure: New directions in research. *Human Biology, 71,* 583–605.

Ehrlich, P. (2000). *Human natures.* Washington, DC: Island Press.

Ewen, S. (1976). *Captains of consciousness: Advertising and the social roots of the consumer culture.* New York: McGraw-Hill.

Ferraro, K. F., & Kelley-Moore, J. A. (2003). Cumulative disadvantage and health: Long-term consequences of obesity? *American Sociological Review, 68,* 707–729.

Fleming-Moran, M., & Coimbra, C. E., Jr. (1990). Blood pressure studies among Amazonian native populations: A review from an epidemiological perspective. *Social Science Medicine, 31,* 593–601.

Gergen, K. J., & Gergen, M. M. (1999). The new aging: Self construction and social values. In K. W. Schaie & J. Hendricks (Eds.), *The evolution of the aging self: The societal impact on the aging process* (pp. 281–306). New York: Springer Publishing.

Gould, S. J. (1977). *Ontogeny and phylogeny.* Cambridge, MA: Belknap Press of Harvard University Press.

Grow, V. K., & Ryan, R. (1999). The relation of psychological needs for autonomy and relatedness to vitality, well-being, and mortality in nursing homes. *Journal of Applied Social Psychology, 29,* 935–954.

Gubrium, J. (1999). Commentary: Deconstructing self and well-being in later life. In K. W. Schaie & J. Hendricks (Eds.), *The evolution of the aging self: The societal impact on the aging process* (pp. 47–61). New York: Springer Publishing.

Holstein, J., & Gubrium, J. (1995). Deprivatization and the construction of domestic life. *Journal of Marriage and Family, 57,* 894.

Holstein, J., & Gubrium, J. (2000). *Constructing the life course.* Lanham, MD: Alta Mira Press.

Jussim, K., & Harber, K. D. (2005). Teacher expectations and self-fulfilling prophecies: Knowns and unknowns, resolved and unresolved controversies, *Personality and Social Psychology Review, 9,* 131–155.

Kanter, R. (1977). *Men and women of the corporation.* New York: Basic Books.

Katz, S. (1994). *Disciplining old age: The formation of gerontological knowledge.* Charlottesville: University of Virginia Press.

Katz, S. (2006). From chronology to functionality: Critical reflections on the gerontology of the body. In J. Baars, D. Dannefer, C. Phillipson, & A. Walker (Eds.), *Aging, globalization and inequality: The new critical gerontology* (pp. 123–137). Amityville, NY: Baywood.

Kohli, M. (1986). Social organization and subjective construction of the life course. In A. Sorensen, F. E. Weinert, & L. R. Sherrod (Eds.), *Human development and the life course: Multidisciplinary perspectives* (pp. 271–292). Hillsdale, NJ: Erlbaum.

Kohn, M., & Slomczymski, K. (1990). *Social structure and self direction: A comparative analysis of the United States and Poland.* New York: Blackwell.

Kozol, J. (2005). *Savage inequalities: Children in America's schools.* New York: Crown.

Kuypers, J. A., & Bengtson, V. L. (1984). Perspectives on the older family. In W. H. Quinn & G. A. Houghston (Eds.), *Independently aging: Family and social systems perspectives* (pp. 3–19). Rockville, MD: Aspen Systems.

Lane, H. (1976). *The wild boy of Aveyron.* Cambridge, MA: Harvard University Press.

Langer, E., & Rodin, J. (1976). The effects of choice and enhanced personal responsibility for the aged: A field experiment in an institutional setting. *Journal of Personality and Social Psychology, 34,* 191–198.

Laslett, P. (2004). *The world we have lost: Further explored.* London: Routledge.

Lerner, R. M., & Walls, T. (1999). Revisiting *Individuals as producers of their development:* From dynamic interactionism to developmental systems. In J. Brandstadter & R. M. Lerner (Eds.), *Action and self-development: Theory and research through the life span* (pp. 3–36). Thousand Oaks, CA: Sage.

Lucas, S. R., & Good, A. D. (2001). Race, class, and tournament track mobility. *Sociology of Education, 74,* 139–156.

Ma, X. H., Muzumdar, R., Yang, X. M., Gabriely, I., Berger, R., & Barzilai, N. (2002). Aging is associated with resistance to effects of leptin on fat distribution and insulin action. *Journals of Gerontology, Ser. B, 57,* 225–231.

Maclean, C. (1978). *The wolf children.* New York: Hill and Wang.

Marmot, M. (2004). *The status syndrome: How social standing affects our health and longevity.* New York: Time Books.

Mascolo, M. F., Fischer, K. W., & Neimeyer, R. A. (1999). The dynamics of codevelopment of intentionality, self and social relations. In J. Brandstadter & R. M. Lerner (Eds.), *Action and self-development: Theory and research through the life span* (pp. 133–166). Thousand Oaks, CA: Sage.

Maxwell, B., & Jacobson, M. (1989). *Marketing disease to Hispanics: The selling of alcohol and tobacco.* Piscataway, NJ: UMDNJ-Robert Wood Johnson Medical School.

Montagu, A. (1989). *Growing young.* New York: McGraw-Hill.

Morss, J. (1990). *The biologising of childhood: Developmental psychology and the Darwinian myth.* Hillsdale, NJ: Erlbaum.

Newton, M. (2003). *Savage girls and wild boys.* New York: St. Martin's Press.

Perry, B., & Svalavitz, M. (2006). *The boy who was raised as a dog: And other stories from a child psychiatrist's notebook: What traumatized children can teach us about loss, love and healing.* New York: Basic Books.

Portmann, A. (1961). *Animals as social beings.* New York: Viking Press.

Reese, H. W., & Worton, W. F. (1970). Models of development and theories of development. In L. R. Goulet & P. B. Baltes (Eds.), Life-Span developmental psychology: Research and theory. New York: Academic Press.

Riley, M. W. (1978). Aging, social change and the power of ideas. *Daedaelus, 107,* 39–52.

Rist, R. (1979). *Desegregated schools: Appraisals of an American experiment.* New York: Academic Press.

Rogoff, B. (2002). How can we study cultural aspects of human development? *Human Development, 45,* 209–210.

Rogoff, B. (2003). *The cultural nature of human development.* New York: Oxford University Press.

Rosenthal, R. (1991). Teacher expectancy effects: A brief update 25 years after the Pygmalion experiment. *Journal of Research in Education, 1,* 3–12.

Rowe, J. W., & Kahn, R. L. (1998). *Successful aging.* New York: Pantheon.

Schaie, K. W. (2005). *Developmental influences on adult intelligence: The Seattle Longitudinal Study.* New York: Oxford University Press.

Schaie, K. W., & Baltes, P. B. (1996). *Intellectual development in adulthood: The Seattle Longitudinal Study.* Cambridge, England: Cambridge University Press.

Schor, J. (2004). *Born to buy: The commercialized child and the new consumer culture.* New York: Scribner.

Shattuck, R. (1994). *The forbidden experiment: The story of the wild boy of Aveyron.* New York: Kodashana International.

Thomas, W. (1996). *Life worth living: How someone you love can still enjoy life in a nursing home.* Acton, MA: VanderWyk and Burnham.

Health and Well-Being

PART I

2

To Act or Not to Act: Using Statistics or Feelings to Reduce Disease Risk, Morbidity, and Mortality

HOWARD LEVENTHAL, TAMARA J. MUSUMECI, AND
ELAINE A. LEVENTHAL

GOALS OF PSYCHOLOGICAL RESEARCH ON HEALTH BEHAVIORS

It has been estimated that the contribution of behavioral factors to health outcomes is equal to the contribution of environmental, genetic, and miscellaneous factors combined (Institute for the Future, 2003). The set of behaviors to which variation in health and illness is attributed is large and heterogeneous. It includes lifestyles for disease prevention and action for early detection such as screening and medical check-ups (primary prevention), behaviors for disease management and prevention of disease progression (secondary prevention), and behaviors for adapting to and living effectively with chronic illness (tertiary prevention). Although the lists specifying particular behaviors for good health (the do's and don'ts) are impressive in their diversity and length, it would be misleading to exaggerate their clarity and/or validity. Specific behaviors move on and off a list in reaction to cultural change and in response

Acknowledgments: I wish to thank Ron Abeles, Elaine Dannefer, Jonathan Micahel Dannefer, Susan Hinze, Robin Shura Patterson, Peter Uhlenberg, and Warner Schaie for suggestions and comments on an earlier version of this chapter.

Preparation of this chapter was supported by grants from the National Institutes of Health (R24-AG023958), Center for the Study of Health Beliefs and Behaviors.

to data from new epidemiological studies. For example, in the early 1900s, professors of physiology at Yale recommended that members of the football team eat large quantities of beef to ready themselves for competitive sports. Such huge amounts of beef consumption are clearly no longer recommended for athletes, and certainly not for their more sedentary brethren (Chao et al., 2005; Song, Buring, Manson, & Liu, 2004). Some behaviors may be legitimate occupants appearing on both lists of do's and don'ts for health, though for different reasons. Coffee and dark chocolate, taken in moderation, have moved from the don't list to the do list, with qualifications (Kris-Etherton & Keen, 2002; Ross et al., 2006; Salazar-Martinez et al., 2004). Deep in our hearts and taste buds, many of us always knew that red wine, again in moderation, deserved its place of honor on the list of behavioral do's (Stampfer, Kang, Chen, Cherry, & Grodstein, 2005). If excessive weight is bad, how do we rate the behavioral procedures for reducing weight: Should one diet, or should one instead use artificially sweetened beverages? What about exercise? Vigorous exercise is on the positive list because it improves cardiovascular fitness (Tanasescu et al., 2002), but it also appears on the negative list as it can lead to musculoskeletal injuries (Gerson & Stevens, 2004; Hootman et al., 2002).

Given the diversity of behaviors with health implications, how can we define a coherent review of the psychological and behavioral factors affecting health over the life span? Both the wide range and the differences in the contextual, social, and individual factors affecting each of the behaviors requires an overview of the pathways from ecological, cultural, and social context to behavior, and from behavior to health. Second, it calls for a coherent theoretical model for integrating concepts from cultural, social, and psychological variables affecting behavior and recognizing the biological processes impacting health and illness. Figure 2.1 provides a sketch of the pathways leading to the healthy and risky behaviors affecting health and identifies the problems in understanding connections among concepts, both along a specific pathway and across pathways. The figure defines the context for any theory that attempts to address these issues. As behavior, health, and disease are processes or products of the individual organisms, the theoretical model at this level needs both to be sufficiently detailed to be tested at the individual behavioral level and open enough to address relationships of individual behavioral processes to cultural and social contexts and to biological processes. In other words, the theory must provide a set of interrelated concepts to represent *how* cultural, institutional, and interpersonal factors influence individual

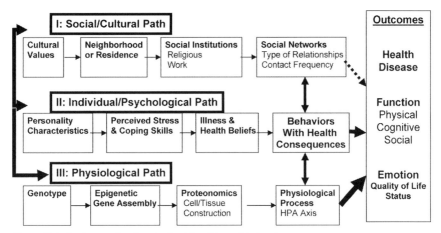

Figure 2.1 Pathways for the study of health and behavior.

psychological processes to affect the particular healthy or risky behavior that is under study. At the interface between psychology and biology, the conceptual structure must help us to understand *how* the behavior affects the biological processes leading to health and/or disease (i.e., how the behaviors get under the skin; Yancura, Aldwin, Levenson, & Spiro, 2006).

Finally, in keeping with the substance of the 20 years of the Penn State series on the role of aging in health, we need to add a life span perspective both to the picture of the pathways and to the theoretical process model at the individual level. The life span issue raises questions such as the following:

1.   Are there environmental and/or behavioral factors in early life (i.e., in utero onward) that affect health and illness in later life? This is both a biological and behavioral issue.
2.   Do behavioral changes in later life produce health benefits? Are the healthy and risky behaviors the same across the life span?
3.   Are the sociopsychological processes involved in the initiation and maintenance of healthy and risky behaviors the same in the early, middle, and later years of life?

As it is impossible to review the enormous number of studies covering all of the behaviors relevant for health in a single volume, let alone in a single chapter, and relate these studies to a common underlying process model, the present chapter will focus on a selected set of the behaviors involved in the prevention and control of chronic conditions such as asthma, cardiovascular disease, diabetes, and hypertension. The first section presents a very brief justification for focusing on chronic conditions and the evidence for healthy and risky behaviors related to these conditions. It refers to both historical observations and recent experimental and longitudinal data.

The second section develops a theoretical model of the psychological processes underlying a subset of behaviors involved in the prevention and control of chronic illnesses: the use of health care and the general lifestyle and specific treatment behaviors involved in the self-management (prevention and control) of chronic conditions. The relevance of these processes for elderly individuals is clear as chronic illnesses are largely conditions of the later years. Thus the data address issues concerning how middle-aged and elderly individuals make health decisions, whether they are willing to modify lifestyle behaviors, and whether they face more external and internal barriers to behavioral change and a reduction of possible health benefits. This section also touches on the relevance of the processes underlying care seeking and adherence to healthy and risky behaviors such as smoking cessation and screening for disease detection. Finally, the section addresses how individual-level variables are related to and are influenced by contextual factors (i.e., culture, social relationships, and the self-concept). The detailed analysis of individual-level processes points to gaps in our understanding of the connections between the individual and the social context.

The closing section comments briefly on intervention strategies for encouraging healthy and reducing risky behaviors, addressing the importance of these studies for both theory and practice. The bidirectional nature of the research process and the need for integrated research teams to achieve bidirectional translation are discussed. The underlying theme throughout is whether the available evidence addresses how variables in a pathway, and in pathways across levels, are connected to one another. In system terms, the issue is the identification of the rules or programs by which the components or variables in a system communicate with one another (Csete & Doyle, 2002).

BEHAVIOR AND THE RISK OF CHRONIC ILLNESS

Although empirical studies support the widely held beliefs that environmental factors and lifestyle behaviors can affect the onset and progression of disease, the validity of these beliefs and the supporting data are often subject to controversy. Our first section provides evidence that awareness of the effect of environment, social context, and behavior on health is not new. We turn next to contemporary evidence linking behavior to health and contrast the evidence from randomized trials with those from longitudinal studies. Finally, we address gaps in the data: the lack of theory and evidence linking social context to individual action and individual action to the physiological processes responsible for health outcomes.

Some History on Healthy and Risky Behaviors

Braudel's (1979) fascinating but sobering review of the cycle of expansion and contraction in world and European populations (the world population expanded from an estimated 333,000,000 in the 14th century to about 800,000,000 in 1800, and to 4,000,000,000 in 1970) points to broad contextual factors as determinants of life span and mortality (e.g., climate change, agricultural practices, and expanding trade). Ecological factors of this type are not typically found in models of health behavior. Cultural practices, such as cigarette smoking, have been a source of contention over decades. Although regarded nowadays as a risk to health by both smokers and nonsmokers (U.S. Public Health Service, 1967), this was not always the case (Borgatta, 1968). The benefits and risks of tobacco were well advertised during its introduction and the early decades of its use in 16th- and 17th-century Europe, and the argument continued into the 20th century (Eysenck, 1980; Warner, Goldenhar, & McLaughlin, 1992).

An obesity epidemic is currently a major source of concern as it is associated with both an overall increase in the incidence of diabetes and the occurrence of adult-onset diabetes (type 2) among adolescents, an effect not observed in earlier decades of the 20th century. The consequences of diabetes are severe in terms of individual suffering, reduced quality of life, increased mortality (e.g., cardiac disease, blindness, and kidney failure), and economic burden due to increased health care costs. Obesity is linked to two sets of behaviors that are shaped by economics, culture, and social context: (a) eating quantities of inexpensive, available foods that are high in processed sugars and saturated fats and (b) limited physical activity (Brownell & Horgen, 2004; Kant, 2000; Troiana, Briefel, Marroll, & Bialostosky, 2000). The evidence is also clear that health benefits accrue from consuming a more costly, balanced, and nutritious diet and engaging in physical activity, which requires a safe venue (Bauman, 2004; Temple, 2000; Willett, 1994). Although the evidence is more varied, there is reason to believe that social connectedness and interpersonal support in contrast to social isolation and loneliness confers health benefits (Cohen & Wills, 1985; Cutrona & Russell, 1990), as do personal characteristics such as conscientiousness, reality-based coping skills, and effective management of emotional distress (Friedman & Booth-Kewley, 1987; Hampson, Goldberg, Vogt, & Dubanoski, 2007), though it is not always clear how these factors transform into health benefits. There is also evidence that behavioral styles, such as interpersonal hostility, may be related to risk for cardiovascular disease (Davis, Matthews, & McGrath, 2000; Guyll & Contrada, 1998).

Scientific Evidence for Behaviors Beneficial and/or Risky for Health

Empirical evidence for the benefits and risks of specific behaviors comes from three sources: correlations between a behavior and a health criterion in cross-sectional data, associations between a behavior and a health criterion in longitudinal data, and evidence from clinical trials. The quality of the evidence for an association is generally presumed to be stronger in the longitudinal than the cross-sectional studies, and strongest in the clinical trials. Each of the three types of evidence exhibit weaknesses, however, which are often unrecognized, and these weaknesses are exploited by the individuals who benefit financially when people act contrary to the scientific evidence, and by the individuals justifying their risky behaviors (e.g., smoke, drink to excess, eat mass quantities of high-calorie foods). When people compare scientific evidence to subjective evidence for health decisions and behaviors, the statistical evidence of science often comes in second best.

Clinical Trials: The Gold Standard for Causal Inference

Clinical trials are considered the gold standard for inferring that a treatment effected (i.e., caused) benefit (or harm) to health. The two features of a trial that are critical for causal inference are (a) the implementation of both the experimental intervention and the control condition prior to the assessment of the health outcome defining treatment efficacy and (b) random assignment of participants to conditions to reduce selection biases associated with participant characteristics such as age, education, gender, motivation for change, preferences for one or another treatment, skills for self-management, and so on. Trials provide the most powerful support for the antecedent aspect of the causal analysis for evaluating the efficacy of a behavioral intervention on health outcomes (Sackett, Rosenberg, Gray, Haynes, & Richardson, 1996). The randomized trials comparing lifestyle versus standard care treatment conditions, conducted by the Finnish Diabetes Prevention Study Group (Lindstrom, Louheranta, & Mannelin, 2003; Tuomilehto et al., 2001) and by the United States (Knowler et al., 2002), are two examples of the evidence needed to demonstrate that behavioral change will improve health outcomes for some people. Both trials reported that 58% fewer individuals at high risk for diabetes became diabetic following participation in a lifestyle intervention in comparison to the high-risk individuals given standard care. These effects were significant over multiple years (7 years in the Finnish trial), and the benefits for the high-risk participants in the lifestyle condition of the U.S. trial (58% fewer of 1,079 participants became diabetic in the 2.8-year postintervention period) also exceeded the benefits of participants given medication (31% of 1,073 participants prescribed metformin became diabetic).

Longitudinal Data: Social Class, Race, Religion, and Health/Mortality

The advantages of the clinical trial can be highlighted by comparing the diabetes prevention clinical trials to studies examining the relationship of risk to health outcomes in cross-sectional and longitudinal data. For example, examinations of the association of social stratification and age with health (House et al., 1992) in the Social Structures and Aging series and Kaplan's (1992) work "Health and Aging in the Alameda County Study" reveal clear associations between social-level variables (e.g., socioeconomic status [SES]) and health outcomes. One cannot tell, however, whether the income and living conditions associated with lower levels of SES are the determinants of poor health or whether poor health leads to low income and poor living conditions; the antecedence is ambiguous. And in the absence of random assignment, it is impossible to rule out the wide range of biological, behavioral, and cognitive differences among the individuals at different SES levels that may be responsible for differences in health outcomes. It is also unclear precisely what aspects of SES affect health and how they do so; does SES affect access to quality diet, to facilities and/or safe locations for physical activity, or access to health care, or are people at lower SES levels exposed to social influences that shape risky and discourage healthy behaviors, or are they exposed to chronic life stressors that gradually undermine physical health? The mechanisms are unclear.

Not all longitudinal data suffer from multiple problems in interpretation. For example, some data show a bidirectional effect of behavior, for example, an overall decline in smoking by English physicians after Doll and Hill's (1950) early publications linking smoking to lung cancer, followed 20 years later by reductions in lung cancer mortality. A similar effect can be seen between the number of men in the United States who quit smoking after the publication of the surgeon general's report (U.S. Public Health Service, 1964)—in contrast to the increase in smoking among women during the same time period (1965–1985)—and a lagging increase in rates of lung cancer. The increase in smoking among women followed changes at the sociocultural level (e.g., mass marketing campaigns targeting women by connecting smoking to the growing women's movement as well as by linking it to weight loss; U.S. Department of Health and Human Services, 2001). The data across and within the sexes provide strong evidence for a causal role of smoking and lung cancer.

Although the changes in social/cultural level variables over time are antecedent to critical health outcomes, thereby strengthening their causal role, the data do not identify *how* specific social influences and economic factors affected the behavior of particular groups of men and women. Thus the data on smoking do not tell us whether media messages or interpersonal influences, or a combination of the two, affected the cessation or uptake of smoking, nor do they identify the specific media messages, social contacts, and communications that were influential. Indeed, the harm and benefits of smoking behavior could be confined to particular subsets of individuals within each sex, and it is possible that the individuals who respond to media and social influence differ on factors such as their behavioral propensities or biological vulnerability, which in turn affect resistance to smoking-related disease. Although we do not support the following hypothesis, it is possible that individuals who are biologically vulnerable to harm from smoking are also more responsive to social factors encouraging the behavior, and conversely, that the biologically least vulnerable are more responsive to communications urging cessation (Eysenck, 1980).

Comparing Clinical Trials to Longitudinal Studies

Though we agree with those who believe that randomized clinical trials are superior to longitudinal descriptive studies for identifying healthy and risky behaviors and, by implication, are superior to descriptive data that are cross-sectional, we are not entirely happy with a blanket endorsement of the clinical trial. For example, although the diabetes prevention trials show that lifestyle changes can improve an objective health outcome, it is not clear *which* lifestyle behaviors provided the critical benefits, that is, was it exercise, a specific change in diet, or weight loss? It also is not clear which specific interventions were responsible for the behavioral changes such as the initiation and maintenance of exercise that led to weight loss. These are not trivial questions; clinical trials are not laboratory experiments that isolate and manipulate a single independent variable. The contrast between the diabetes prevention trials and the Hypertension Optimal Treatment (HOT) trial illustrates these points. HOT focused on a relatively simple intervention, that is, taking 75 Mg of aspirin daily in addition to a daily calcium channel blocker (Hansson et al., 1998), and found that adding aspirin resulted in 15% fewer major cardiovascular events ($p = .03$) and 36% fewer myocardial infarctions ($p = .002$) among the 18,790 participants randomly assigned to aspirin. There was, however, no advantage for reductions of stroke. The intervention promoting the use of aspirin and the behavior itself are simple in contrast to the lifestyle changes in the diabetes trials. In addition, the end points defining the benefits of aspirin were multiple and were identified by physiological models of aspirin's physiological effects, that is, how it gets under the skin. A recent review showing high agreement between longitudinal studies and randomized trials for pharmacological interventions requiring little or no complex behavioral management speaks to the virtue of simplicity in intervention studies (Concato, Shah, & Horwitz, 2000).

Gaps in the Empirical Picture

Although our review of the evidence from both clinical trials and population studies is highly selective, it is representative of what is known about the relationship between behavior and health, and the data strongly support the hypothesis that behavioral changes can be of major benefit to health. The two substantial gaps in the empirical picture concern how the ecological and social context affects individual action and how individual actions affect the physiological processes that influence hard health outcomes.

How Do Social Factors Affect Individual Behavior?

Both the recent community studies (House et al., 1992; Kaplan, 1992) and Braudel's (1979) historical observations agree that the poor, undereducated, very young are most likely the victims of mortality from environmental hazards and are most vulnerable to starvation and infectious disease. The studies fail, however, both to specify the exact aspects of socioeconomic gradient associated with specific health behaviors at the individual or psychological level and how these factors influence behavior. For example, do individuals with more education engage in preventive health actions with greater frequency because their employment provides the resources (e.g., financial support, time, place) for action, because they understand risk, or because they have the skills and resources to reorganize daily life patterns to insert exercise and diet change, or is the cross-level effect observed because educational achievement is associated with a time orientation that places greater emphasis on future time and does not discount future rewards (Chapman, 1998)?

Another feature that is missing in the network of findings that is needed to understand how social context affects individual behavior is the minimal data on public understanding and use of scientific evidence in guiding health actions. Cultural norms for behavioral prevention and control of chronic illness will not reflect scientific evidence unless these data enter into the public domain. Behaviors that have been validated as healthy or useless in so-called objective clinical trials or longitudinal studies may fail to be seen as such by laypersons (H. Leventhal, Rabin, Leventhal, & Burns, 2001). For example, juries ignored the statistics for both the effectiveness of prostate antigen testing (PSA) and treatments for prostate cancer when ruling against a physician who failed to recommend PSA testing on the basis of established statistical evidence (Merenstein, 2004). The huge market for alternative or complementary treatments provides ample evidence of public readiness to accept and adopt untested, unproven, and potentially hazardous prevention and treatment procedures because these procedures fit common-sense understandings of health, disease, and treatment (Cassileth, 1998; Gunther, Patterson, Kristal, Stratton, & White, 2004). Examples include the belief that natural remedies are more efficacious and safer than medications (Conrad, 1985; Durante, Whitmore, Jones, & Campbell, 2001) given that the natural are viewed as superior as they are not seen as artificial or chemical (Kaptchuk & Eisenberg, 1998). Haber (2004) suggested that the 19th-century view of aging as a disease, combined with common-sense perceptions of biological processes, opens the gates to marketers, who earn millions by marketing nonsense such as imbibing a growth hormone that will allow us to "gain muscle, enhance sex life, decrease wrinkles, prevent disease, and reverse the aging process" (Klatz & Kahn, 1998 as cited in Haber, 2004). Life-extending treatments have spawned a multi-billion-dollar industry, for which there is neither evidence of effectiveness nor reason to believe that such evidence will be forthcoming (Olshansky, Hayflick, & Carnes, 2002; U.S. General Accounting Office, 2001; for history, see Binstock, 2004). Furthermore, from the perspective of the culture and the individual, many behaviors are adopted and adhered to for reasons unrelated to health, though they pose significant health risks or benefits. What is abundantly clear is that the beliefs and perceptions of possible benefits associated with specific behaviors both prior to initiation and throughout maintenance are often far more significant determinants of initiating and sustaining behaviors than the actual risks and benefits defined by scientific study.

Limitations aside, population data are important for identifying inequalities in health across factors such as area of residence (e.g., nations, states, postal zones), ethnicity, income and/or education, and age as these data set the stage for research to identify the specific conditions leading to adverse health outcomes. Controlling for a few behaviors, such as smoking, and indices, such as weight, social relationships (e.g., marital status, frequency of social contacts), and acute and chronic stress (e.g., number of negative events in a lifetime or prior 3 years), can create the impression that the residual effects relating illness to SES reflect a direct, causal relationship of SES. These indices are not, however, direct causes of disease and physical well-being. An indicator like social class houses a composite of variables, some of which may have direct causal links to multiple illnesses and others to specific conditions. What is most clearly missing is *how* the cultural and social beliefs about illness, health care institutions, and providers, in conjunction with rules of behavior subsumed under ethnicity and SES, are communicated, perceived, and understood by individuals, thereby affecting their behavior.

How Does the Behavior Get Under the Skin?

The second challenge in knowledge visible in many behavioral studies in community settings concerns how specific health behaviors influence the physiological pathways leading to disease and mortality. Given the constraints on data collection (e.g., difficulties and costs of obtaining physiological measures on large samples and recruiting representative samples of individuals willing to participate in time-demanding protocols), longitudinal studies in community settings frequently combine different physical health factors to form a health index. For example, House and colleagues (1992) combined 10 different factors to form an index of health (e.g., acute fractures to chronic illnesses such as arthritis, cardiovascular disease, strokes, and cancers) and therefore are unable to identify the specific environmental factors and behaviors responsible for particular illnesses. It is possible, for example, that the greater number of illnesses experienced in midlife (44–65 years of age) by occupants of the lower SES strata is due to injuries and/or arthritic complications caused by occupational risks or other factors affecting the chronic illnesses in the index. Furthermore, combinations of factors, such as smoking and unhealthy diet, may relate to elevated levels of chronic illnesses across SES.

The clinical trials on daily use of aspirin and the longitudinal data on smoking are superior to the community studies in suggesting specific pathways by which behaviors get under the skin. The clarity differs, however, by behavior. In general, it is clear that the more specific the behavior (e.g., cigarette smoking or daily use of aspirin versus weight loss and exercise), the more certain the pathway for some, if not all, diseases. By-products of tobacco (over 5,000) and the pathways by which they attack the respiratory and cardiovascular systems and instigate several cancers are reasonably well specified. Though not all of the pathways for the benefits of daily use of aspirin are fully specified, many are well articulated (Fuster, Dyken, Vokonas, & Hennekens, 1993; Hayden, Pignone, Phillips, & Mulrow, 2002; Patrono, Rodriguez, Landolfi, & Baigent, 2005). On the other hand, obesity represents a risk for multiple diseases, and the physiological pathways are worked out for a few (e.g., diabetes and some cardiovascular disease), but less so for many cancers (Krauss, Winston, Fletcher, & Grundy, 1998; Kumanyika, 1993; Lazar, 2005; McTigue, Garrett, & Popkin, 2002).

The knowledge gap in both the clinical trials and the longitudinal studies is at the input end, that is, few adequately describe the factors involved in securing study participation and adherence to treatment. A review of the methods used in the working group study for diabetes prevention might suggest to the casual reader that the investigators understood the processes producing the lifestyle changes responsible for the movement from prediabetic to diabetic; the impression, however, is deceptive. The 16 one-on-one counseling sessions combined educational inputs and cognitive behavioral procedures to create an inclusive recipe for implementation of many ingredients, some of which might have been unnecessary. In addition, those that were critical and possibly sufficient to bring about change may only be effective for a highly select volunteer population. The deficit in this and other randomized behavioral trials is the lack of evidence as to how specific features of the intervention altered specific processes involved in adherence to particular prescribed behaviors, and how these specific behaviors altered the physiological process underlying the development of disease.

Concluding Remarks

The historical record, longitudinal descriptive studies, and the clinical trial support the obvious conclusion that behavioral factors have a substantial and clear impact on the health of populations and subsamples within populations. It is less clear, however, precisely which behavior and/or what dose or level of the behavior is responsible for the benefit. The concept of responsibility is unclear as a behavior may (a) impact known physiological pathways affecting health outcomes (taking an aspirin), (b) act through pathways as yet unidentified, or (c) have complex, indirect effects by creating the platform for effective behaviors, but not in itself have direct health benefits (e.g., a well-structured, orderly lifestyle allowing consistent performance of health behaviors such as taking the aspirin or antihypertensive pill every morning; avoiding excessive alcohol; not smoking). Although the social context is clearly critical for producing behavioral change in both the community and clinical trial, there is much to learn as to how specific contextual factors affect specific individual actions.

CARE SEEKING AND SELF-MANAGEMENT OF CHRONIC ILLNESS

Studies of the behavioral factors involved in seeking health care and the management of chronic illnesses provide examples of increasingly well defined pathways concerning both the social and psychological antecedents of behaviors in association with potentially clear views of the physiological pathways responsible for disease and health outcomes. By treating care seeking and self-management of chronic illness as health and risk behaviors, we are ignoring Kasl and Cobb's (1966) classic distinction between health behavior and illness behavior. This distinction was helpful in freeing investigators to examine in detail the effects of a wide range of behaviors affecting disease onset and prevention, as distinct from investigations of behaviors affecting disease management and progression. We believe, however, that the division of the research enterprise into health (e.g., primary prevention) and illness behaviors (secondary prevention) has outlived its usefulness and has had at least two negative effects. The first has been the development of separate models for the examination of the social and psychological factors involved in health and illness behavior, ignoring the commonalities among their determinants. The failure to examine the role of symptoms and illness as triggers for health-motivated primary prevention is likely a consequence of the separation of health and illness models. A second effect has been a tendency to separate the psychological–behavioral studies of primary prevention from the investigation of behavioral pathways related to clinical disease progression. This division is unfortunate as there is no sharp separation between the physiological processes involved in primary prevention, disease progression, and mortality. These issues will be elaborated on following the examination of the issues in care seeking and illness management.

Psychological Processes Underlie Care Seeking and Self-Management Behaviors

People seek medical services to satisfy clearances for insurance, in response to messages from mass media, to get inoculations needed for travel, for follow-up appointments for ongoing treatment, and for annual physicals and/or inoculations for flu or pneumonia. Scheduled visits are but part of the care-seeking picture; the other part is the patient-initiated visit that may be spontaneous or urgent or a deliberate decision to check on a specific symptom or change in function. Two sets of factors play a critical role in the generation of patient-initiated visits, one at the individual level and another at the social level. How they are connected is less well understood.

Symptoms as Cues to Action

Changes in somatic experience and function, for example, the appearance of symptoms, unpleasant feelings, or dysfunctions such as unsteadiness, inability to sleep, and fatigue, are the factors that are within the individual's skin that influence patient-initiated care seeking. New symptoms are by far the most powerful predictor of visits for medical care (Berkanovic, Telesky, & Reeder, 1981; Ory, DeFriese, & Duncker, 1998). The overwhelming importance of symptoms as cues to action is illustrated by the findings of Cameron, Leventhal, and Leventhal (1993). They used a complex longitudinal design to describe how the occurrence and inter-pretation of symptoms affect patient-initiated care seeking. One hundred and eleven pairs of older adult participants, each pair matched on age, gender, and medical history (222 individuals in all), were interviewed five times at 3-month intervals over a yearlong time frame. If either member of the pair arranged for a nonroutine or non-physician-scheduled medical visit, both the patient and the non-care-seeking matched partner were interviewed. As expected, care-seeking participants reported significantly more symptoms than their matched controls (7.15 vs. 4.79). The more striking statistic was the difference between the percentage of users re-porting new symptoms in comparison to the nonusers; 100% (all 111 users) versus 30% (33 of 111 nonusers).

The finding that 30% of those not seeking care were symptomatic is consistent with findings of other studies. Scambler, Scambler, and Craig (1981) estimated that less than half of symptomatic individuals seek health care, and Sorofman, Tripp-Reimer, Lauer, and Martin (1990) reported that medical consultations were sought for only 30% of the symptoms reported among a sample of adults who recorded daily symptoms for 28 days—the same percentage as that for Cameron et al. (1993). A com-parison between Cameron et al.'s (1993) 33 control patients with new symptoms with the 111 care seekers showed that the care seekers reported their symptoms to be more severe, and more important, to be *increasing in severity and unresponsive to efforts at control* during the time preced-ing care seeking. The potency of symptoms as cues to action increases with the appraisals that the symptoms are severe, on a trajectory of increasing severity and nonresponse to efforts to control the symptoms.

Heuristics and Symptom Interpretation

These three factors—(a) is it severe? (b) does it have a worsening tra-jectory?, and (c) are the symptoms unresponsive to treatment?—are common-sense if–then rules or questions that give meaning to somatic experience when answered (Brownlee, Leventhal, & Leventhal, 2000). These common-sense if–then rules or heuristics are the factors that con-nect perceptions (symptoms) to disease prototypes, and these *interpre-tations* guide the self-regulation process. If an elderly male experiences chest pain that is severe and of sudden onset (location and pattern), it will likely evoke the prototype for a heart attack and encourage rapid action (e.g., immediately seeking care; Bunde & Martin, 2006). On the other hand, *if* the somatic experience is of relatively mild, chronic breathlessness and swollen legs, it may *then* be processed as a problem with the lungs and legs due to overexertion or advancing age, the net result being inaction, that is, failure to seek care. Heuristics give meaning to somatic experience and create representations of illness threats. Understanding how heuristics operate in relation to illness and treatment prototypes is critical for developing interventions to improve chronic illness management.

Four sets of heuristics are involved in the question-asking process that gives meaning to somatic experience (see Table 2.1). Heuristics reflect a person's (a) anatomical representation of the body, (b) prior biological disease experiences, (c) social behavioral schemata; and (d) comparisons made between oneself and others. When evaluating novel symptoms, people rely on different combinations of these heuristics to help determine whether they need to seek care and what kind of care to seek. Patient-initiated health care visits are neither one-time decisions nor exclusively private decisions; a decision to visit a practitioner is one of many decisions involved in health management, and some of the prior, and perhaps the final, decisions are embedded in social exchanges. The initial, appraisal phase of a somatic change can be rapid or slow, depending on the severity of the cue, the rapidity and direction of change, and its total duration (Mora, Robitaille, Leventhal, Swigar, & Leventhal, 2002). Slower and less severe somatic changes prompt individuals to rely on heuristics based on life experiences such as stress–illness (i.e., is it illness or stress?) and age–illness (i.e., is it illness or is it age?). These heuristics provide a tentative classification for symptom cause as an indicator of illness or an alternative explanation.

For adults who have not yet experienced a chronic condition, the heuristics are most likely to assess changes against an internal framework for acute illness. This appraisal phase is visible in Western (Matthews, Siegel, Kuller, Thompson, & Varat, 1983; Safer, Tharps, Jackson, & Leventhal, 1979) and non-Western cultures. How the changes are interpreted by the individual in his or her cultural context can determine what the individual identifies as illness (i.e., that "I am sick or possessed"). Affective factors come into play, which, along with cognitive heuristics, determine if and from whom further advice and treatment are sought (see Bunde & Martin, 2006). If the heuristic-based self-assessment fails to confirm the acute model, one or more alternative models will likely be activated, some of which may be threatening, for example, the possibility of cancer or heart disease. A threatening alternative will stimulate some level of concern or fear, and the affective process

Table 2.1

FOUR TYPES OF HEURISTICS FOR EVALUATING AND RESPONDING TO SOMATIC CHANGE

HEURISTICS REFLECTING BASIC MENTAL OPERATION AND HUMAN ANATOMY		
HEURISTIC	**CUE –> PATIENT THOUGHTS**	**PATIENT THOUGHTS –> ACTIONS**
Location	Breathlessness	Likely a lung issue (not heart)
Duration	Symptom exceeds expected time	It's lasted "too long" –> better check it out
Severity	Pain: Disruption of physical function Disruption of mental function	Mild disruption = no need for care Major disruption = seek care

LEARNED HEURISTICS BASED ON UNIVERSAL SOMATIC EXPERIENCE OF BIOLOGICAL FEATURES OF DISEASE		
HEURISTIC	**CUE –> PATIENT THOUGHTS**	**PATIENT THOUGHTS –> ACTIONS**
Symmetry rule	I have a symptom I have an illness	Look for an illness Look for symptoms
Acute vs. chronic (timeline)	Symptoms some of the time Symptoms all of the time	Use treatment some of the time Use treatment all of the time
Rate of change (temporal trajectory)	Symptoms changing quickly Symptoms changing slowly	Better get help before it is unbearable! Not a big deal, can deal with it later.
Pattern (conceptual fit)	Pain in chest, radiation over left side of body –> must be heart GI distress, bloating, moving pain –> must be gut	Heart related = need to seek outside help Not heart related = it will clear, wait it out
Novelty	Symptom is new Symptom is familiar	Need to seek outside help Must be part of my ____, no need for help
Control (responded to care)	Symptom responds to patient treatment Symptom does not respond to patient treatment	Hurts less now, must not be serious Must be serious, better seek outside help

(continued)

Table 2.1

FOUR TYPES OF HEURISTICS FOR EVALUATING AND RESPONDING TO SOMATIC CHANGE (*CONTINUED*)

HEURISTICS BASED ON SOCIAL BEHAVIORAL SCHEMATA, LIFE-EXPERIENCE BASED AND REINFORCED		
HEURISTIC	**CUE –> PATIENT THOUGHTS**	**PATIENT THOUGHTS –> ACTIONS**
Age–illness	Is it age or is it illness?	If aging, accept it If illness, seek care
Gender stereotypes	Chest pain: I'm male: likely heart attack I'm female: likely stress	Likely a heart attack: seek care Likely stress: nothing medicine can do, wait and see
Stress–illness	Is it stress or is it illness?	If stress, nothing medicine can do and it will go away If illness, seek care
Feel good = am well	No symptoms and in a good mood	I must be healthy
HEURISTICS BASED ON SOCIAL COMPARISONS		
HEURISTIC	**CUE –> PATIENT THOUGHTS**	**PATIENT THOUGHTS –> ACTIONS**
Similar exposures (cause)	Gastric distress: We ate the same thing We ate different things	We're both sick, thus not serious Only I'm sick, could be serious
Similar vulnerabilities (similarity and contrast tests)	Temperament same as sister and she had cancer	Symptom is not like sister's, no need for care Symptom is like sister had, better seek care
Prevalence	Everyone has it Only I have it	Less serious, no need to seek care More serious, better seek care

will bring additional coping strategies into play. For example, concerns or fears associated with threats of cancer and heart disease appear to delay care seeking for middle-aged adults, but not for individuals over

65 years of age (E. A. Leventhal, Easterling, Leventhal, & Cameron, 1995; E. A. Leventhal, Leventhal, Schaefer, & Easterling, 1993).

Bidirectionality and Common Sense Self-Management

The bidirectionality hypothesis is a central assumption of the Common-Sense Model of Illness Self-Regulation (CSM) (H. Leventhal, Nerenz, & Steele, 1984; Meyer, Leventhal, & Gutmann, 1985; see Figure 2.2). The experience of disease-related biological changes, symptoms, moods, and physical and mental dysfunctions represents a pathway from biology to psychology that plays a critical role in behavioral self-management. Every human being is familiar with the signs and symptoms of illness—the aches and pains, feverishness, and fatigue of upper respiratory and gastrointestinal conditions as well as toothaches, earaches, and injuries. The model also assumes that a host of self-management processes are associated with these experiences and that the behavioral strategies and tactics acquired from a lifetime of illness management can be consistent and inconsistent with the procedures required for the optimal management of chronic illnesses.

One component of the pathway from biology to psychological experience is well known to physicians, pharmacists, adherence

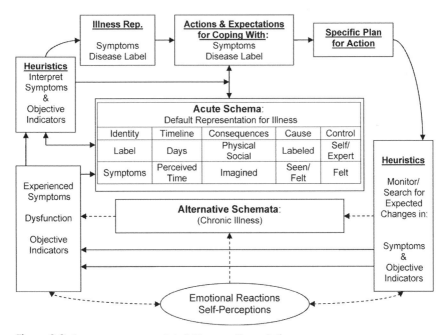

Figure 2.2 Common-sense model of illness self-regulation.

researchers, and pharmaceutical companies: so-called treatment side effects. Contingent on how they are perceived by the patient, physical changes produced by treatment can disrupt adherence if the changes are interpreted as signs that the treatment is harmful, or they can enhance adherence if interpreted as signs of treatment efficacy. The complexity of this interpretive process was revealed to us during an early study that examined the interaction among somatic cues and treatment adherence among elderly patients with hypertension (Meyer et al., 1985). This study led to the discovery of the *symmetry rule*: that concrete experiences generate a search for abstract labels (i.e., symptoms and functional changes lead to a search for a diagnosis), and abstract labels lead to a search for concrete experience (i.e., a label or diagnosis will lead to a search for and finding of symptoms). The combination of the concrete symptoms and abstract label forms the identity of a condition. When asked if they agreed that "people can't tell when their blood pressure is up," 80% of people (40 of 50) in the continuous treatment group strongly agreed with the statement (patients were classified as in continuous treatment if they had no history of having dropped out of treatment; it was one of four groups). On the other hand, when asked at another point in the interview, "Do you think you can tell when your blood pressure is up?" 92% (46 of 50) agreed, a far higher percentage than reported by 50 non-hypertensive control patients (48% felt they could tell), and higher than patients new to treatment (71% of 65 cases).

The paradox of their conflicting agreements did not faze the participants in the continuing care group as there is likely little reason why they should disagree with what their physicians say about people in general. The physician has seen many patients, and it is entirely possible that other people cannot tell when their blood pressure is up, even though "I [the patient] can!" The source of patients' confidence in their personal experience is evident from an examination of the symptoms they report as signs of hypertension: headache (24% of 50), dizziness (17%), warm face (22%), nervousness (16%), and assorted other symptoms. These symptoms are experienced with physical exertion and emotional stress, occasions likely associated with temporary, though not chronic, elevations in blood pressure (Stewart, Janicki, & Kamarck, 2006). These symptoms are reported by nonhypertensive study participants given false elevated blood pressure readings in carefully controlled laboratory settings (Baumann, Cameron, Zimmerman, & Leventhal, 1989).

The association of symptoms with the label, that is, the diagnosis of hypertension, has important behavioral consequences. First, it affected adherence to medication among the 50 patients in the continuing care group: 70% of the patients (32/46) who reported symptoms said that medication treatment affected their symptoms. These patients were adherent to medication, and these adherent patients had better blood pressure control. The 30% (14/46) who reported that treatment did not affect their symptoms were nonadherent and in poor control. The second behavioral effect was observed in an inception sample, a group of 65 patients who were new to treatment. Some of these patients told their doctor that they could tell their blood pressure was elevated by monitoring symptoms; some did not. Among those who told their doctors, 60% had dropped out of treatment 9 months later; only 25% dropped out among the patients who did not tell their doctors that they could tell when their blood pressure was elevated by monitoring symptoms. Communicating the belief in the efficacy of monitoring puts the patient at odds with the doctor, a disagreement that, in this case, appears to have led to nonadherence.

The need to label somatic experiences and the search for somatic experiences to make sense of labels involve the very same heuristics used in the decisions to seek care. When somatic changes are attributed to stress (Cameron, Leventhal, & Leventhal, 1995) or to age (Prohaska, Keller, Leventhal, & Leventhal, 1987), rather than to illness, the interpretation will slow or block care seeking for newly experienced conditions and affect the need to act for the management of existent chronic conditions. A vivid picture of the operation of these heuristics can be seen in the contrast between care-seeking behavior following myocardial infarction (heart attack) and the absence of care seeking during flares of congestive heart failure. Bunde and Martin (2006) conducted intensive interviews with 433 patients (mean age = 60 years) 8 days, on average, following a myocardial infarct (MI). They found that swift use of care following an MI was associated with a series of cognitive heuristics, or mental shortcuts, for interpreting symptom patterns. Care seeking was more rapid for the novel symptom of sweating (*novelty* heuristic; see Mora et al., 2002), and for symptoms *location* and *pattern*, which encouraged attribution to cardiac disease. If, however, the experience of symptom location and pattern was interpreted as gastrointestinal distress, care seeking was slowed. Care seeking was also slowed in response to an affective or emotional heuristic, feelings of depression, and more specifically, feelings of fatigue; its effect was independent of that for the cognitive heuristics. Finally, and as expected, a prior history of MI sped care seeking.

Bunde and Martin's (2006) quantitative findings contrast with the qualitative findings for patients with congestive heart failure (CHF;

Horowitz, Rein, & Leventhal, 2004). Life expectancy for patients with this severe coronary disease is limited; most die within 5 years after diagnosis. Inappropriate self-management can result in episodes of cardiac decompensation and risk of death. Decompensation occurs due to failure to detect and monitor signs of fluid buildup and use diuretics. Interviews with these patients show that they do not understand they have heart problems. They are told they have heart problems (CHF) and report, "When you hear about having heart problems, you're supposed to feel maybe a pain in your left arm, maybe a pain in your chest or pressure." Neither the location nor the pattern of CHF symptoms fit the patient's model of cardiac symptoms. Regarding location, CHF symptoms of breathlessness suggest that the problem is located in the lungs, while the symptom of swollen feet suggests that there is a problem with the feet. Relying on the pattern heuristic is also problematic for patients with CHF as the pattern of symptoms does not match the classic cardiac symptoms of chest pain and pressure. CHF patients in this study reported that they did not seek care because the symptoms "just didn't seem to me like anything came together," and "I had to struggle in order to talk. . . . I guess it would have been more clear to me if I had chest pain and then I would have said, okay, I'll call."

Interpretive processes are present across multiple chronic conditions; they are not unique to hypertension and cardiovascular disease. Asthma, a chronic condition punctuated by severe episodes, involves the patient in a problem-solving game similar to that for congestive heart failure and hypertension. Although many asthmatics know which of their symptoms are likely due to asthma and which are not (Mora, Halm, Leventhal, & Ceric, in press), severe attacks are difficult to control, and death may occur if the patient fails to use medications on a daily basis to control chronic underlying pulmonary inflammation. For many with asthma, medications are to be used during asymptomatic periods to reduce airway inflammation and sensitivity to stimulants that trigger attacks. Optimal management requires that patients treat their asthma as a chronic condition, something that is there all the time.

Baseline interviews with 198 asthmatics hospitalized during severe attacks showed that 80% of the sample believed they definitely (66%) or probably (14%) "will always have asthma" (Halm, Mora, & Leventhal, 2006). The abstract conceptualization these patients have of their asthma does not, however, correspond to their experience. When asked, "Do you think you have asthma all of the time or only when you're having symptoms?" 53% said they had asthma "only when they had symptoms" or "some of the time when they had symptoms" (4%). In other words, 57% of these patients linked their asthma to symptoms, and only 40% held a chronic belief, stating that they had asthma all of the time, even when they did not have symptoms. Not surprisingly, daily maintenance inhalers to control airway inflammation were used all or most of the time by only 45% of the patients who felt asthma was episodic, in comparison to 70% of the patients who perceived it as there all of the time (chronic). Although the effect of these divergent views of the asthma experience shrank somewhat 6 months following discharge, it was still the case that use of inhalers was less among patients who saw asthma as episodic or acute (63% used inhalers) versus those who perceived it as there even when they were asymptomatic, that is, as truly chronic (80% used inhalers as prescribed).

Labels Integrate Experience Over Time

The reports of the illness representations and self-management behavior of the patients in the CHF and asthma studies make clear the importance of linking a symptomatic condition with an abstract, diagnostic label. The diagnostic label provides a conceptual framework for linking experiences that vary over time and connecting experiences to specific actions. Lacking the overarching concept of CHF, these patients failed to see the connection between the episodes of frighteningly severe decompensation that led them to the emergency room and the persistent fatigue, minor breathlessness, and swelling of legs that mark the very same disease underlying the severe episodes. Forming connections between the severe episodes and chronic symptoms is likely further hampered by the logical attributions of the latter to aging; a fundamental and chronic feature of the self is linked to a chronic symptom of the disorder. The separation of acute episodes from chronic symptoms creates confusion, if not outright disbelief, in response to recommendations that the use of diuretics to treat low-level chronic symptoms will help to avoid severe episodes.

Prototypes Underlie Representations of Illness and Representations of Treatments

The conceptual framework and the empirical data provide a bidirectional view of the connection between biological processes and the psychological system. As the stimuli having access to consciousness from biological processes are generally ambiguous, their interpretation and meaning depend on psychological operations; these operations involve heuristics used for decoding the information. Heuristics test the fit between the evidence and a set of underlying models. The basic distinction, visible in the studies focused on care seeking, is between sickness and wellness. Attributing symptoms and functional declines to stress or to age removes them from the illness side of the equation and reduces the likelihood of seeking traditional medical care. The second distinction made when the heuristics point to illness is whether the illness is acute or chronic. Both the hypertension and asthma data suggest that the default model, "I have high blood pressure and/or asthma when I have symptoms," is for acute, rather than chronic, illness. The chronic side of the equation is more complex as multiple illness schemas or prototypes are in the chronic category; MI or heart attack is clearly one, and CHF may or may not be one.

Although heuristics and prototypes involved in common-sense problem solving may operate in a consistent and logical manner, they will not lead to valid self-diagnoses or use of treatment if the logical operations begin with faulty premises. Treating symptoms and disease as equivalent, the symmetry assumption may be consistent with lifelong experience with head colds, injuries, and gastric distress but is an inappropriate interpretation of the relationship of symptoms to chronic illnesses. For example, strong heart beats, warm faces, and headache can indicate elevations in blood pressure during physical exertion and stress but are inappropriate indicators of elevations of resting levels of systolic and diastolic pressure. That which is stable and chronic is not the same as the short-term state. The same applies to asthma: The salient attack reflects an interaction of an attack trigger with chronic inflammation but is neither identical to the chronic inflammation, nor does it require the same treatment; control of the chronic inflammation often calls for daily use of maintenance medications (e.g., inhaled corticosteroids), while control of attacks requires the use of quick relievers (e.g., beta agonists).

Treatments, self-selected or prescribed activities for both prevention and management, are related to disease models and have models of their own. As with disease labels, labeling treatments can have marked effects on expectations for treatment efficacy and treatment risks, in addition to linking the treatment to specific experiences. For example, inhaled corticosteroids used to maintain low levels of pulmonary inflammation and quick relief medications used to control attacks are linked to asthma; they are part of the perceived controllability of the disease representation. However, the abstract labels that create specific expectations for asthma treatment can also connect these medications to medications unrelated to asthma. For some patients, the word *steroid* in the label corticosteroid may link this inhaler medication to the dangerous steroids used by athletes to increase muscle mass. Making this connection raises concerns about medication safety and may be one of the factors responsible for the widespread underuse of these medications (Boulet, 1998; van Grunsven et al., 1998).

Labels can create links among diseases and treatments that can have surprising effects. For example, the media and medical practitioners have linked use of aspirin to protection against cardiovascular disease: daily low-dose aspirin is viewed by many as an effective way to prevent cardiovascular disease (Patrono et al., 2005). But common sense also recognizes that aspirin is a painkiller and places it in that category, along with other medications such as acetaminophens. Painkillers of the latter type are preferred by people susceptible to gastric distress or risk of uncomfortable, though not life-threatening, bleeding (e.g., nosebleeds due to low blood platelet levels). It is unlikely, however, that many asthmatics with histories of moderate to severe asthma recognize that acetaminophens, but not aspirin, will exacerbate asthma attacks (McKeever et al., 2005; Shaheen, Sterne, Songhurst, & Burney, 2000). In sum, there is probably little reason to expect that everyday observation will create a negative link between the representations of asthma and those of the specific painkiller acetaminophens. Concocting labels and descriptions that relate specific treatments to larger health themes is a cornerstone of medication marketing. Substances labeled as natural and having ancient or mystical pedigrees are seen as nonchemical and therefore safe. Although the first implication is clearly false, given that natural substances may not be manufactured but are clearly chemical, their safety depends on the properties of the substance and how it will interact with a person's physiology and other prescribed treatments (Niggemann & Gruber, 2003). Labels are also chosen to suggest links to particular ailments. In sum, marketing in the $73,000,000,000 health food and alternative medicine industry relies on common-sense modeling to sell its products.

Concluding Remarks on Common-Sense Perceiving and Thinking

It is important to be clear about the precise referents for common-sense models and common-sense perceiving and thinking and the role of these processes in more comprehensive biobehavioral theory. The phrases refer specifically to people's everyday ways of perceiving and thinking about current and future illness threats. Individuals engage in an ongoing process in an effort to make sense of their somatic experience. They rely on the underlying illness and treatment prototypes of illnesses, their domains (e.g., symptoms and labels, timelines, consequences, causes, control), and heuristics to test the fit of ongoing somatic experience to these existing prototypes. These processes define control systems, that is, set points or targets, against which to evaluate a changing landscape. Common-sense models also include larger strategies for self-management. Some of these strategies of special significance for the aging individual will be discussed briefly in the following section.

It is critical to recognize that common-sense models may or may not overlap with the actual biological processes they are designed to manage. The common-sense models guiding the behavior of many patients with hypertension and diabetes are not valid representations of the underlying biology of these diseases; the consequence can be poor management. Common-sense justifications for risky behaviors (e.g., "smoking calms my nerves," "high-fat foods are comforting") are equally false. In addition, common-sense thinking may or may not be sensitive to and accurately represent the origins of its contents. People may or may not be aware of the influence of media, observations of friends, and experiences of family members on (a) how they represent illnesses and treatment and (b) the heuristics they use for evaluating their own somatic experiences. In addition, they may be only partially aware of the way in which environmental events and their own behavior affect learning, habit formation, and later action. Common-sense conceptions of these processes may have important effects for preferences and resistances to specific treatments. Thus much remains to be explored.

LEVELS AND THEIR CONNECTIONS: SELF/ PSYCHOLOGICAL, SOCIAL, AND BIOLOGICAL

We have described common-sense perceiving and thinking as a problem-solving process focused on interpreting, giving meaning to, and managing somatic changes that portend future risk to health or are current signs of illness. As this problem-solving process takes place within the perceived self, the individual's representation of his or her physical and self-competencies will affect how illness threats are represented and managed. As self and health threats are interrelated, these processes can in turn lead to revised perceptions of the durability and competence of the physical self and its ability to perform specific tasks and social roles (Epstein, 1973).

Relationships of Facets of the Self and Health Behaviors

Two aspects of the self-concept that have been examined extensively are *self-efficacy*, or the perception that one is able to perform a specific action in an efficacious manner (Bandura, 1989, 2004), and beliefs respecting control or the perception of personal control over and responsibility for daily events (Langer & Rodin, 1976); both are concerned with the skill component of the problem-solving process. Both efficacy and control are dynamic concepts; that is, they are beliefs that affect behavior and are affected by behavior, though some investigators have treated them as fixed traits. It is easier, however, to identify studies that demonstrate how efficacy affects behavior than to identify studies that examine how behavior affects efficacy. The path from efficacy to behavior has been examined with regard to the effects of level of self-efficacy on taking medication (e.g., Barclay et al., 2007), healthy eating (e.g., Shields & Brawley, 2006), and exercising (e.g., Renner & Schwarzer, 2005).

A critical barrier for understanding the conditions under which behavior will lead to changes in self-efficacy among elderly individuals (Maibach & Murphy, 1995) can be seen in the difficulties faced by investigators attempting to recruit older adults into exercise programs to improve strength and health; recruitment rates are often less than 50% of the individuals approached (see the review by H. Leventhal et al., 2001). Those elderly who participate develop a sense of self-efficacy for exercise the more frequently they exercise and the more positive affect and social support they experience while exercising (e.g., Dechamps, Lafont, & Bourdel-Marchasson, 2007; McAuley, Jerome, Marquez, Elavsky, & Blissmer, 2006). Exercise is related to improved balance and cognitive performance at all ages and can benefit the frail as well as the more healthy elderly (King, Rejeski, & Buchner, 1998).

In addition to the relative paucity of studies that have explicitly examined how feedback from the problem-solving level, that is, feedback from illness management, affects self-efficacy or other self-perceptions, there also is little empirical data showing how self-perceptions (e.g., self-assessments of health as excellent vs. poor) and feelings of vulnerability to specific diseases affect the construction and content of illness and treatment representations. Available data indicate that the relationship between perceptions of the self on one hand, and specific health threats and procedures for maintaining health on the other, is domain-specific as well as bidirectional. For example, an individual's self-efficacy for regulating diet is ineffective for regulating exercise and vice versa (Baldwin et al., 2006). Domain-specific self-perceptions have been reported in studies of participation in rehabilitation programs following MI (Schwarzer & Fuchs, 1995), for example, efficacy for the initiation and maintenance of exercise (Sallis, Hovell, & Hofstetter, 1992) is separate from efficacy for the regulation of a healthy diet (Schwarzer & Fuchs, 1995).

The differentiation of efficacy across domains and changes in self-efficacy over time are consistent with its conceptualization as a dynamic factor, rather than as a trait, and with the importance of defining and assessing efficacy as a domain-specific factor. Investigators have questioned, however, whether efficacy is merely a correlate or a causal factor in the chain between prior and later action, that is, whether efficacy has a functional relationship to subsequent performance. Heggestad and Kanfer (2005) showed that prior behaviors build self-efficacy and that prior behavior, and not the individual's self-reports of efficacy, are causally related to subsequent behavior. Whether their findings will hold for maintenance of a health behavior versus the initiation of new health behaviors, and whether efficacy can affect success for some health behavior changes and not others (Vancouver & Kendall, 2006), has yet to be determined. Finally, in contrast to the domain specificity reported in investigations of self-efficacy, Heidrich, Forsthoff, and Ward (1994) showed that broadly defined self-perceptions (i.e., the discrepancy between ideal and perceived self) can mediate adjustment to a severe health threat; this discrepancy mediated patients' representations of cancer to social adjustment and depression. Future studies will be needed to determine whether such self-ideal discrepancies are also domain-specific.

Psychological Strategies of the Aging Self

Investigators have examined a number of cognitive and affective strategies visible with advancing age. Two such factors are the belief that conservation of resources is critical for maintaining health and the readiness to relinquish goals that are perceived as unattainable. Both factors appear to be related to the elderly individual's experience and interpretation of the biological and social changes experienced in the later years of life, and both affect motivation for the initiation, cessation, and/or maintenance of healthy and risky behaviors.

Age-Related Biological Change

E. A. Leventhal and Crouch (1997) suggested that biological changes in the later years of life, such as reduced control of sympathetic activation due to declines in parasympathetic control, reduced immune competence, and loss of muscle mass, lead, respectively, to reductions in the automatic processes responsible for the control of emotional distress, increased vulnerability to and slower recovery from illness, and greater susceptibility to falls. They hypothesized that the experience of these changes leads to the development of a strategy for the conservation of resources as a way of avoiding threats to the physical self, and this strategy can influence a wide range of health and social behaviors. One manifestation of the conservation strategy is more rapid seeking of medical care by elderly individuals than by middle-aged individuals. Rapid care seeking recruits expert resources to address both the reality of physical symptoms and dysfunction and to terminate the worry and sense of physical depletion that can result from living with emotional distress over a prolonged period of time (E. A. Leventhal et al., 1995; E. A. Leventhal et al., 1993). The loss of muscle mass and loss of feedback from the feet due to diabetic neuropathy, which contribute to unsteadiness and falls, will further encourage conservation and discourage an active lifestyle, resulting in the relinquishment of social roles and the onset of depressive affect (Vileikyte, Rubin, & Leventhal, 2004).

Self-Regulation Strategies, Activity Replacement, and Goal Setting

The effects of conservation of resources to avoid self-depletion were documented by Duke, Leventhal, Brownlee, and Leventhal (2002) among community-dwelling elderly who were forced to give up a vigorous physical activity (e.g., jogging, tennis) or intense social activity due to a severe illness. The subsequent replacement of vigorous and/or intense activities with less vigorous (e.g., walking) ones was positively associated with an optimistic outlook (Carver, Scheier, & Weintraub, 1989), satisfaction with support from one's social network, and having social obligations. Replacement of demanding activities with less demanding ones was less likely, however, among elderly who were committed to a strategy of conservation of resources for maintaining health. Finding replacement was nontrivial for quality of life: Those who replaced reported more positive affect a year later. Being able to disengage and replace unattainable with reachable goals has been found to be critical for adjustment in the later years of life in multiple studies by Wrosch, Scheier, Carver, and Schulz (2003). They hypothesized that elderly people high on internal control are less likely to disengage, even though the goals they are seeking are unattainable due to their limited lifetimes, and that failing to disengage will lead to a syndrome of emotional distress, reduced quality of life, and negative effects for health. By contrast, elderly low on control will more readily yield the unattainable and identify and work toward more reachable goals. Interestingly, they propose that internal control beliefs will be beneficial for giving up and replacing goals among younger persons.

Affective Management, Cognitive Decline, and Health Behaviors

For the elderly, bad news risks chronic stress, and good news is a balm; not surprisingly, the elderly rely on affective cues, for example, feeling good, as an indicator of good health (Benyamini, Leventhal, & Leventhal, 1999) and feelings of chronic stress as a sign of weakening resources and risk to health. A lifelong search for positive inputs leads to a strategy to seek positive feelings and to evaluate positive feelings as a sign of good health. This hypothesis is consistent with Carstensen's (1992; Carstensen & Charles, 1998) proposal of a transition in the later years from the acquisition and use of knowledge to solve problems of work and career toward a focus on emotionally satisfying close relationships: the social emotional selectivity theory. This broad hypothesis appears to describe age-related changes for many elderly and is consistent with two well-documented biobehavioral changes of the life span. The first such change is the decline beginning at 20 years of age among a broad array of cognitive competencies related to working memory (e.g., digit symbol test, spatial skills, computation span, etc.). This decline contrasts with the trajectory of crystallized skills, such as vocabulary, which increase gradually until the sixth decade of life and remain relatively stable afterward (Park et al., 2002). The decline in cognitive agility, for example, working memory skills, would seem one possible factor underlying the shift from knowledge acquisition and problem-solving skills toward interpersonal contacts; if you still possess the language competencies for communication but cannot perform complex novel tasks, motivation and active engagement in new learning and problem solving are likely to decline.

While loss of cognitive competency may account for declines in felt efficacy and reduced motivation to engage in knowledge-based tasks, it seems insufficient to account for an increased focus on social relationships that are emotionally satisfying. The second possible contributor to social emotional selectivity is the age-related decline in the reported intensity of emotional experience (Magai, 2001), a change that likely creates the risk of social disengagement and loss of interest in daily life. The emotional satisfaction that derives from participating in close social relationships can counter the age-related decline in emotional affectivity, and the maintenance of the verbal communication skills essential for maintaining these relationships can in turn help to sustain cognitive competency (Holtzman, et al., 2004). An orientation toward and search for sources of positive affect that underlies the emotional selectivity aspect of Carstensen's (1992) interpersonal hypothesis may also reflect the value of positive affect as a screen capable of minimizing the sense of debilitation produced by the experience of negative affects related to onset of multiple chronic conditions and age-related declines in physical strength. As the threat of cancers and cardiac diseases increases in the later years and the end of life looms closer, the search for close, meaningful relationships that create positive affects may provide an effective screen from those less pleasant emotions. These affective relationships and the complementary withdrawal from information acquisition and work will also serve to shield the elderly from social comparisons with more active individuals and from participating in tasks that would make reductions in cognitive capacities painfully visible.

Social Context, Self, Self-Regulation, and Individual Health Behaviors

As we stated earlier, multilevel models examining individual health beliefs and behavior nested under different levels of social and institutional factors do not tell us which health behaviors are affected by community- or social-level variables, nor do these models identify the processes by which contextual variables affect behavior. Factors such as postal zone, SES, whether the community is traditional or contemporary, religious affiliation, and attendance at religious services subsume a host of specific variables ranging from access to care through diet, physical activity, and other healthy and risky behaviors (e.g., physical activity, smoking, and alcohol use) that may be responsible for their association with indices of morbidity and mortality (Idler, 2004; Krause, 2004). The studies of care seeking and illness management provide valuable clues as to the processes connecting these levels.

Connecting Social and Individual Levels

For over three decades, investigators have examined how social influences affect decisions and use of health care (Dimsdale et al., 1979; Roghmann & Haggerty, 1973). Consistent with earlier studies, more recent findings show that direct communication plays a role in care-seeking decisions (Oberlander, Pless, & Dougherty, 1993; Sanders, 1982). Cameron et al. (1993) found that 92% of the participants discussed their somatic changes with another person, typically their spouse. There was no indication, however, as to whether these exchanges occurred prior to the decision that one was ill, in which case it would act as a message encouraging the appraisal of oneself as at risk, or after the decision was made that one was likely ill. Zola's (1973) analysis of lay networks suggests that much social influence occurs both before and after illness decisions are made. For example, he found that lay networks often engage in *sanctioning*, that is, the well member in a network indicating that it is reasonable to seek medical attention for a given complaint as they would do so if they were in that position. Sanctioning was more common among Irish American than Italian American patients, while symptoms in combination with an interpersonal crisis were more likely to lead to care seeking among Italian American than Irish American patients. Care seeking was also more likely for both Italian American and Irish American patients if symptoms threatened social or personal relationships, while for Anglo American patients, care seeking was enhanced if symptoms interfered with vocational or physical activities. It is likely that these decisions follow a strong suspicion that one may be or definitely is ill (Apple, 1960; Zola, 1973).

Friends and family members do not always promote care seeking. They may encourage a wait-and-see attitude or outright avoidance of care seeking (Albrecht & Goldsmith, 2003; Dakof & Taylor, 1990; Martin, Davis, Baron, Suls, & Blanchard, 1994; Rook, 1984), and under certain circumstances, which are as yet unclear, it has been found that strong social networks have encouraged delays in seeking care (Berkanovic et al., 1981; Granovetter, 1978; Liu & Duff, 1972) or discouraged it altogether (Suls & Goodkin, 1994). Factors encouraging delay may be differences in the way family members interpret symptoms or unwarranted expressions of certainty in the invulnerability of the complaining individual. If family members report having experienced similar symptoms and survived in good health, these experiences may reduce the current sufferer's perceptions of the seriousness of his or her condition (Croyle & Jemmott, 1991). Likewise, being surrounded by supportive others may lower the sufferer's sense of ambiguity and reduce anxiety and concern about his or her well-being and lessen motivation to seek care. It is also possible that a large active support network may encourage the individual to remain active, despite the presence of symptoms, and encourage avoidance if the individual is too fearful of possible diagnoses and treatments. Suls and Goodkin (1994) also suggested that family members may discourage the use of care because they distrust or dislike the health care system and health practitioners. Lay consultation is a time-consuming process. However astute the lay consultants might be, the very act of discussing the presence and potential meanings of symptoms requires time and delays entry into the health care delivery system (Suls, Martin, & Leventhal, 1997). Research is needed to examine how the social context shapes the individual's representations of health threats, treatments and the treatment system, and the final decision to seek or delay and avoid the use of professional care.

It would be a mistake to view the available evidence as supporting a simple, unidirectional flow of influence, that is, from social network to individual. As reported by Cameron et al. (1993), individuals experiencing symptoms and physical dysfunction actively seek information and support from family members and friends, and family members and friends may independently seek information they then communicate to or screen from the eyes and ears of the ill individual (Brashers, Goldsmith, & Hsieh, 2002). How a somatic event is represented by a symptomatic or ill person will affect the meaning he or she assigns the event, the type of advice sought, and the persons from whom advice is sought. An individual's common-sense model of his or her symptoms is one such moderator. For example, if a person experiencing gastric distress and vomiting wonders if he or she has consumed contaminated food, the person will select a comparison person who has eaten the same or similar meals at the same places: If this comparison person is experiencing the same symptoms, it confirms the tainted food hypothesis for both parties (H. Leventhal, Hudson, & Robitaille, 1997).

On the other hand, if the individual is frightened because he or she believes that gastric distress is caused by esophageal cancer, the person will seek out and share concerns with a person more capable of providing reassuring evidence (H. Leventhal et al., 1997). In this example, social comparison is a heuristic for interpreting and/or clarifying the meaning of symptoms, and the underlying hypothesis (e.g., food poisoning vs. cancer) affects the person selected for comparison. Depending on the patient's needs, for example, acquiring skills to master a treatment, the target for comparison can be someone with mastery (an upward comparison), or someone doing less well (a downward comparison), if the patient's perception of self in relation to his or her views of disease and treatment has damaged self-confidence, creating a need to bolster self-esteem (Taylor & Lobel, 1989).

In addition to affecting the meaning of social comparisons, common-sense models of illness also can affect how we respond to others when they are ill. If we believe that diseases such as cancer or AIDS are infectious and have serious and uncontrollable consequences, we may be reluctant to shake hands with and/or be near someone who is infected. Indeed, if we believe these diseases are infectious and asymptomatic in their most virulent stages, we may be threatened by and motivated to avoid individuals perceived as carriers. Our reactions and recommendations are determined by our cognitive representation of the other's symptoms and our affective response to the other's state of illness.

In summary, the evidence indicates that lay referral networks are important moderators of decisions and the duration of delay in seeking health care. The moderating effects, however, are neither unidimensional nor unidirectional, and the processes linking social and individual processes are underexplored and not well understood. There is still much to be learned about how an individual's representation of problems (i.e., threats to health and procedures for management) are affected by the social context and whether the effect is mediated by shared heuristics or the interpretation of information generated by self-testing. There is a difference between hierarchical models, in which individual processes are nested under social factors, and models that describe *how* the levels are connected. How the factors at each level communicate with one another is the critical question. The communication is clearly bidirectional, though the direction of influence is likely to be more substantial from the cultural and social levels to the individual level. The data from care seeking provide limited insight into the substance of these bidirectional processes.

Connecting Psychological and Biological Processes

Many health psychologists have focused on the search for so-called direct pathways from behavior to health; details of these studies are covered in fine reviews of the stress–illness hypothesis (Cohen et al., 1998; Cohen, Tyrrell, & Smith, 1991; Cohen & Williamson, 1991; Kemeny, 2003; Schneiderman, Antoni, Saab, & Ironson, 2001; Taylor, Repetti, & Seeman, 1997). Although many interesting findings have emerged from these investigations, the stress to illness pathways that have been described generally terminate on an intermediate biomarker, rather than an outcome such as disease onset, morbidity, or mortality. It is simpler to elaborate the steps in the pathways from psychological through biological processes to such outcomes when focusing on treatment. As we have indicated throughout this chapter, treatment adherence is clearly an early and critical step in these pathways. For example, if a medication that is 100% effective is taken less than half the time by more than half of the patients using it, it will appear to be less effective than a medication that is 75% effective but taken exactly as prescribed by all users (Sackett & Haynes, 1976). Adherence is a necessary antecedent for behavior to get under the skin, and it is influenced by multiple contextual, social, and economic factors, ranging from access to treatment (Collins, Kriss, Davis, Doty, & Holmgren, 2006) to trust in the health care system and practitioners, the complexity of the treatment regimen, and whether the treatment is added to a set of treatments for other comorbid conditions (see H. Leventhal, Zimmerman, & Gutmann, 1984). Because adherence has a marked impact on outcomes, use of medication (metformin), exercise, and diet were meticulously recorded in the Diabetes Working Group trial (Knowler et al., 2002). Once adherence is documented, there is less mystery as to how a behavior gets under the skin as the biological pathways leading from adherence to clinical disease and mortality are relatively well defined for treatments such as antihypertension medication (e.g., diuretics, beta blocker, or ace inhibitors) and metformin for the control of blood sugar.

Three factors that affect the understanding of the ways in which a behavior gets under the skin are the remoteness of the health outcomes from the initiation of behavioral change, the number of pathways by which treatments work, and the availability of biomarkers to detect treatment effects. Each of these factors affects our ability to map the steps in the pathways leading to hard health outcomes for adherence to behaviors such as exercise and diet as multiple complex pathways are involved in moving these behaviors under the skin. The unexpected complexity of the pathways from treatment to chronic illness outcomes can also appear, however, with medication. For example, clinical trials examining the effects of lipid-lowering drugs (e.g., statins) for the prevention of cardiovascular disease and complications such as strokes have shown that these drugs are more or less equally effective for lowering blood lipid levels, but some protect against strokes and others do not. Califf and DeMets (2002) labeled the expectation that all drugs (e.g., statins) will have common outcomes as the *class effect*. The class effect contains a key message: The detailed knowledge of the multiple pathways involved in lipid management is currently insufficient to predict the effect of interventions using specific medications with well-defined molecular structures. Thus, despite their complexities, the pathways to disease that begin with medication adherence for the control of existent disease or for people at high risk, as in the diabetes trials (Knowler et al., 2002), are generally better understood than pathways involved in reduction of risk by exercise and diet. These latter pathways are better defined than the pathways involved in relationships to future disease of personality traits, such as hostility, and perceived stress, either lifetime or recent (Baum & Posluszny, 1999; Cohen et al., 1998; Krantz, Grunberg, & Baum, 1985).

BEHAVIORAL CHANGE AND REDUCTION OF HEALTH RISK IN THE ELDERLY

A question lurking in the background throughout this review is whether health benefits will accrue from behavioral changes made in the later years of life. Whether the answer will be a yes or a no depends on the definition of a health benefit, the nature of the behavioral change, and the interplay between the two. Two broad classes of benefits can be used as criteria for evaluating change: (a) reductions in mortality and increased life span and (b) improved function and quality of life. Behavioral changes can also be placed in either of two broad categories: (a) lifestyle behaviors, for example, diet, physical activity, stress management, social behaviors, and so on, and (b) treatment behaviors, for example, screening for disease detection, life-saving treatment, and adherence to treatment for control of chronic conditions. It unlikely that any single behavioral change will have a positive effect for all the health benefits that one might enumerate; such a broad-based effect is even less likely when one considers the multiple chronic illnesses associated with advanced age. For example, the set of behaviors including access to health care for cardiac screening and early detection of blocked arteries, followed by coronary artery bypass surgery, an effective and cost-effective treatment (Russell, 1992), can prevent early death and morbidity, but it will not increase overall life span relative to individuals unaffected by coronary disease and may not improve daily function and enhance quality of life. Thus the interactions among behaviors and outcomes present a complex picture that will defy simple answers.

Qualifications aside, a limited number of generalizations are possible. First, it is clear that behavioral changes can generate health benefits in elderly individuals. Adherence to treatments known to be effective can delay and, in many cases, prevent the onset of complications for asthma (e.g., use of inhaled corticosteroids can prevent decompensation and possible death), diabetes (e.g., heart disease, kidney damage, blindness, and amputations), and hypertension (e.g., MI and stroke) and can delay death and improve function and quality of life for congestive heart failure (Sisk et al., 2006). Our chapter focused on treatment adherence because of the clear evidence of benefits for the (a) delay and avoidance of complications and (b) maintenance of function and quality of life. Though the benefits are more easily observed among individuals at risk, lifestyle changes can also benefit the elderly. Benefits of lifestyle change were clear for individuals over 60 years of age ($n = 648$) who participated in the three arms of the diabetes prevention trial and were at high risk to become diabetic; the benefit of lifestyle relative to placebo was larger, and the difference of lifestyle to medication was significantly larger among participants in the over 60 years of age group than for participants in the two younger age groups. However, data from a longitudinal study of blood sugar monitoring found that individuals over 65 years of age were less likely than younger patients to initiate self-monitoring (Soumerai et al., 2004). Thus the elderly may be less likely to take advantage of available procedures for self-management, even though they may benefit more from doing so.

Given the evidence that lifestyle changes can produce health benefits for elderly individuals with chronic illness, one might be tempted to ask whether lifestyle changes will produce health benefits for elderly individuals who are not chronically ill or at high risk for chronic illness. The question is somewhat moot as nearly all elderly are dealing with one or more chronic illnesses, whether or not these illnesses are classified as problems. This is often the case with mild levels of osteoarthritis or incipient diabetes, which is potentially serious but currently not life threatening, or as would be the case with cardiac disease, a disease that is stable but of potential and immediate threat to life. Physical activity at mild to moderate levels is likely the one lifestyle behavior that can generate health benefits for elderly individuals with most any chronic condition. As we have already indicated, physical activity reduces the risk of onset and the risk of complications of diabetes, hypertension, and coronary disease. An additional benefit of physical activity is increased muscle mass and improvement in balance, both factors critical for sustaining physical function and avoiding falls, which can lead to incapacitating injuries. Fall-related injuries among the elderly are of major concern as they compromise the performance of activities of daily living, disrupt independence, lead to social isolation, and are associated with accelerated physical and mental decline. Despite the demonstrated health benefits of mild to moderate physical activity for elderly individuals, it is difficult to persuade and recruit them to physical activity programs. The difficulty of recruiting the elderly into clinical trials to evaluate the benefits of physical activity programs has created biases in the participating samples, which can raise some doubts as to the universality of the health benefits of such programs. Existent data suggest, however, that, excluding those for whom physical activity will be harmful, the greatest benefit may accrue to those elderly who are at greatest risk.

FINAL COMMENTS

Two themes were central to this brief examination of the relationships among health behaviors and physical health. First, it is clear that some behaviors are associated with substantial risk to health, while others are clearly related to benefit. Randomized trials, longitudinal studies, and historical data agree in showing that situational factors and human actions have a major impact on disease risk and that changes in behavior can produce positive gains in health. Two extremely clear examples of behavioral health relationships are seen in the risks of multiple chronic conditions (e.g., cancers at multiple sites and cardiovascular disease), of cigarette smoking and the benefits of quitting, and the benefits of increases in exercise and dietary change for controlling the onset and risks associated with diabetes. Second, we focused on the factors underlying the initiation and maintenance of behavior, as distinct from factors that predict behavior and health outcomes (e.g., personality traits). Third, we emphasized that an explanatory model should describe how people interpret and respond to somatic and functional changes and how the experience of the anticipated effects of coping responses creates representations of health threats and representations both of self and professional treatments. We used the term *representation*, rather than the word *belief*, as the former encompasses an array of both perceptual/experiential and abstract cognitive factors, while the term *belief* suggests abstract, verbal concepts. The model of behavior advanced here is an example of a hierarchical control system model for managing anticipated and ongoing threats to health.

Fourth, the model describing the control system for managing anticipated and ongoing threats to health is nested within two sets of contextual factors: (a) definitions and roles of the self and (b) the perceptions and beliefs respecting the social and cultural context. The self and context are also conceptualized as bilevel: They involve experience and concepts derived from experience, for example, roles or enactments by the self (e.g., commuting to office, lecturing, advising students) and the self label or concept encompassing these enactments (e.g., professor). Fifth, we argue that far too little attention has been paid to the communication processes among the control systems for managing health, the self, and the social context. The bidirectional processes involved in how specific cultural practices and values or self roles and concepts affect management of illness threats and how management of illness threats affects cultural practices and values or roles and self-concepts are underexamined. A systems analysis requires examination of the processes integrating these levels; multilevel models that nest self in culture and nest health management in person traits and cultural values may tell us where to look for cross-level connections but do not describe the processes involved in cross-level communication. Understanding how processes at the cultural/social, person, and problem-solving levels affect biological processes requires detailed models of the mechanisms and dynamics at each level and an understanding of precisely how these dynamics impact biological pathways. The studies of seeking medical care and self-management of chronic conditions provide a view of the processes underlying these behaviors: the heuristics and disease prototypes (e.g., acute, chronic, etc.) that impact behaviors, with direct effects on biological processes and measurable disease outcomes.

Finally, we support the hypothesis that behavioral change in the later years can generate clear health benefits for the elderly. Available data suggest that the benefits of behavioral changes in the later years can enhance function and slow, and perhaps prevent, the comorbidities of

chronic conditions such as kidney failure, blindness, and amputation associated with diabetes, disability due to falls, and stroke and cardiovascular
complications from hypertension. These suggestions must be tempered,
however, by recognition that health behavior change in the elderly is
understudied and suffers from recruitment problems. It is unclear if
the proportion of elderly refusing to participate, often greater than 50%
of those approached for inclusion, would experience the same, less, or
greater benefits from participation. As individuals at greatest risk can
benefit more, we suspect that more inclusive studies would find greater
benefits from late life participation in behavioral change programs. Studies to demonstrate potential benefit need to consider new approaches
to recruitment, simplifying and reducing barriers to participation, and
new approaches to study design (H. Leventhal, Weinman, Leventhal,
& Phillips, 2008). In summary, there are many reasons to believe that
theoretically informed clinical trials have an important role to play both
in advancing systems-based sociopsychological theory and in developing effective and efficient interventions for improving the health of the
elderly.

REFERENCES

Albrecht, T. L., & Goldsmith, D. J. (2003). Social support, social networks, and health. In
A. M. Dorsey, K. I. Miller, R. Parrott, & T. L. Thompson (Eds.), *Handbook of health
communication* (pp. 263–284). Mahwah, NJ: Erlbaum.

Apple, D. (1960). How laymen define illness. *Journal of Health and Human Behavior,
1*, 219–225.

Baldwin, A. S., Rothman, A. J., Hertel, A. W., Linde, J. A., Jeffery, R. W., Finch, E. A.,
et al. (2006). Specifying the determinants of the initiation and maintenance of behavior change: An examination of self-efficacy, satisfaction, and smoking cessation.
Health Psychology, 25, 626–634.

Bandura, A. (1989). Self-regulation of motivation and action through internal standards
and goal systems. In L. A. Pervin (Ed.), *Goal concepts in personality and social psychology* (pp. 19–85). Hillsdale, NJ: Erlbaum.

Bandura, A. (2004). Health promotion by social cognitive means. *Health Education and
Behavior, 31*, 143–164.

Barclay, T. R., Hinkin, C. H., Castellon, S. A., Mason, K. I., Reinhard, M. J., Marion, S. D.,
et al. (2007). Age-associated predictors of medication adherence in HIV-positive adults:
Health beliefs, self-efficacy, and neurocognitive status. *Health Psychology, 26*, 40–49.

Baum, A., & Posluszny, D. M. (1999). Health psychology: Mapping bio-behavioral
contributions to health and illness. *Annual Review of Psychology, 50*, 137–163.

Bauman, A. E. (2004). Updating the evidence that physical activity is good for health:
An epidemiological review 2000–2003. *Journal of Science and Medicine in Sport,
7*(Suppl. 1), 6–19.

Baumann, L., Cameron, L. D., Zimmerman, R., & Leventhal, H. (1989). Illness representations and matching labels with symptoms. *Health Psychology, 8*, 449–469.

Benyamini, Y., Leventhal, E. A., & Leventhal, H. (1999). Self-assessments of health: What do people know that predicts their mortality? *Research on Aging, 21*, 477–500.

Berkanovic, E., Telesky, C., & Reeder, S. (1981). Structural and social psychological factors in the decision to seek medical care for symptoms. *Medical Care, 19*, 693–709.

Binstock, R. H. (2004). Anti-aging medicine and research: A realm of conflict and profound societal implications. *Journals of Gerontology, Ser. A, 59*, 523–533.

Borgatta, E. F. (1968). Some notes on the history of tobacco use. In E. F. Borgatta & R. R. Evans (Eds.), *Smoking, health and behavior* (pp. 3–11). Chicago: Aldine.

Boulet, L. P. (1998). Perception of the role and potential side effects of inhaled corticosteroids among asthmatic patients. *Chest, 113*, 587–592.

Brashers, D. E., Goldsmith, D. J., & Hsieh, E. (2002). Information seeking and avoiding in health contexts. *Human Communication Research, 28*, 258–271.

Braudel, F. (1979). *The perspective of the world: Civilization and capitalism 15th–18th century.* New York: Harper and Row.

Brownell, K. D., & Horgen, K. B. (2004). *Food fight: The inside story of the food industry, America's obesity crisis, and what we can do about it.* Chicago: McGraw-Hill.

Brownlee, S., Leventhal, E. A., & Leventhal, H. (2000). Regulation, self-regulation and construction of the self in maintaining physical health. In M. Boekartz, P. R. Pintrich, & M. Zeidner (Eds.), *Handbook of self-regulation* (pp. 369–416). San Diego, CA: Academic Press.

Bunde, J., & Martin, R. (2006). Depression and prehospital delay in the context of myocardial infarction. *Psychosomatic Medicine, 68*, 51–57.

Califf, R. M., & DeMets, D. L. (2002). Principles from clinical trials relevant to clinical practice: Part I. *Circulation, 106*, 1015–1021.

Cameron, L., Leventhal, E. A., & Leventhal, H. (1993). Symptom representations and affect as determinants of care seeking in a community dwelling adult sample population. *Health Psychology, 12*, 171–179.

Cameron, L. C., Leventhal, E. A., & Leventhal, H. (1995). Seeking medical care in response to symptoms and life stress. *Psychosomatic Medicine, 57*, 37–47.

Carstensen, L. L. (1992). Social and emotional patterns in adulthood: Support for the socioemotional selectivity theory. *Psychology and Aging, 7*, 331–338.

Carstensen, L. L., & Charles, S. T. (1998). Emotion in the second half of life. *Current Directions in Psychological Science, 7*, 144–149.

Carver, C. S., Scheier, M. F., & Weintraub, J. K. (1989). Assessing coping strategies: A theoretically based approach. *Journal of Personality and Social Psychology, 56*, 267–283.

Cassileth, B. R. (1998). *The alternative medicine handbook: The complete reference guide to alternative and complementary therapies.* New York: W. W. Norton.

Chao, A., Thun, M. J., Connell, C. J., McCullough, M. L., Jacobs, E. J., Flanders, W. D., et al. (2005). Meat consumption and the risk of colorectal cancer. *Journal of the American Medical Association, 293*, 172–182.

Chapman, G. B. (1998). Sooner or later: The psychology of inter-temporal choice. *Psychology of Learning and Motivation, 38*, 83–114.

Cohen, S., Frank, E., Doyle, W. J., Skoner, D. P., Rabin, B. S., & Gwaltney, J. M., Jr. (1998). Types of stressors that increase susceptibility to the common cold in healthy adults. *Health Psychology, 17*, 211–213.

Cohen, S., Tyrrell, D. A. J., & Smith, A. P. (1991). Psychological stress and susceptibility to the common cold. *New England Journal of Medicine, 325*, 606–612.

Cohen, S., & Williamson, G. M. (1991). Stress and infectious disease in humans. *Psychological Bulletin, 109*, 5–24.

Cohen, S., & Wills, T. A. (1985). Stress, social support, and the buffering hypothesis. *Psychological Bulletin, 98*, 310–357.

Collins, S. R., Kriss, J. L., Davis, K., Doty, M. M., & Holmgren, A. L. (2006). *Squeezed: Why rising exposure to health care costs threatens the health and financial well-being of American families*. New York: The Commonwealth Fund.

Concato, J., Shah, N., & Horwitz, R. I. (2000). Randomized, controlled trials, observational studies, and the hierarchy of research designs. *New England Journal of Medicine, 342*, 1887–1892.

Conrad, P. (1985). The meaning of medications: Another look at compliance. *Social Science and Medicine, 20*, 29–37.

Croyle, R. T., & Jemmott, J. B., III. (1991). Psychological reactions to risk factor testing. In J. A. Skelton & R. T. Croyle (Eds.), *Mental representation in health and illness* (pp. 85–107). New York: Springer Verlag.

Csete, M. E., & Doyle, J. C. (2002). Reverse engineering of biological complexity. *Science, 295*, 1664–1669.

Cutrona, C. E., & Russell, D. W. (1990). Type of social support and specific stress: Toward a theory of optimal matching. In B. R. Sarason, I. G. Sarason, & G. R. Pierce (Eds.), *Social support: An interactional view* (pp. 319–366). New York: John Wiley.

Dakof, G. A., & Taylor, S. E. (1990). Victims' perceptions of social support: What is helpful from whom? *Journal of Personality and Social Psychology, 58*, 80–89.

Davis, M. C., Matthews, K. A., & McGrath, C .E. (2000). Hostile attitudes predict elevated vascular resistance during interpersonal stress in men and women. *Psychosomatic Medicine, 62*, 17–25.

Dechamps, A., Lafont, L., & Bourdel-Marchasson, I. (2007). Effects of Tai Chi exercises on self efficacy and psychological health. *European Review of Aging and Physical Activity, 4*(1), 25–32.

Dimsdale, J. E., Eckenrode, J., Haggerty, R. J., Kaplan, B. H., Cohen, F., & Dornbusch, S. (1979). The role of social supports in medical care. *Social Psychiatry, 14*, 175–180.

Doll, R., & Hill, A. B. (1950). Smoking and carcinoma of the lung: Preliminary report. *British Medical Journal, 2*, 739–748.

Duke, J., Leventhal, H., Brownlee, S., & Leventhal, E. (2002). Giving up and replacing activities in response to illness. *Journals of Gerontology, Ser. B, 57*, P367–P376.

Durante, K. M., Whitmore, B., Jones, C. A., & Campbell, N. (2001). Use of vitamins, minerals, and herbs: A survey of patients attending family practice clinics. *Clinical and Investigative Medicine, 24*, 242–249.

Epstein, S. (1973). The self-concept revisited: Or a theory of a theory. *American Psychologist, 28*, 404–416.

Eysenck, H. J. (1980). *The causes and effects of smoking*. Beverly Hills, CA: Sage Publications.

Friedman, H. S., & Booth-Kewley, S. (1987). The "disease-prone personality": A meta-analytic view of the construct. *American Psychologist, 42*, 539–555.

Fuster, V., Dyken, M. L., Vokonas, P. S., & Hennekens, C. (1993). Aspirin as a therapeutic agent in cardiovascular disease. *Circulation, 87*, 659–675.

Gerson, L. W., & Stevens, J. A. (2004). Recreational injuries among older Americans, 2001. *Injury Prevention, 10,* 134–138.

Granovetter, M. (1978). Thresholds models of collective behavior. *American Journal of Sociology, 83,* 1420–1443.

Gunther, S., Patterson, R. E., Kristal, A. R., Stratton, K. L., & White, E. (2004). Demographic and health-related correlations of herbal and specialty supplement use. *Journal of the American Dietetic Association, 104,* 27–34.

Guyll, M., & Contrada, R. J. (1998). Trait hostility and ambulatory cardiovascular activity in males and females. *Health Psychology, 17,* 30–39.

Haber, C. (2004). Life extension and history: The continual search for the fountain of youth. *Journals of Gerontology, Ser. A, 59,* 515–522.

Halm, E. A., Mora, P., & Leventhal, H. (2006). No symptoms, no asthma: The acute episodic disease belief is associated with poor self-management among inner city adults with persistent asthma. *Chest, 129,* 573–580.

Hampson, S. E., Goldberg, L. R., Vogt, T. M., & Dubanoski, J. P. (2007). Mechanisms by which childhood personality traits influence adult health status: Educational attainment and health behaviors. *Health Psychology, 26,* 121–125.

Hansson, L., Zanchetti, A., Carruthers, S. G., Dahlof, B., Elmfeldt, D., Julius, S., et al. (1998). Effects of intensive blood-pressure lowering and low-dose aspirin in patients with hypertension: Principal results of the hypertension optimal treatment (HOT) randomised trial. *Lancet, 351,* 1755–1763.

Hayden, M., Pignone, M., Phillips, C., & Mulrow, C. (2002). Aspirin for the primary prevention of cardiovascular events: A summary of the evidence for the U.S. Preventive Services Task Force. *Annals of Internal Medicine, 136,* 161–172.

Heggestad, E. D., & Kanfer, R. (2005). The predictive validity of self-efficacy in training performance: Little more than past performance. *Journal of Experimental Psychology: Applied, 11,* 84–97.

Heidrich, S. M., Forsthoff, C. A., & Ward, S. E. (1994). Psychological adjustment in adults with cancer: The self as mediator. *Health Psychology, 13,* 346–353.

Holtzman, R. E., Rebok, G. W., Saczynski, J. S., Kouzis, A. C., Doyle, K. W., & Eaton, W. W. (2004). Social network characteristics and cognition in middle-aged and older adults. *Journals of Gerontology, Ser. B, 59,* 278–284.

Hootman, J. M., Macera, C. A., Ainsworth, B. E., Addy, C. L., Martin, M., & Blair, S. N. (2002). Epidemiology of musculoskeletal injuries among sedentary and physically active adults. *Medicine and Science in Sports and Exercise, 34,* 838–844.

Horowitz, C. R., Rein, S. B., & Leventhal, H. (2004). A story of maladies, misconceptions and mishaps: Effective management of heart failure. *Social Science and Medicine, 58,* 631–643.

House, J. S., Kessler, R. C., Herzog, A. R., Mero, R. P., Kinney, A. M., & Breslow, M. J. (1992). Social stratification, age, and health. In K. W. Schaie, D. Blazer, & J. S. House (Eds.), *Aging, health behaviors, and health outcomes* (pp. 1–32). Hillsdale, NJ: Erlbaum.

Idler, E. (2004). Religious observance and health: Theory and research. In K. W. Schaie, N. Krause, & A. Booth (Eds.), *Religious influences on health and well-being of the elderly* (pp. 20–43). New York: Springer Publishing.

Institute for the Future. (2003). *Health and healthcare 2010: The forecast, the challenge.* Retrieved September 1, 2006, from http://www.iftf.org/features/library.html#2003

Kant, A. K. (2000). Consumption of energy-dense, nutrient-poor foods by adult Americans: Nutritional and health implications: The Third National Health and Nutrition Examination Survey, 1988–1994. *American Journal of Clinical Nutrition, 72*, 929–936.

Kaplan, G. A. (1992). Health and aging in the Alameda County study. In K. W. Schaie, D. Blazer, & J. S. House (Eds.), *Aging, health behaviors, and health outcomes* (pp. 69–88). Hillsdale, NJ: Erlbaum.

Kaptchuk, T. J., & Eisenberg, D. M. (1998). The persuasive appeal of alternative medicine. *Annals of Internal Medicine, 129*, 1061–1065.

Kasl, S. V., & Cobb, J. (1966). Health behavior, illness behavior and sick-role behavior. *Archives of Environmental Health, 12*, 531–541.

Kemeny, M. A. (2003). The psychobiology of stress. *Current Directions in Psychological Science, 12*, 124–129.

King, A. C., Rejeski, W. J., & Buchner, D. M. (1998). Physical activity interventions targeting older adults: A critical review and recommendations. *American Journal of Preventative Medicine, 15*, 316–333.

Klatz, R., & Kahn, C. (1998). *Grow young with HGH, the amazing medical plan to reverse aging.* New York: Harper Perennial.

Knowler, W. C., Barrett-Connor, E., Fowler, S., Hamman, R. F., Lachin, J. M., Walker, E. A., et al. (2002). Reduction in the incidence of type 2 diabetes with lifestyle intervention or metformin. *New England Journal of Medicine, 346*, 393–403.

Krantz, D. S., Grunberg, N. E., & Baum, A. (1985). Health psychology. *Annual Review of Psychology, 36*, 349–383.

Krause, N. (2004). Religion, aging, and health: Exploring new frontiers in medical care. *Southern Medical Journal, 97*, 1215–1222.

Krauss, R. M., Winston, M., Fletcher, B. J., & Grundy, S. M. (1998). Obesity: Impact on cardiovascular disease. *Circulation, 98*, 1472–1476.

Kris-Etherton, P. M., & Keen, C. L. (2002). Evidence that the antioxidant flavonoids in tea and cocoa are beneficial for cardiovascular health. *Current Opinion in Lipidology, 13*, 41–49.

Kumanyika, S. K. (1993). Special issues regarding obesity in minority populations. *Annals of Internal Medicine, 119*, 650–654.

Langer, E. J., & Rodin, J. (1976). The effects of choice and enhanced personal responsibility for the aged: A field experiment in an institutional setting. *Journal of Personal and Social Psychology, 34*(2), 191–198.

Lazar, M. A. (2005). How obesity causes diabetes: Not a tall tale. *Science, 307*, 373–375.

Leventhal, E. A., & Crouch, M. (1997). Are there differences in perceptions of illness across the lifespan? In K. J. Petrie & J. A. Weinman (Eds.), *Perceptions of health and illness: Current research and applications* (pp. 77–102). Amsterdam, Netherlands: Harwood Academic.

Leventhal, E. A., Easterling, D., Leventhal, H., & Cameron, L. (1995). Conservation of energy, uncertainty reduction, and swift utilization of medical care among the elderly: II. *Medical Care, 33*, 988–1000.

Leventhal, E. A., Leventhal, H., Schaefer, P., & Easterling, D. (1993). Conservation of energy, uncertainty reduction, and swift utilization of medical care among the elderly. *Journals of Gerontology, Ser. B, 48*, 78–86.

Leventhal, H., Hudson, S., & Robitaille, C. (1997). Social comparison and health: A process model. In B. Buunk & F. X. Gibbons (Eds.), *Health, coping and well being: Perspectives from social comparison theory* (pp. 411–432). Hillsdale, NJ: Erlbaum.

Leventhal, H., Nerenz, D., & Steele, D. (1984). Illness representations and coping with health threats. In A. Baum & J. Singer (Eds.), *A handbook of psychology and health* (Vol. 4, pp. 219–252). Hillsdale, NJ: Erlbaum.

Leventhal, H., Rabin, C., Leventhal, E. A., & Burns, E. (2001). Health risk behaviors and aging. In R. Birren & W. Schaie (Eds.), *Handbook of the psychology of aging* (5th ed., pp. 186–214). San Diego, CA: Academic Press.

Leventhal, H., Weinman, J., Leventhal, E., & Phillips, L. A. (2008). Health psychology: The search for pathways between behavior and health. *Annual Review of Psychology, 59,* 477–505.

Leventhal, H., Zimmerman, R., & Gutmann, M. (1984). Compliance: A self-regulation perspective. In W. D. Gentry (Ed.), *Handbook of behavioral medicine* (pp. 369–436). New York: Guilford Press.

Lindstrom, J., Louheranta, A., & Mannelin, M. (2003). The Finnish Diabetes Prevention Study (DPS): Lifestyle intervention and 3-year results on diet and physical activity. *Diabetes Care, 26,* 3230–3236.

Liu, W. T., & Duff, R. W. (1972). The strength in weak ties. *Public Opinion Quarterly, 36,* 361–366.

Magai, C. (2001). Emotions over the lifespan. J. Birren & K. W. Schaie (Eds.), *Handbook of the psychology of aging* (pp. 339–426). San Diego, CA: Academic Press.

Maibach, E., & Murphy, D. A. (1995). Self-efficacy in health promotion research and practice: Conceptualization and measurement. *Health Education Research, 10,* 37–50.

Martin, R., Davis, G. M., Baron, R. S., Suls, J., & Blanchard, E. B. (1994). Specificity in social support: Perceptions of helpful and unhelpful provider behaviors among irritable bowel syndrome, headache, and cancer patients. *Health Psychology, 13,* 432–439.

Matthews, K. A., Siegel, J. M., Kuller, L., Thompson, M., & Varat, M. (1983). Determinants of decisions to seek medical treatment by patients with acute myocardial infarction symptoms. *Journal of Personality and Social Psychology, 44,* 1144–1156.

McAuley, E., Jerome, G. J., Marquez, M. S., Elavsky, S., & Blissmer, B. (2003). Exercise self-efficacy in older adults: Social, affective and behavioral influences. *Annals of Behavioral Medicine, 25,* 1–7.

McKeever, T. M., Lewis, S. A., Smit, H. A., Burney, P., Britton, J. R., & Cassano, P. A. (2005). The association of acetaminophen, aspirin, and ibuprophen with respiratory disease and lung function. *American Journal of Respiratory and Critical Care Medicine, 171,* 966–971.

McTigue, K. M., Garrett, J. M., & Popkin, B. M. (2002). The natural history of the development of obesity in a cohort of young U.S. adults between 1981 and 1998. *Annals of Internal Medicine, 136,* 857–864.

Merenstein, D. (2004). Winners and losers. *Journal of the American Medical Association, 291,* 15–16.

Meyer, D., Leventhal, H., & Gutmann, M. (1985). Common-sense models of illness: The example of hypertension. *Health Psychology, 4,* 115–135.

Mora, P. A., Halm, E. A., Leventhal, H., & Ceric, F. (in press). Elucidating the relationship between negative affectivity and symptoms: The role of illness-specific affective responses. *Annals of Behavioral Medicine.*

Mora, P., Robitaille, C., Leventhal, H., Swigar, M., & Leventhal, E. A. (2002). Trait negative affect relates to prior week symptoms, but not to reports of illness episodes, illness symptoms and care seeking among older people. *Psychosomatic Medicine, 64,* 436–449.

Niggemann, B., & Gruber, C. (2003). Side-effects of complementary and alternative medicine. *Allergy, 58,* 707–716.

Oberlander, T. F., Pless, I. B., & Dougherty, G. E. (1993). Advice seeking and appropriate use of a pediatric emergency department. *Archives of Pediatrics and Adolescent Medicine, 147,* 863–867.

Olshansky, S. J., Hayflick, L., & Carnes, B. A. (2002). No truth to the fountain of youth. *Scientific American, 286,* 92–95.

Ory, M. G., DeFriese, G. H., & Duncker, A. P. (1998). The nature, extent and modifiability of self-care behaviors in later life. In G. H. DeFriese & M. G. Ory (Eds.), *Self care in later life research, program, and policy issues* (pp. 1–23). New York: Springer Publishing.

Park, D. C., Lautenschlager, G., Hedden, T., Davidson, N., Smith, A. D., & Smith, P. (2002). Models of visuospatial and verbal memory across the adult life span. *Psychology and Aging, 17,* 299–320.

Patrono, C., Rodriguez, L. A. G., Landolfi, R., & Baigent, C. (2005). Low-dose aspirin for the prevention of atherothrombosis. *New England Journal of Medicine, 353,* 2373–2383.

Prohaska, T. R., Keller, M. L., Leventhal, E. A., & Leventhal, H. (1987). Impact of symptoms and aging attribution on emotions and coping. *Health Psychology, 6,* 495–514.

Renner, B., & Schwarzer, R. (2005). The motivation to eat a healthy diet: How intenders and non-intenders differ in terms of risk perception, outcome expectancies, self-efficacy, and nutrition behavior. *Polish Psychological Bulletin, 36,* 7–15.

Roghmann, K. J., & Haggerty, R. J. (1973). Daily stress, illness and use of health services in young families. *Pediatric Research, 7,* 520–526.

Rook, K. S. (1984). The negative side of social interaction: Impact on psychological well-being. *Journal of Personality and Social Psychology, 46,* 1097–1108.

Ross, G. W., Abbott, R. D., Petrovitch, H., Morens, D. M., Grandinetti, A., Tung, K., et al. (2006). Association of coffee and caffeine intake with the risk of Parkinson disease. *Journal of the American Medical Association, 284,* 2674–2679.

Russell, L. B. (1992). Opportunity costs in modern medicine. *Health Affairs, 11*(2), 162–169.

Sackett, D. L., & Haynes, R. B. (1976). *Compliance with therapeutic regimens.* Baltimore: Johns Hopkins University Press.

Sackett, D. L., Rosenberg, W., Gray, J. A., Haynes, B. R., & Richardson, W. S. (1996). Evidence based medicine: What it is and what it isn't. *British Medical Journal, 312,* 71–72.

Safer, M. A., Tharps, Q. J., Jackson, T. C., & Leventhal, H. (1979). Determinants of three stages of delay in seeking care at a medical clinic. *Medical Care, 17,* 11–29.

Salazar-Martinez, E., Willett, W. C., Ascherio, A., Manson, J. E., Leitzmann, M. F., Stampfer, M. J., et al. (2004). Coffee consumption and risk for type 2 diabetes mellitus. *Annals of Internal Medicine, 140,* 1–8.

Sallis, J. F., Hovell, M. F., & Hofstetter, C. R. (1992). Predictors of adoption and maintenance of vigorous physical activity in men and women. *Preventative Medicine, 21,* 237–251.

Sanders, G. S. (1982). *Social comparison and perceptions of health and illness.* Hillsdale, NJ: Erlbaum.

Scambler, A., Scambler, G., & Craig, D. (1981). Kinship and friendship networks and women's demand for primary care. *Journal of the Royal College of General Practitioners, 26,* 746–750.

Schneiderman, N., Antoni, M. H., Saab, P. G., & Ironson, G. (2001). Health psychology: Psychosocial and biobehavioral aspects of chronic disease management. *Annual Review of Psychology, 52,* 555–580.

Schwarzer, R., & Fuchs, R. (1995). Self-efficacy and health behaviors. In M. Connor & P. Norman (Eds.), *Predicting health behaviour* (pp. 163–196). Buckingham, England: Open University Press.

Shaheen, S. O., Sterne, J. A. C., Songhurst, C. E., & Burney, P. G. J. (2000). Frequent paracetemol use and asthma in adults. *Thorax, 55,* 266–270.

Shields, C. A., & Brawley, L. R. (2006). Preferring proxy-agency: Impact on self-efficacy for exercise. *Journal of Health Psychology, 11,* 904–914.

Sisk, J. E., Hebert, P. L., Horowitz, C. R., McLaughlin, M. A., Wang, J. J., & Chassin, M. R. (2006). Effects of nurse management on the quality of heart failure care in minority communities. *Annals of Internal Medicine, 145,* 273–283.

Song, Y. A., Buring, J. E., Manson, J. E., & Liu, S. (2004). Prospective study of red meat consumption and type 2 diabetes in middle-aged and elderly women. *Diabetes Care, 28,* 2108–2114.

Sorofman, B., Tripp-Reimer, T., Lauer, G. M., & Martin, M. E. (1990). Symptom self-care. *Holistic Nursing Practice, 4,* 45–55.

Soumerai, S. B., Mah, C., Zhang, F., Adams, A., Barton, M., Fajtova, V., et al. (2004). Effects of health maintenance organization coverage of self-monitoring devices on diabetes self-care and glycemic control. *Archives of Internal Medicine, 164,* 645–652.

Stampfer, M. J., Kang, J. H., Chen, J., Cherry, R., & Grodstein, F. (2005). Effects of moderate alcohol consumption on cognitive function in women. *New England Journal of Medicine, 352,* 245–253.

Stewart, J. C., Janicki, D. L., & Kamarck, T. W. (2006). Cardiovascular reactivity to and recovery from psychological challenge as predictors of 3-year change in blood pressure. *Health Psychology, 25,* 111–118.

Suls, J., & Goodkin, F. (1994). Medical gossip and rumor: Their role in the lay referral system. *Health Psychology, 13,* 103–113.

Suls, J., Martin, R., & Leventhal, H. (1997). Social comparison, lay referral, and the decision to seek medical care. In B. Buunk & F. X. Gibbons (Eds.), *Social comparisons, health, and coping* (pp. 195–226). Hillsdale, NJ: Erlbaum.

Tanasescu, M., Leitzmann, M. F., Rimm, E. B., Willett, W. C., Stampfer, M. J., & Hu, F. B. (2002). Exercise type and intensity in relation to coronary heart disease in men. *Journal of the American Medical Association, 288,* 1994–2000.

Taylor, S. E., & Lobel, M. (1989). Social comparison activity under threat: Downward evaluation and upward contacts. *Psychological Review, 96*, 569–575.

Taylor, S. E., Repetti, R. L., & Seeman, T. (1997). Health psychology: What is an unhealthy environment and how does it get under the skin? *Annual Review of Psychology, 48*, 411–447.

Temple, N. J. (2000). Antioxidants and disease: More questions than answers. *Nutrition Research, 20*, 449–459.

Troiana, R. P., Briefel, R. R., Marroll, M. D., & Bialostosky, K. (2000). Energy and fat intakes of children and adolescents in the United States: Data from the National Health and Nutrition Examination Surveys. *American Journal of Clinical Nutrition, 72*, 1343S–1353S.

Tuomilehto, J., Lindstrom, J., Eriksson, J. G., Valle, T. T., Hamalainen, H., Ilanne-Parikka, P., et al. (2001). Prevention of type 2 diabetes mellitus by changes in lifestyle among subjects with impaired glucose tolerance. *New England Journal of Medicine, 344*, 1343–1350.

U.S. Department of Health and Human Services. (2001). *Women and smoking: A report of the surgeon general* (Stock No. 017-023-00207-4). Washington, DC: U.S. Government Printing Office.

U.S. General Accounting Office. (2001). *Health products for seniors: Anti-aging products pose potential for physical and economic harm* (GAO Publication No. GAO-01-1129). Washington, DC: Author.

U.S. Public Health Service. (1964). *Smoking and health: Report of the Advisory Committee to the Surgeon General of the Public Health Service* (PHS Publication No. 1103). Washington, DC: U.S. Government Printing Office.

U.S. Public Health Service. (1967). *The health consequences of smoking* (PHS Publication No. 1696). Washington, DC: U.S. Government Printing Office.

Vancouver, J. B., & Kendall, L. N. (2006). When self-efficacy negatively relates to motivation and performance in a learning context. *Journal of Applied Psychology, 91*, 1146–1153.

van Grunsven, P. M., van Schayck, C. P., van Kollenburg, H. J. M., van Bosheide, K., van den Hoogen, H. J. M., Molema, J., et al. (1998). The role of "fear of corticosteroids" in nonparticipation in early intervention with inhaled corticosteroids in asthma and COPD in general practice. *European Respiratory Journal, 11*, 1178–1181.

Vileikyte, L., Rubin, R. R., & Leventhal, H. (2004). Psychological aspects of diabetic neuropathic foot complications: An overview. *Diabetes/Metabolism Research and Review, 20*(Suppl. 1), 13–18.

Warner, K. E., Goldenhar, L. M., & McLaughlin, C. G. (1992). Cigarette advertising and magazine coverage of the hazards of smoking: A statistical analysis. *New England Journal of Medicine, 326*, 305–309.

Willett, W. C. (1994). Diet and health: What should we eat? *Science, 264*, 532–537.

Wrosch, C., Scheier, M. F., Carver, C. S., & Schulz, R. (2003). The importance of goal disengagement in adaptive self-regulation: When giving up is beneficial. *Self and Identity, 2*, 1–20.

Yancura, L. A., Aldwin, C. M., Levenson, M. R., & Spiro, A. (2006). Coping, affect, and the metabolic syndrome in older men: How does coping get under the skin? *Journals of Gerontology, Ser. B, 61*, 295–303.

Zola, I. (1973). Pathways to the doctor: From person to patient. *Social Science and Medicine, 7*, 577–689.

3

Religion, Health, and Health Behavior

NEAL KRAUSE

A growing number of studies suggest that older people who are more involved in religion tend to enjoy better physical and mental health than older adults who are not involved in religion (Schaie, Krause, & Booth, 2004). Some of the most compelling studies in this area focus on the relationship between church attendance and mortality. This research indicates that older individuals who go to church on a regular basis tend to live longer than older people who do not attend church as often (McCullough, 2001). Although this research has made important contributions to the literature, it suffers from three interrelated problems.

First, researchers are becoming increasingly aware that religion is a complex multidimensional phenomenon. For example, the Fetzer Institute/National Institute on Aging Working Group (1999) developed survey questions to assess 12 different dimensions of religion. Because comprehensive studies on the relationship between multiple facets of religion and health have not been conducted, researchers have yet to isolate the particular dimension (or dimensions) of religion that may enhance and maintain better health.

Acknowledgment: The research discussed in this chapter was supported by a grant from the National Institute on Aging (RO1 AG014749).

73

Second, studies that focus on church attendance alone are important, but they leave significant questions unanswered about the causal mechanisms that are at work because church attendance is a complex construct in its own right that encompasses a number of different factors. For example, when people attend formal church services, they typically listen to sermons, participate in group prayers, sing hymns, perform rituals (e.g., communion, baptism), and interact with their fellow church members. Any (or all) of these factors could explain the relationship between religion and health. So when studies show that frequent church attendance is associated with outcomes like mortality, it is not clear what these findings mean. This leads to the third and final problem in the literature.

So far, researchers have shown that various facets of religion are associated with health. This is an important first step. But it is now time to take the literature to the next level by conducting studies that are designed to explain *how* the potentially health-enhancing effects of religion arise. A number of theoretical explanations have been offered, and research indicates that these explanations have some validity. For example, some investigators maintain that religious involvement has important health-related effects because it helps people deal more effectively with stressful life events and other forms of adversity (Pargament, 1997). Other researchers argue that social relationships that are formed with fellow church members may be an important factor (Krause, 2006). And yet other scholars suggest that prayer or forgiveness may have something to do with it (Dosey, 1993; McCullough, Pargament, & Thoresen, 2000).

The goal of this chapter is to explore another potentially important factor that may help explain the link between religion and health behavior. The basic rationale for exploring this relationship is simple and relatively straightforward, or so it may seem initially. Essentially, this perspective specifies that people who are more involved in religion tend to have better health because they are more likely to engage in positive health behaviors (e.g., maintaining a good diet), while avoiding negative or undesirable health behaviors (e.g., alcohol abuse; Hill, Burdette, Ellison, & Musick, 2006). But what appears to be a relatively straightforward proposition may not be as simple as it first seems. The challenges that arise in studying religion and health behavior are examined in this chapter by exploring five issues.

First, like religion, health behavior encompasses a broad conceptual domain that contains many different factors. This raises the possibility that religion may affect some, but not all, health behaviors. However, literature will be reviewed that suggests that religion may influence a wide range of health behaviors. But as this review will also reveal, no one has evaluated all health behaviors in the same study.

Second, although research is needed to assess the influence of a range of religious factors on a number of different health behaviors, other types of studies are needed as well. Consistent with the issue that was raised earlier, it is time to think about building more focused conceptual models that provide a more in-depth examination of how specific components of religion may influence a given health behavior. Conducting this type of research is important because it can show precisely how the potentially beneficial effects of religion arise. An effort will be made to illustrate the advantages of this more focused strategy by exploring the ways in which social relationships in the church influence the adoption of beneficial health behaviors.

Third, a case will then be made for focusing explicitly on the influence of denominational preference. Most research on religion and health has been conducted in the United States, where the wide majority of people are Christian. When researchers assess the relationship between religion and health with these data, they typically pool all Christians into a single sample. But the Christian faith is not a single, tightly unified system of beliefs and practices. Instead, it is fractured into a bewildering array of denominations, which have their own unique views of how best to pursue their faith. As a result, it is difficult to study religion and health behavior without taking denominational differences into consideration.

Fourth, an effort will be made to move beyond the discussion of theoretical and conceptual issues to the evaluation of empirical data. However, it would be impossible to provide a comprehensive evaluation of the interface between all the different facets of religion and all the various types of health behavior because the necessary data do not exist. Consequently, a more circumscribed approach will be presented that takes a more in-depth look at the empirical relationship between several different types of social relationship in the church and one specific health behavior (the consumption of alcoholic beverages).

Finally, a small cluster of studies will be reviewed that challenge the notion that religion always encourages the use of beneficial health behaviors. Instead, as this research will reveal, greater involvement in religion may also be associated with health behaviors that are not beneficial.

STAKING OUT THE CONTENT DOMAIN
OF HEALTH BEHAVIOR

It is hard to find a good definition of *health behavior* in the literature. Nevertheless, Gochman (1982), one of the pioneers in the field, defines *health behavior* in the following way:

> those personal attributes, such as beliefs, expectations, motives, values, and perceptions, and other cognitive elements; personality characteristics, including affect and emotional states and traits; and overt behavior patterns, actions, and habits, that relate to health maintenance, to health restoration, and health improvement. (p. 168)

It is difficult to get a firm grasp on such a broad definition. However, investigators who study the relationship between religion and health behavior would probably be most interested in the last segment because it refers specifically to behavior: Health behavior is the "overt patterns, actions, and habits that relate to health maintenance, to health restoration, and health improvement."

But instead of struggling with the development of a good verbal definition of health behavior, it is easier to get a handle on this unwieldy domain by listing some of the specific types of health behavior. The various types of health behavior can be partitioned into two broad categories: positive and negative health behavior. Positive health behaviors are those that are either thought or known to maintain, restore, and improve health. Included among positive health behaviors are things like engaging in regular exercise, getting regular medical check-ups, taking vitamin supplements, and adhering to safety regulations (e.g., wearing seat belts while driving or riding in a car). Negative health behaviors are those that are either thought or known to exert an adverse effect on health. Included here are things like consuming excessive amounts of alcohol, using tobacco, and using illegal drugs or abusing prescription drugs.

There is another way to think about the health behavior domain that has rarely been examined in the literature on religion and health. Instead of thinking in terms of single health behaviors, some investigators prefer to focus on health lifestyles (Cockerham, 2000). Rather than referring to one particular type of health behavior, the study of lifestyles involves assessing patterns or clusters of health behaviors. So, for example, researchers might devise measures that identify people who not only maintain a good diet, but who also avoid smoking and engage in regular exercise, as well. Unfortunately, there is no agreed on operational definition of a healthy lifestyle.

RESEARCH ON RELIGION AND HEALTH BEHAVIOR

Research on religion and health behavior is incomplete. There are three reasons for this state of affairs. First, the wide majority of researchers examine either the use of alcohol or tobacco, whereas far less attention has been given to other health behaviors. Second, many investigators focus solely on the relationship between the frequency of church attendance and health behavior. But as the discussion provided earlier reveals, there is far more to religion than attending worship services. Third, a good deal of the literature on religion and health behavior has been conducted with either adolescents or young adults, especially college students. As a result, it is difficult to know whether the findings from this work can be generalized to older people. Studying the factors that shape health behaviors among older people is important because this knowledge can be used to confront some of the most pressing challenges that face our society. Research indicates that older people consume a disproportionately large amount of health care resources (Federal Interagency Forum on Aging Related Statistics, 2004). Moreover, a number of studies consistently show that engaging in positive health behaviors, such as regular exercise, can restore and maintain health across the life course (U.S. Department of Health and Human Services, 1992). Therefore identifying the factors that are associated with beneficial health behaviors in late life may provide a good way to hold down rapidly escalating health care costs.

Even though there are limitations in research on religion and health behavior, a number of noteworthy insights have emerged from the work that has been done so far. To begin with, a fairly large number of studies suggest that greater involvement in religion is associated with either the moderate use of alcohol or the avoidance of alcoholic beverages altogether (Herd, 1996; Hill et al., 2006). In fact, researchers have been studying religion and alcohol use for at least 50 years (Skolnick, 1958). But more recently, a number of investigators have explored the relationship between religion and alcohol use with samples that are composed solely of older people. For example, a nationwide survey of older people that was conducted by Krause (2003) revealed that older people who are affiliated with fundamentalist denominations are more likely to abstain from the use of alcohol than older adults who belong to either moderate or liberal denominations. This study is unique because it explores a facet of religion that has not been assessed by other investigators. Researchers have argued for decades that one of the primary functions of religion is to help people find a sense of meaning in life (Berger, 1990). The study by Krause (2003) suggested that older people who feel that religion has helped them derive a deeper sense of meaning in life are more likely to avoid using alcohol than older adults who have not been able to find a sense of meaning in life through religion.

A number of others studies suggest that religion is associated with the avoidance of tobacco, as well. For example, Idler and Kasl (1997) reported that older adults who attend worship services more often have a lower probability of having ever smoked. This study also revealed that older people who go to church more often have significantly higher levels of physical activity and lower levels of alcohol consumption.

Fortunately, researchers are beginning to explore the relationship between religion and other kinds of health behaviors. For example, based on data from a nationwide survey, Benjamins (2005) found that older adults who attend religious services frequently and who belong to mainline Protestant denominations are more likely to report that they had their cholesterol checked. In another study, Benjamins and Brown (2004) found that older men and women who feel that religion is important in their lives are more likely to use a range of preventive health practices, including breast self-examinations, flu shots, mammograms, pap smears, prostate screening, and cholesterol screening.

One recent study of religion and health behavior stands out from the rest (Hill et al., 2006). This research was conducted by Hill et al. (2006). These investigators examined the influence of the frequency of church attendance on 12 health behaviors. Their findings revealed that regular attendance at worship services (especially weekly attendance) is associated with avoiding tobacco, drinking alcoholic beverages moderately, engaging in strenuous exercise, seat belt use, vitamin use, the utilization of preventive health care (e.g., physical and dental examinations), sleeping well, walking, and infrequent attendance in establishments that serve alcohol. But, unfortunately for the purposes of the current chapter, the sample in this study consisted of adults of all ages who reside in Texas.

In a longer version of this study, Hill, Burdette, Ellison, and Musick (2007) explored the relationship between greater involvement in religion and healthy lifestyles. A measure of healthy lifestyles was formed by summing the total number of beneficial health behaviors adopted by study participants. Their findings revealed that more frequent church attendance is associated with more healthy lifestyles. This appears to be the first time that the relationship between religion and healthy lifestyles has been examined in the literature.

Taken as a whole, the literature reviewed in this section suggests that greater involvement in religion is associated with the use of a relatively broad array of health behaviors. But what is lacking in this work is a clear sense of precisely how these beneficial health practices arise. As the discussion in the next section will reveal, social relationships in the church may have something to do with it.

SOCIAL RELATIONSHIPS IN THE CHURCH AND HEALTH BEHAVIOR

As Hill et al. (2006) pointed out, many religions adhere to the notion that the body is the temple of God. As a result, various religious groups encourage the use of certain types of health behaviors, while discouraging the practice of others. For example, the Seventh Day Adventist Church strongly encourages the pursuit of sound dietary practices, while the Southern Baptist Church has a strict prohibition against the use of alcohol. But a key issue that arises at this juncture involves precisely how these religious teachings and beliefs are transmitted to rank-and-file church members.

At least part of the answer may be found in Stark and Finke's (2000) comprehensive theory of religion. Among the constructs they explore is something they refer to as *religious explanations*. These are religious models of reality, or religious worldviews, that typically contain rules that influence attitudes and guide behavior. The impact of social relationships on the decision to adopt sanctioned behavior is underscored in one of the key propositions in their theoretical perspective. More specifically, Stark and Finke (2000) argued that "an individual's confidence in religious explanations is strengthened to the extent that others express their confidence in them" (p. 107). Simply put, religious rules and teachings are transmitted and reinforced through social interaction with like-minded religious others.

The emphasis on the social underpinnings of religion is hardly without precedent in the literature. James Mark Baldwin was one of the founding fathers of psychology and an early president of the American Psychological Association. Writing in 1902, he captured the social essence of this perspective on religion when he argued that "the fact is constantly recognized that religion is a social phenomenon. No man is religious by himself, nor does he choose his god, nor devise his offering, nor enjoy his blessings alone" (p. 325).

But the references to the social underpinnings of religion that have been reviewed up to this point are vague because social relationships in the church may take many different forms. As a result, it is hard to derive testable propositions from this work. In the discussion that follows, an effort will be made to identify several key types of church-based social relationships.

Recall that Stark and Finke (2000) proposed that religious belief systems are strengthened to the extent that others express confidence in them. These researchers then delved more deeply into how this sense of confidence arises. Stark and Finke (2000) argued that "confidence in religious explanations increases to the extent that people participate in religious rituals" (p. 107). Cast within the context of the current chapter, this means that church teachings about health behaviors are likely to be adapted and reinforced through participation with other people in formal church activities. In effect, these shared religious activities may be construed as a kind of formal social relationship. Included among church rituals is attendance at worship services. But there may be more to it than this. In particular, attendance at Bible study and prayer groups also provides the opportunity for further reinforcement of church teachings related to health behaviors.

The literature reviewed up to this point specifies that the establishment of formal social ties in the church through things like attendance at worship services and Bible study groups provides a forum for the transmission of religious teachings about health behaviors. But this does not exhaust all the ways in which religious messages about health behavior may be passed along. In particular, informal social relationships among rank-and-file church members may play a role, as well. To see why this may be so, it is helpful to turn to two specific types of church-based social relationships, which have been discussed by Krause and colleagues (Krause, 2002; Krause, Ellison, & Wulff, 1998). The first type is called *spiritual support*, and the second involves *negative interaction* in the church.

As research by Krause (2002) revealed, fellow church members often informally discuss their religious beliefs and practices among themselves. In fact, Krause pointed out that a good deal of this interaction is intended to encourage others to adopt and maintain various religious beliefs and practices. Krause (2002) called this interaction *spiritual support*. More specifically, spiritual support is assistance that is intended to increase the religious commitment, beliefs, and behavior of a fellow church member. There are a number of ways in which members of a congregation can exchange spiritual support. For example, they may share their own religious experiences with fellow church members or show them how to apply religious teachings in daily life. Cast in the context of the current chapter, fellow church members may also informally encourage the use of beneficial health behaviors as well as the avoidance of those health behaviors that are viewed as undesirable by their church.

But informal influences on health behavior may not always take a positive tone in the church. As Krause et al. (1998) demonstrated, social relationships in the church may also become unpleasant, as fellow church members become critical of each other and reject one another. In fact, research by these investigators revealed that informal negative interaction in the church may erode a person's sense of psychological well-being. But the effects of negative interaction in the church may not always be undesirable. As Rook, Thuras, and Lewis (1990) pointed out some time ago, significant others may resort to the use of negative interaction to get a focal person to engage in beneficial health behaviors. For example, a close friend at church may criticize an older person for consuming too much alcohol. If the older person takes this criticism to heart and curbs his or her intake of alcohol, then an initially negative encounter may ultimately have a positive effect on his or her health and well-being.

Taken as a whole, the argument developed in this section specifies that formal as well as informal social relationships in the church may play an important role in transmitting church doctrine about health behavior. With respect to formal relationships, attendance at worship services, Bible study, and prayer groups may provide a forum for the reinforcement of church teachings about health behavior, while informal spiritual support and informal negative interaction with fellow church members may have a similar effect. There do not appear to be any studies in the literature that empirically evaluate the influence of formal and informal social relationships in the church on health behavior.

Exploring the Influence of Denominational Preference

The model of social relationships in the church and health behavior that has emerged up to this point is helpful, but it is incomplete because it overlooks another construct that influences both church-based social relationships and health behavior. That construct is denominational preference. Ultimately, the decision to adopt a health behavior begins with a cluster of beliefs. These beliefs underscore the benefits of the health behavior and specify that practicing it is consistent with the basic tenets of the church. These specific beliefs constitute the substance of what is transmitted through formal and informal social relationships in the church. Despite the straightforward appeal of this observation, it is surprising to find that specific beliefs about a given health behavior are not explicitly measured in most studies. Instead, investigators either ignore beliefs about health behaviors altogether, or they use denominational preference as a proxy measure of them (Benjamins, 2005). Information on denominational preference is typically used to create a nominal-level variable that specifies whether a study participant is a member of a fundamentalist, moderate, or liberal congregation (Smith, 1987). If specific religious beliefs promote health behaviors, then these beliefs should be measured directly. It is risky to use denominational preference as a proxy because an investigator can never be certain that he or she is studying the influence of specific religious beliefs per se, or the effect of some other facet of denominational preference that is correlated with them.

CHURCH-BASED SOCIAL RELATIONSHIPS AND ALCOHOL USE

Empirical Evidence

Developing a sound theoretical rationale for the relationship between religion and health behavior is helpful, but evaluating at least some of the intervening mechanisms empirically is even better. The purpose of this section is to briefly present data from a nationwide survey of older people that focused on social relationships in the church and alcohol use. After providing a brief overview of the data source and measures, the findings will be reviewed, and additional theoretical insights will be derived from them.

Sample

The data come from a nationwide survey, conducted by Krause (2002), of older Whites and older African Americans. The study population was defined as all household residents who were either White or Black,

English-speaking, and at least 66 years of age. Residents of Alaska and Hawaii were excluded. The population was restricted to older adults who were currently practicing Christians, older individuals who were Christian in the past but no longer practiced any religion, and older people who were not affiliated with any faith at any point in their lifetimes. The sampling frame consisted of all eligible people contained in the Medicare Beneficiary Eligibility List maintained by the Centers for Medicare and Medicaid Services. The study was longitudinal, but only data from the baseline survey are presented here. Interviewing for the baseline survey took place in 2001. Harris Interactive (New York) conducted all data collections. A total of 1,500 interviews were completed successfully. All interviewing took place in the homes of study participants. The overall response rate was 62%.

Older Blacks were oversampled so that sufficient statistical power would be available to study race differences in religion. However, issues involving race are not examined in the analyses presented subsequently. The sample comprised 748 older Whites and 752 older African Americans.

The analyses presented subsequently focus on spiritual support from fellow church members as well as participation in Bible study and prayer groups. When the baseline interviews were conducted, 374 older adults indicated that they attended church no more than twice a year. However, it did not make sense to ask people questions about things like spiritual support and attendance at Bible study groups if they rarely went to church. Therefore the 374 low or nonattending individuals were excluded from the analyses.

After using listwise deletion to deal with item nonresponse, the analyses presented subsequently are based on the responses of 875 older people. Preliminary analysis revealed that the average age of the people in this sample was 74.6 years (SD = 6.2 years). Approximately 47% were White, 37% were men, and 49% were married at the time the interview took place. Finally, the older people in this study reported that they had completed an average of 11.5 years of schooling (SD = 3.4 years).

Measures

Table 3.1 contains the core survey measures. The procedures used to code these indicators are provided in the footnotes of this table.

Alcohol use. Study participants were asked whether they ever drink beer, wine, or liquor. Preliminary analysis revealed that 29.8% of the

Table 3.1

CORE STUDY MEASURES

1. Alcohol use
   A. Do you ever drink beer, wine, or liquor?[a]
2. Denominational preference[b]
3. Frequency of church attendance
   A. How often do you attend religious services?[c]
4. Attending Bible study groups
   A. How often do you attend Sunday school or Bible study groups?[c]
5. Attending prayer groups
   A. How often do you participate in prayer groups that are not part of regular worship services or Bible study groups?[c]
6. Spiritual support[d]
   A. Not counting Bible study groups, prayer groups, or church services, how often does someone in your congregation share his or her own religious experiences with you?
   B. Not counting Bible study groups, prayer groups, or church services, how often does someone in your congregation help you to lead a better religious life?
   C. Not counting Bible study groups, prayer groups, or church services, how often does someone in your congregation help to know God better?
7. Private prayer
   A. How often do you pray by yourself?[e]

---

[a]This variable is scored in the following manner (coding in parentheses): currently drinks alcohol (1); does not drink alcohol (0). [b]Computed variable, which is scored in the following manner: fundamentalist (1); moderate or liberal (0). [c]These variables are scored in the following manner: several times a week (9); every week (8); nearly every week (7); 2–3 times a month (6); about once a month (5); several times a year (4); about once or twice a year (3); less than once a year (2); never (1). [d]These items are scored in the following manner: very often (4); fairly often (3); once in a while (2); never (1). [e]This variable is scored in the following manner: several times a day (8); once a day (7); a few times a week (6); once a week (5); a few times a month (4); once a month (3); less than once a month (2); never (1).

---

older study participants drank alcohol. A binary measure was created from these data, where a score of 1 denoted older study participants who drink and a score of 0 represented older people who do not consume alcohol.

Denominational preference. The participants in this study were asked a detailed series of questions (not shown in Table 3.1) about their denominational preference. These data were coded with the scheme devised by Smith (1987). This scheme classifies Christian churches as being either fundamentalist, moderate, or liberal. On the basis of the work of Herd (1996), it is anticipated that fundamentalists will be more likely than either moderates or liberals to avoid the use of alcohol. Therefore a binary measure was developed that contrasted fundamentalists (scored 1) with both moderates and liberals (scored 0). Preliminary analysis revealed that 55% of the study participants attended fundamentalist congregations.

Formal social interaction in the church. Three indicators were used to assess formal interaction with people at church. The first reflected the frequency of attendance at worship services, the second assessed how often older people attended Bible study groups, and the third involved how often older study participants attended prayer groups. A high score on any of these items denoted more frequent attendance.

Informal social relationships in the church. As shown in Table 3.1, three items were used to assess how often older study participants received informal spiritual support from the people in their congregations. These items were devised by Krause (2002). The indicators measured, for example, how often a fellow church member encouraged an older person to live according to his or her religious beliefs. It should be emphasized that study participants were specifically asked not to count spiritual support they might have received in Bible study groups, prayer groups, or during worship services. This helped to ensure that the spiritual support indicators measured something that is conceptually distinct from formal social interaction in the church. A high score on the spiritual support items meant that older people received spiritual support from fellow church members more often. The internal consistency reliability estimate for the composite formed from these items was .847.

Private prayer. Items that measure various facets of religion are often correlated fairly highly (Idler et al., 2003). Consequently, it is important to control for core measures of religion when exploring the relationship between things like spiritual support and alcohol use. Doing so helps ensure that any findings reflect the influence of spiritual support and not some other component of religion that is correlated with it. A measure of the frequency of private prayer was included in the analysis for this purpose. A high score on this indicator stood for more frequent private prayer.

Demographic control variables. The relationships between alcohol use and the variables listed in Table 3.1 were estimated after the effects of age, sex, education, marital status, and race were controlled statistically. Age and education were scored continuously in years, whereas sex (1 = man; 0 = woman), race (1 = White; 0 = Black), and marital status (1 = married; 0 = not married) were represented with binary indicators.

Results

The relationship between religion and alcohol use was assessed with a hierarchical logistic regression analysis. A hierarchical analysis was performed because denominational preference is an overarching or master status variable that may influence a number of the other measures of religion in this study. For example, research reveals that fundamentalists (i.e., evangelicals) are more likely to attend church, pray, and attend Bible study and prayer groups than either moderates or liberals (Barna, 2002). As a result, denominational preference may influence alcohol use indirectly through these various measures of involvement in religion. Therefore, to derive a deeper appreciation for the influence of denominational preference, the analyses were conducted in three steps. The first step contained the demographic control variables as well as the denominational preference indicator. Then, based on the rationale provided previously, the measures of church attendance and attendance at Bible study and prayer groups, and the frequency of private prayer, were entered into the model. Following this, spiritual support was entered in the third step. The decision to enter spiritual support last was based on the premise that strong informal relationships in the church are more likely to develop among older people who go to church more often and who are more deeply involved in formal church activities like Bible study and prayer groups.

The findings from the analyses are presented in Table 3.2. Before turning to the substantive results, it is important to briefly discuss the coefficients contained in the table. Three coefficients are presented. In addition to unstandardized logistic regression coefficients and odds ratios, the table also provides standardized logistic regression coefficients. Because some readers are not likely to be familiar with standardized estimates in logistic regression, it is important to briefly discuss why they are useful and how they were derived. One problem with logistic regression arises from the fact that it is difficult to determine whether the impact of one independent variable is greater than another. Comparing odds ratios will not help because these coefficients are influenced by the metric of the independent variable. Fortunately, Selvin (1991) provided a simple

Table 3.2

RELIGION AND ALCOHOL USE (N = 875)

INDEPENDENT VARIABLE	MODEL 1 b[a]	MODEL 1 B[b]	MODEL 1 ODDS RATIO	MODEL 2 b	MODEL 2 B	MODEL 2 ODDS RATIO	MODEL 3 b	MODEL 3 B	MODEL 3 ODDS RATIO
Age	−.034*	−.210	.967	−.034	−.210	.967	−.041**	−.253	.960
Sex	1.299***	.626	3.667	1.173***	.565	3.232	1.199***	.578	3.317
Education	.134***	.460	1.144	.150***	.515	1.162	.152***	.522	1.164
Marital status	.066	.033	1.068	.131	.066	1.140	.134	.067	1.144
Race	.302	.151	1.352	.204	.102	1.226	.134	.067	1.144
Fundamentalist	−.745***	−.370	.475	−.508***	−.253	.601	−.427***	−.212	.652
Prayer				−.078	−.101	.925	−.050	−.065	.952
Church attendance				.001	.002	1.001	.039	.060	1.040
Bible study				−.105**	−.328	.900	−.096**	−.299	.909
Prayer group				−.025	−.069	.976	−.012	−.033	.988
Spiritual support							−.109**	−.293	.896
−2 Log likelihood	907.481			887.720			878.750		

[a]Unstandardized logistic regression coefficient. [b]Standardized logistic regression coefficient computed by multiplying the unstandardized logistic regression coefficient by the standard deviation of the independent variable.
*p < .05. **p < .01. ***p < .001.

way of deriving standardized estimates in logistic regression analyses. This procedure involves multiplying the unstandardized logistic regression coefficient by the standard deviation of the independent variable. Cast within the context of the present study, this estimate reflects the change in log odds of consuming alcohol for a one-standard-deviation increase in a given independent variable.

The data from the first step in the hierarchical analysis are presented in the second, third, and fourth columns of Table 3.2 (Model 1). Consistent with research reviewed earlier, the findings in Model 1 reveal that fundamentalists are much less likely to consume alcohol than either moderates or liberals ($b = -.745$; $p < .001$). In fact, as the odds ratio reveals, fundamentalists are about 53% less likely to drink than others.

The data in the fifth, sixth, and seventh columns of Table 3.2 (Model 2) were obtained after church attendance, private prayer, and attendance at Bible study and prayer groups were added to the model. Two findings from this step in the analysis are noteworthy. First, the data suggest that older people who attend Bible study groups more often are less likely to consume alcohol than older adults who do not attend Bible study groups as frequently ($b = -0.105$; $p < .01$). But in contrast, neither attendance at worship services, attendance at prayer groups, or private prayer appear to have much of an effect. The second important finding has to do with the change in the size of the effect of denominational preference. The data indicate that the effect of this construct is smaller in Model 2 ($b = -.508$; $p < .01$) than in Model 1 ($b = -.745$; $p < .001$). Put another way, including the indicators of formal interaction in the church reduces the impact of denominational preference on alcohol use by about 32%. And the bulk of this reduction is due to the mediating influence of attending Bible study groups.

The final model in Table 3.2 (Model 3) was estimated after the effects of informal spiritual support were added to the analyses. These data, which appear in columns 8, 9, and 10, suggest that greater spiritual support is associated with a lower odds of consuming alcohol ($b = -0.109$; $p < .01$). Comparing the findings in Model 1 and Model 3 reveals that including formal and informal interaction in the church reduces the effect of denominational preference by about 43%. This means that fundamentalists are less likely to drink than others, and nearly half of this relationship can be explained by the fact that fundamentalists are more likely to attend Bible study groups and that they are more likely to receive informal spiritual support from the people they worship with. Consistent with the theoretical rationale that was developed earlier, this means that religion is associated with the decision to drink, and a good deal of this influence operates through the formal and informal social ties that are formed in the church. This helps further reinforce the notion that relationships formed in the church are a major factor in religious life.

The findings that have been presented are useful, but they are limited. Three shortcomings should be mentioned briefly. First, only one kind of health behavior was evaluated (alcohol use). Consequently, it is not clear if the same findings would emerge with other health behaviors such as diet or exercise. Second, as discussed earlier, negative interaction may play an important role in the transmission of religious teachings about alcohol. However, proper measures of negative interaction involving alcohol use were not available in this study. Third, denominational preference was used as a proxy for specific religious beliefs regarding the use of alcohol. However, as the theoretical rationale that was presented earlier suggests, it is important to evaluate these beliefs directly in the future.

EXPLORING THE NEGATIVE INFLUENCE OF RELIGION ON HEALTH BEHAVIOR

Up until this point, the discussion and data presented highlighted the potentially beneficial influence of religion on health behavior. This is consistent with the image conveyed in the wide majority of studies. However, an intriguing cluster of studies suggests that this perspective may not be entirely accurate and that religion may not always promote health behaviors that are beneficial. Therefore, to accurately and fully portray the influence of religion on health behavior, it is important to briefly review this work. But there are deeper reasons for focusing on this research, as well. Researchers who study religion typically focus solely on its potential benefits, without paying sufficient attention to the potential drawbacks of religion. This may add to the mistaken impression that if people get more involved in religion, they will never get sick, and they will live to a ripe old age. But even casual observation reveals this is not true. Deeply religious people do, indeed, become very ill, and individuals who are very devout do, in fact, die young.

Focusing on the potentially negative facets of religion may help researchers figure out why religion appears to bolster or maintain the health of some people, but not others. One way to approach this issue is to recognize that religious institutions are created and maintained by human beings, and because humans are flawed, so are the institutions they develop. To the extent that this is true, researchers must explore the negative as well as the positive aspects of religion. And it is for this reason that we also need to see if there are ways in which religion influences the adoption of undesirable health behaviors.

During the past several years, findings from several studies have suggested that people who are more involved in religion are more likely to be overweight than individuals who are less involved in religion. For example, Lapane, Lasater, Allan, and Carleton (1997) reported that church members are more likely than people who are not church members to be more than 20% overweight. Similarly, Ferraro (1998) found more obese individuals in states with a higher proportion of Baptists. Finally, a study by Kim, Sobel, and Wethington (2003) revealed that men in conservative Protestant denominations were more likely to have a higher body weight than men who were affiliated with other denominations (but see Ellis & Biglione, 2000). These findings are important because research consistently shows that excess body weight is associated with the risk of developing a number of health problems, including diabetes, heart disease, and cancer (U.S. Department of Health and Human Services, 1992).

Unfortunately, it is difficult to determine what these findings mean. Why are people who are more involved in religion heavier than individuals who are less involved in religion? Cline and Ferraro (2006) offered several potential explanations. They noted, for example, that many religious organizations celebrate major events with food. Unfortunately, the food that is served on these occasions often has a high fat content. In addition, high-fat foods are often served at Sunday school and Bible study groups (e.g., donuts), and people typically consume fairly large amounts of food at church potluck suppers. Presumably, these negative dietary practices are more widespread in conservative or fundamentalist churches, but no studies appear to evaluate this possibility with data on actual food consumption. Regardless of these shortcomings, the studies reviewed in this section provide one way of showing how religion may encourage health behaviors that are not beneficial.

CONCLUSIONS

The purpose of this chapter was to see if the well-documented relationship between religion and health could be explained, at least in part, by health behaviors. More specifically, the goal was to examine the proposition that people who are more involved in religion are more likely to adopt positive health behaviors and avoid negative or undesirable health behaviors than individuals who are less involved in religion. But instead of merely reviewing existing studies, an effort was made to take the field to the next level by asking how the potentially beneficial influence of religion on health behaviors is transmitted. The central thesis in this argument is that the decision to adopt good health behaviors is a social product that arises from the influence exerted by significant others at church. Viewed broadly, this perspective adds further credence to a long-standing principle in classic sociological theory that specifies that the basis of religion may be found in the social ties that develop in the church (Simmel, 1898/1997). Consistent with this view, preliminary data were presented that suggested that the decision to drink alcohol is influenced, at least in part, by formal and informal social relationships in the church. More specifically, the data suggested that older people who participate in Bible study groups as well as older adults who receive informal spiritual support from their fellow church members are more likely to avoid the use of alcohol than older individuals who do not develop or maintain these types of church-based social ties.

But the theoretical perspective developed in this chapter does not go far enough because it is still not entirely clear how significant others at church influence the decision to adopt a given health behavior. The challenge to those who wish to pursue this line of thinking is to delve more deeply into this issue. Fortunately, this work does not have to begin from scratch because a good deal of insight may be found in rich literatures developed in public health and social psychology.

One of the core theoretical perspectives in health behavior is the *theory of reasoned action* (Fishbein, 1967). A central tenet in this framework is that the decision to adopt a health behavior is determined by a person's attitude toward performing the behavior and his or her subjective evaluation of the desirability of the outcome. The emphasis in this theory on attitudes is important because a vast literature has emerged over the past 50 years on the factors that influence attitudes and bring about attitude change (for reviews of this research, see Chaiken, Wood, & Eagly, 1996; Prislin & Wood, 2005). Researchers interested in studying the relationship between social ties in the church and health behavior would be well advised to take advantage of the principles that have emerged from this work. The benefits of doing so can be illustrated by showing how four simple propositions from the literature on attitude change can be used to derive testable hypotheses about the relationship between religion and health behavior.

First, as Chaiken et al. (1996) pointed out, people will be more likely to yield to social influence exerted by a group if they identify with the group and are highly committed to it. People in a congregation are not all equally committed to the faith. If there is variation in commitment, then some people in church may be more likely to adopt church teachings on health behavior than others. This proposition may be evaluated, for example, by testing for a statistical interaction effect between church teachings that discourage the use of alcohol and the level of commitment to religion on the decision to drink.

Second, research reviewed by Prislin and Wood (2005) suggested that conformity to the attitudes of others is motivated by fear of rejection and the desire to obtain the approval of others. This suggests that valuable insight may be obtained by explicitly measuring the need for approval from others at church and assessing whether it is associated with adopting health behaviors that are endorsed by the faith.

Third, as the propositions presented so far reveal, the church may endorse certain health behaviors, but everyone in the congregation may not follow this advice. This raises a whole host of research questions. For example, researchers need to know what happens to those who decide not to comply with church teachings about a given health behavior. Does rejection of church views lead to greater psychological distress, and if it does, under what conditions is it most likely to emerge? For example, must other members of the congregation be aware of noncompliance, or is a person's own realization that he or she is rejecting tenets of the faith sufficient to produce distress?

The fourth proposition that may be derived from the literature on attitude change comes at the issue from the perspective of the person who is trying to get others to adopt a given view. As Chaiken et al. (1996) showed, persuading others to adopt an attitude or behavior reinforces the persuader's own attitudes and behaviors. This means that people at church who encourage others to adopt a health behavior are more likely to find that their effort to change the behavior of others strengthens their own resolve to adopt and maintain the health behavior. Once again, this simple proposition presents a number of research opportunities. We need to know how often people at church try to convince others to adopt health behaviors that are sanctioned by their faith. There do not appear to be any studies in the literature that examine this issue. Then, using data gathered over time, we need to see if encouraging others to adopt a health behavior increases the persuader's own resolve to engage in the same health behavior.

As research on religion and health behavior continues to mature, a series of questions arises about how this knowledge will be used and applied. Lately, a good deal of attention has been given to faith-based human service initiatives (Tangenberg, 2005). Essentially, these programs involve the provision of health services that have explicit religious foundations and overtones. Considerable controversy has arisen over whether faith-based initiatives should be financed with state or federal funds because doing so appears to violate long-standing legal principles involving the separation of church and state. It is obviously not possible to resolve these complex issues here. But researchers would be well advised to keep them in mind because whether they are aware of it or not, the work they are doing on religion and health contributes to this debate, one way or the other.

REFERENCES

Baldwin, J. M. (1902). *Fragments in philosophy and science being: Collected essays and addresses*. New York: Charles Scribner's Sons.

Barna, G. (2002). *The state of the church 2002*. Ventura, CA: Issachar Resources.

Benjamins, M. R. (2005). Social determinants of preventive service utilization: How religion influences the use of cholesterol screening in older adults. *Research on Aging, 27*, 475–497.

Benjamins, M. R., & Brown, C. (2004). Religion and preventive health care utilization among the elderly. *Social Science and Medicine, 58*, 109–118.

Berger, P. L. (1990). *The sacred canopy: Elements of a sociological theory of religion*. New York: Random House.

Chaiken, S., Wood, W., & Eagly, A. H. (1996). Principles of persuasion. In E. T. Higgens & A. W. Kruglanski (Eds.), *Social psychology: Handbook of basic principles* (pp. 702–742). New York: Guilford Press.

Cline, K. M. C., & Ferraro, K. F. (2006). Does religion increase the prevalence and incidence of obesity in adulthood? *Journal for the Scientific Study of Religion, 45*, 269–281.

Cockerham, W. (2000). The sociology of health behavior and health lifestyles. In C. Bird, P. Conrad, & A. Fremont (Eds.), *Handbook of medical sociology* (5th ed., pp. 159–172). Upper Saddle River, NJ: Prentice Hall.

Dosey, L. (1993). *Healing words: The power of prayer and the practice of medicine*. San Francisco: HarperCollins.

Ellis, L., & Biglione, D. (2000). Religiosity and obesity: Are overweight people more religious? *Personality and Individual Differences, 28*, 1119–1123.

Federal Interagency Forum on Aging Related Statistics. (2004). *Older Americans 2004: Key indicators of wellbeing*. Washington, DC: U.S. Government Printing Office.

Ferraro, K. F. (1998). Firm believers? Religion, body weight, and well-being. *Review of Religious Research, 39,* 224–244.

Fetzer Institute/National Institute on Aging Working Group. (1999). *Multidimensional measurement of religiousness/spirituality for use in health research.* Kalamazoo, MI: John E. Fetzer Institute.

Fishbein, M. (1967). *Readings in attitude theory and measurement.* New York: John Wiley.

Gochman, D. S. (1982). Labels, systems, and motives: Some perspectives on future research. *Health Education Quarterly, 9,* 167–174.

Herd, D. (1996). The influence of religious affiliation on sociocultural predictors of drinking among Black and White Americans. *Substance Use and Misuse, 31,* 35–63.

Hill, T. D., Burdette, A. M., Ellison, C. G., & Musick, M. A. (2006). Religious attendance and health behaviors of Texas adults. *Preventive Medicine, 42,* 309–312.

Hill, T. D., Burdette, A. M., Ellison, C. G., & Musick, M. A. (2007). Religious involvement, health behaviors, and healthy lifestyles: Evidence from the survey of Texas adults. *Annals of Behavioral Medicine, 34,* 217–222.

Idler, E. L., & Kasl, S. V. (1997). Religion among disabled and nondisabled persons I: Cross-sectional patterns in health practices, social activities, and well-being. *Journals of Gerontology, Ser. B, 52,* S294–S305.

Idler, E., Musick, M., Ellison, C. G., George, L. K., Krause, N., Levin, J. S., et al. (2003). National Institute on Aging/Fetzer Institute Working Group brief measures of religion and spirituality. *Research on Aging, 25,* 327–365.

Kim, K. H., Sobel, J., & Wethington, E. (2003). Religion and body weight. *International Journal of Obesity and Related Metabolic Disorders, 27,* 469–477.

Krause, N. (2002). Church-based social support and health in old age: Exploring variations by race. *Journals of Gerontology, Ser. B, 57,* S332–S347.

Krause, N. (2003). Race, religion, and abstinence from alcohol in late life. *Journal of Aging and Health, 15,* 508–533.

Krause, N. (2006). Exploring the effects of church-based social support and secular social support on health in late life. *Journals of Gerontology, Ser. B, 61,* S35–S43.

Krause, N., Ellison, C. G., & Wulff, K. M. (1998). Church-based emotional support, negative interaction, and psychological well-being: Findings from a national sample of Presbyterians. *Journal for the Scientific Study of Religion, 37,* 725–741.

Lapane, K. L., Lasater, T. M., Allan, C., & Carleton, R. A. (1997). Religion and cardiovascular disease risk. *Journal of Religion and Health, 36,* 155–163.

McCullough, M. E. (2001). Religious involvement and mortality: Answers and more questions. In T. G. Plante & A. C. Sherman (Eds.), *Faith and health: Psychological perspectives* (pp. 53–74). New York: Guilford Press.

McCullough, M. E., Pargament, K. I., & Thoresen, C. E. (2000). *Forgiveness: Theory, research, and practice.* New York: Guilford Press.

Pargament, K. I. (1997). *The psychology of religion and coping: Theory, research, and practice.* New York: Guilford Press.

Prislin, R., & Wood, W. (2005). Social influence in attitude and attitude change. In D. Albarracin, B. T. Johnson, & M. P. Zanna (Eds.), *The handbook of attitudes* (pp. 671–706). Mahwah, NJ: Erlbaum.

Rook, K. S., Thuras, P. D., & Lewis, M. A. (1990). Social control, health risk taking, and psychological distress among the elderly. *Psychology and Aging, 5,* 327–334.

Schaie, K. W., Krause, N., & Booth, A. (2004). *Religious influences on health and well-being in the elderly*. New York: Springer Publishing.

Selvin, S. (1991). *Statistical analysis of epidemiologic data*. New York: Oxford University Press.

Simmel, G. (1997). A contribution to the sociology of religion. In H. J. Helle (Ed.), *Essays on religion: George Simmel* (pp. 101–120). New Haven, CT: Yale University Press. (Original work published 1898)

Skolnick, J. H. (1958). Religious affiliation and drinking behavior. *Quarterly Journal of Studies on Alcohol, 19*, 452–470.

Smith, T. W. (1987). *Classifying protestant denominations: Methodological report 43*. Unpublished manuscript.

Stark, R., & Finke, R. (2000). *Acts of faith: Explaining the human side of religion*. Berkeley: University of California Press.

Tangenberg, K. M. (2005). Faith-based human services initiatives: Considerations for social work theory and practice. *Social Work, 50*, 197–206.

U.S. Department of Health and Human Services. (1992). *Healthy people 2000: National health promotion and disease prevention objectives*. Boston: Jones and Bartlett.

Commentary: Assessing Health Behaviors Across Individuals, Situations, and Time

DAVID M. ALMEIDA, SUSAN TURK CHARLES, AND SHEVAUN D. NEUPERT

The most common causes of death have changed dramatically in the last century. In developed countries, public health practices and medical advances have reduced the likelihood of contracting and dying from infectious diseases. The earlier top causes of mortality—typhoid, cholera, polio, and tuberculosis—are now rare and often treatable diseases. Instead, causes of death stem predominantly from chronic conditions; to illustrate, a little more than half of all deaths in the United States are the result of cancer or heart-related conditions, including stroke, heart attack, or heart failure (Miniño, Heron, Smith, & Kochanek, 2006). As a result, age at death has also shifted, such that the average life expectancy across all developed countries now nears 80 years (Miniño et al., 2006). These changes have led researchers to recognize the importance of health behaviors for determining physical morbidity and mortality. Behaviors influence trajectories of health across the life span, both preventing illness as well as shaping the course of chronic conditions.

Chapter 2 of this volume, by Howard Leventhal, Tamara J. Musumeci, and Elaine A. Leventhal, and chapter 3 of this volume, by Neal Krause, discuss the importance of understanding health behaviors as well as the factors that shape health behaviors. These preeminent scholars point out the complexities underlying these phenomena. Both chapters discuss social influences that determine health outcomes. Sociocultural forces, including religion and social support networks, interact with individual characteristics (both physical and psychological) to affect a person's perceptions and actions. Both chapters discuss the challenges in studying traits at the person-level as well, addressing the multiple behaviors and experiences unique to the individual that determine his or her actions.

In the present chapter, we highlight the contributions of these scholars and offer a critical analysis for how to expand their models in future research. We review the importance of studying how sociocultural influences shape health-related perceptions and actions and recognize the points raised in these chapters. We also discuss and provide an example of the value of studying day-to-day variation in these perceptions and actions. In addition to understanding how people engage simultaneously in both health-promoting and health-damaging behaviors, we emphasize the need to examine how these behaviors fluctuate on a daily basis as well as how both individual characteristics and daily experiences interact to affect health behaviors.

TO ACT OR NOT TO ACT: HEALTH BEHAVIORS AS DETERMINED BY BETWEEN- AND WITHIN-PERSON FACTORS

Leventhal and his colleagues begin their chapter by dispelling any notion that studying health behaviors is easy; even the definition of the phenomenon is elusive. The authors note that researchers have identified health behaviors and then later dismissed them, as in the example of the once-encouraged habit of eating foods high in saturated fats prior to exercise. In addition, researchers now advocate for other healthy behaviors that were heretofore unknown. After this description, Leventhal et al. then proceed to discuss the many determinants of these behaviors. The reader quickly gets the idea: studying the determinants of health behavior is even more complex than identifying them. They argue that the traditional division of primary versus secondary health prevention is artificial and misleading, and because health and illness run along a continuum, so, too, should these behaviors be studied as continuous processes that exist throughout the course of health and illness. They next present the requisites of any theory of health behavior (see Figure 2.1 in Leventhal et al., this volume) to describe processes determining health behavior. These necessary requirements include both macro-level social processes and more micro-level individual factors. The pathways encompassing larger contextual factors include sociocultural variables such as cultural mores, neighborhoods, and social networks. Another set of pathways stems from individual characteristics, such as personality traits and coping strategies. Finally, they describe biological pathways that influence health behaviors, including genes, physiological reactivity, and cell physiognomy. Each of these pathways is associated with the other, leading to an array of relationships that influence and determine health and behavior related to functional, emotional, and physical health outcomes.

Leventhal et al. assert that the requisites of a solid theory of health behavior encompass multiple sociocultural, interpersonal, and intrapersonal constructs. Researchers can apply a developmental perspective to each of these constructs to inform age differences in health behaviors. For example, social processes include cultural values, and these values can be defined as cohort-specific beliefs and practices. Whereas modern young women have been raised to believe that exercise is valuable, and modern young men have been instructed in the value of planning balanced and nutritious meals, these same messages may not have been given to older cohorts. For older women, exercise was often limited to dance, and meal planning was relegated to the mostly female home economics courses. In addition, the necessary ingredients for optimal health include unique profiles for people who vary in health status, a construct within the pathway of micro-level factors. For example, vigorous exercise and pushing boundaries of physical abilities is often encouraged for healthy young adults, reinforced by Nike commercials to "just do it" and by the saying that "no pain means no gain." For a person with a predisposing heart condition, this same recommendation could have lethal consequences.

Within-Person Variability and Its Relation to Illness Perception

Theories of health behavior rarely include within-person processes, yet we think their inclusion would further explain functional, emotional, and physical health outcomes. Most theories seek to explain how people vary from one another, with this variation shaped by both larger social influences and individual factors such as knowledge, motivation, and physiognomy. Yet differences in behaviors also occur within an individual; not all days are the same, and some people vary in their daily patterns of symptom perceptions and health behaviors more than others. Methodological advances in technology and statistical models now allow people to assess within-person variability more easily and efficiently than in the past.

In their chapter, Leventhal et al. describe the many factors that determine how people perceive their symptoms and when they decide to seek help in the authors' common-sense model of illness and self-regulation. They discuss how aging is associated with sometimes rapid and accurate health care seeking (E. A. Leventhal, Easterling, Leventhal, & Cameron, 1995; E. A. Leventhal, Leventhal, Schaefer, & Easterling, 1993), but sometimes with greater delays out of misconception of age-related changes in individuals' physical health (Prohaska, Keller, Leventhal, & Leventhal, 1987).

We maintain that theories of health behavior and health promotion would benefit from incorporating models of within-person variability. The common-sense model is no exception. For example, the common-sense model states that bidirectionality characterizes the association between emotional experience and the perception of physical symptoms (Leventhal, Nerenz, & Steele, 1984; Meyer, Leventhal, & Gutmann, 1985). This bidirectionality does occur, but we propose that studying the daily fluctuations of this bidirectional relationship yields further information about different types of illnesses. For example, in a study of over 1,000 adults ranging from 25 to 74 years of age, we found that negative emotions were related to transient physical symptoms, but these relationships (and the direction of these relationships) depended on the type of symptom studied (Charles & Almeida, 2006). For symptoms that were related to diffuse pain, the relationship from pain symptoms and emotional distress was bidirectional: Pain was reported more frequently on days following a day characterized by high levels of negative affect, but high levels of negative affect were also more likely to follow days after which people reported frequent pain experiences. In contrast, other symptoms shared a strong concurrent association with negative affect but no lagged associations. These influences depended on more stable factors as well, as evidenced by the effects being stronger among people with high levels of neuroticism.

Within-Person Variability in the Developmental Context

Researchers often focus on static factors accounting for age differences in health and health behaviors. Age is related to the types of health problems encountered and how people perceive and react to these conditions, as research by Leventhal and others has clearly shown (e.g., E. A. Leventhal et al., 1995). Age also is related, however, to daily processes that may interact with these between-subject factors. By combining these factors, we can form a more complete picture of how people engage in activities that influence their health on a daily basis.

Older age is related to benefits when engaging in health promotion and responding to health problems. First, older adults have gained experience, both from their own interactions with health problems and health behaviors and from those of their friends and families. Unfortunately, however, their expertise may not always come into play with the type of health problems they encounter. Although older adults may respond to acute disease processes better than younger adults based on years of experience, they may be poor at recognizing and responding to chronic conditions. Chronic conditions are more likely to develop in older age, so their health-related expertise needs to be understood in this new context. For example, a sprained ankle may require restricted activity to give the ligaments time to heal. For older adults, joint pain may instead be the result of osteoarthritis. For this condition, light exercise is often recommended by the attending physician to strengthen the muscles supporting the joints. If older adults treat their chronic pain from osteoarthritis as they had their acute pain conditions, they may not engage in the necessary exercise and rehabilitation exercises that could potentially improve their conditions.

The decision to seek medical care may also vary according to the seemingly transient nature of the symptoms. Some symptoms of chronic conditions exhibit unstable patterns of symptoms. People with rheumatoid arthritis, for example, have symptoms with intermittent recurrence patterns. Someone who notices that pain is gradually decreasing may interpret their symptoms as an acute problem that is improving, and several rounds of pain recurrence may need to occur before a person notices this pattern and recognizes the possibility of a potential underlying chronic condition. The different types of symptoms evolving from chronic conditions, as opposed to acute events, may be one reason why many older adults often misinterpret their symptoms and delay treatment relative to younger adults (Prohaska et al., 1987).

Other studies find that older adults seek medical treatment more rapidly than do younger adults (e.g., E. A. Leventhal et al., 1995). Perhaps this discrepancy may be explained by understanding both the types of symptoms and the context in which these symptoms are experienced. Age differences in chronic versus acute natures of symptoms, as described previously, may delay care seeking for older adults. Older adults are more likely to experience symptoms from chronic conditions, and misinterpreting the initial symptoms of an underlying chronic condition may delay the seeking of medical treatment. On the other hand, life circumstances may allow older adults to seek health care more rapidly and perceive symptoms more accurately. Older adults report fewer daily stressors in their lives (Almeida & Horn, 2004) and lower levels of negative affect (Charles, Reynolds, & Gatz, 2001). The experience of higher levels of stress and negative affect are often coupled with health symptoms (e.g., Mallers, Almeida, & Neupert, 2005), and people coming home after a long day experiencing aches, pains, and fatigue may dismiss these symptoms as the result of overwork and negative mood. Someone whose day is filled with fewer activities may notice fatigue, aches, and pains and not attribute their symptoms to external factors. In addition, retirement may allow older adults to test whether taking a day of rest alleviates symptoms; middle-aged adults may not have as many opportunities to test this hypothesis. Given this explanation, age differences may arise from the structure of the day more than chronological age. An overscheduled older adult may look similar in her delay of treatment to a younger adult, and a younger adult who has more free time may appear more similar to an older adult than to his or her more distracted peer.

In summary, Leventhal and colleagues beautifully elucidate the prospect and challenge of using a process model of health behavior to describe the dynamic linkage between cultural/social, psychological/ behavioral, and biological levels. While the assessment of these multiple levels of information is becoming more common, perhaps the most critical issue for integrating concepts and data across levels is not differences in access; it is the limited conceptualization and empirical examination of the processes involved in cross-level communication We maintain that studying within-person variation will help translate this communication and refine theories of health promotion and health care. Age differences occur both in the more commonly studied social and traitlike characteristics, but also in the seemingly minor, but no less important, fluctuations of daily life. Studying each of these processes as well as interactions between them will enrich our understanding regarding how health care and health promotions change across the adult life span.

RELIGION, HEALTH, AND HEALTH BEHAVIOR: ADVANTAGES OF COMBINING BETWEEN- AND WITHIN-PERSON SOURCES OF VARIATION

The chapter by Neil Krause provides a wonderful complement to the Leventhal et al. chapter by offering a multilevel framework for understanding the links between religion (cultural level), alcohol use (behavioral level), and mortality (biological level). Krause contends that communication across cultural and behavioral levels occurs via social interactions that foster both social learning and peer pressure. The key to understanding communication across these levels is to capture and explain variation at each of these levels. First, there is variation across religious denominations in teaching and sanctions regarding alcohol use. Krause's analyses show that fundamentalists were more likely to abstain from alcohol than individuals from other denominations. Next, variation across religious activities accounts for differences in denominational affiliation. Indeed, Krause's analyses demonstrate that social ties to other church members (e.g., attending prayer groups) mediate association between type of denomination and alcohol use.

It is important to note that Krause's findings illuminate *between-person differences* in religious activities and health behaviors. As we have argued, much can be gained by looking for *within-person variation* in health behaviors. First, most health behaviors are not static, but rather ebb and flow with proximal situational determinants that often follow daily, weekly, and even monthly rhythms. Keeping with the alcohol use exemplar, Del Boca, Darkes, Greenbaum, and Goldman (2004) found a great degree of temporal variability in alcohol use among first-year college students. Students drank more on the weekend, after exams, and on holidays (New Year's Eve, spring break). Such time-related situational triggers, such as religious holidays, would illuminate conditions when religious activities limit alcohol use. Second, static between-person designs are unable to assess if and how individuals select themselves into groups and activities. It is possible that abstainers are more likely to choose to be with like-minded individuals at Bible study. Bible study in turn may serve to maintain abstention from alcohol. In other words, cross-level communication between culture and behavior is often a two-way conversation.

The "birds of a feather" notion also holds among those individuals who consume a lot of alcohol. During a regular semester week, college students who take a spring break trip typically drink 33% more alcohol than their peers who stay at home. During spring break week, this difference increases to 50% more alcohol for students on a trip compared to homebound students (Rankin & Maggs, 2006). This example illustrates that health behaviors may be determined by interplay of selection and socialization factors that can only be unpacked with within-person designs.

RELIGION AND HEALTH: A DAILY HEALTH PERSPECTIVE

Within-person designs also allow researchers to view health behaviors as daily adaptation. We now briefly describe some of our own findings on how religious activities predict adaptation or reactivity to daily stressors. *Stressor reactivity* is the likelihood that an individual will show psychological or physical reactions to daily stressors (Almeida, 2005). Thus stressor reactivity is not defined as health, but is operationalized as the within-person slope between stressors and health. Reactivity, therefore, is a dynamic process that links stressors and health over time. Differences in reactivity depend on the resources of individuals and their environments (e.g., education, income, children in the household) that limit or enhance the possibilities and choices for coping with daily experiences. Aspects of religious activity may be related to allocation of such resources. In the following analyses, we assess if church attendance, religious identification, religious coping, and spirituality modify how daily stressors affect daily psychological and physical health.

Sample and Procedure

Data are from the National Study of Daily Experiences (NSDE). Respondents were 1,031 adults, aged 25–74 years (562 women, 469 men), all of whom had previously participated in the Midlife in the United States Survey (MIDUS). Over the course of eight consecutive evenings, respondents completed short telephone interviews about their daily experiences, including time use, physical and psychological health, and daily stressors (for a complete description, see Almeida, 2005).

Daily physical symptoms were assessed using a shortened version of Larsen and Kasimatis's (1991) symptoms checklist. The scale assessed health symptoms in five categories: (a) headaches, backaches, and muscle soreness; (b) cough, sore throat, fever, chills, or other cold and flu symptoms; (c) nausea, poor appetite, or other stomach problems; (d) chest pain or dizziness; and (e) other physical symptoms or discomforts. Each day, respondents indicated how frequently they experienced each symptom over the past 24 hours on a 5-point scale from 1 (*none of the time*) to 5 (*all of the time*). Summed scores across the five items were computed for each day. This scale has been used effectively in previous studies (Charles & Almeida, 2006; Neupert, Almeida, & Charles, 2007).

Daily psychological distress was measured using 10 items designed specifically from the MIDUS. Respondents were asked questions concerning how much of the time during a particular day they felt worthless, hopeless, nervous, restless or fidgety, that everything was an effort, and so sad that nothing could cheer them up. They rated their response on a 5-point scale 1 (*none of the time*) to 5 (*all of the time*). Scores across the 10 items were summed for each day. This scale has also demonstrated good reliability and validity in previous studies (Kessler et al., 2002; Mroczek & Kolarz, 1998).

Daily stressors were assessed through the semistructured Daily Inventory of Stressful Events (DISE; Almeida, Wethington, & Kessler, 2002). The inventory consisted of a series of seven stem questions asking whether certain types of daily stressors (i.e., arguments, potential arguments, work stressors, home stressors, network stressors, discrimination stressors, and other stressors) had occurred in the past 24 hours. For each daily interview, individuals who responded affirmatively to the stem questions received a value of 1 for the relevant stressor domain. Scores of 0 were assigned to domains where no stressors were experienced on that day. The present analyses utilized an index of stressor exposure, where days without any stressors occurring received a score of 0 and days with one or more stressors occurring received a score of 1.

Religion variables were assessed in the baseline MIDUS interview (Ryff, Singer, & Palmersheim, 2004), and included items related to church attendance ("How often do you attend church"), religious coping ("When you have decisions to make in your daily life, how often do you ask yourself what would your religious beliefs suggest you do?"), religious identification ("How important is religion in your daily life?"), and spirituality ("How spiritual are you?"). All items were rated on a 4-point scale ranging from 1 (*not at all*) to 4 (*very*).

Analyses

Multilevel modeling using SAS Institute's (1997) Proc Mixed was implemented to examine emotional and physical reactivity to daily stressors. In this framework, individual change/variability is represented through a two-level hierarchical model (Hawkins, Guo, Hill, Battin-Pearson, & Abbott, 2001). At Level 1, each person's variability is represented by an individual regression equation that depends on a set of parameters (intercept and slope). These individual parameters become the outcome variables in a Level 2 model, where they may depend on some person-level characteristics.

Multilevel modeling is frequently used to model intraindividual variability, that is, people's variability around their own average. This technique was especially useful in the current study because we sought to examine interindividual differences (e.g., spirituality) in intraindividual covariation (e.g., the within-person relationship between stressors and psychological distress). For example, to examine spirituality differences in emotional reactivity to stressors, the following model was formulated:

$$\text{Level 1: DISTRESS}_{it} = \beta_{0it} + \beta_{1it} (\text{STRESSOR EXPOSURE}_{it}) + r_{it}, \quad (1)$$

$$\text{Level 2: } \beta_{0i} = \gamma_{00} + \gamma_{01} (\text{SPIRITUALITY}_{i}) + u_{0i}, \quad (2)$$

$$\beta_{1i} = \gamma_{10} + \gamma_{11} (\text{SPIRITUALITY}_{i}) + u_{1i}. \quad (3)$$

In Equation 1, the intercept (β_{0it}) is defined as the expected level of psychological distress for person i on days when no stressors occurred (i.e., STRESSOR = 0). The slope (β_{1it}) is the expected change in psychological distress associated with days when stressors occur. The error term (r_{it}) represents a unique effect associated with person i (i.e., fluctuation around the mean). Equation 2 tests for spirituality differences in the average level of psychological distress, with the intercept (γ_{00}) representing the average level of psychological distress for someone with an average level of spirituality (religion variables were centered around their grand mean). Equation 3 tests for spirituality differences in the within-person association between stressor exposure and psychological distress, with the intercept (γ_{10}) representing the average relationship between stressors and psychological distress. Interindividual fluctuations from the level and slope are represented by u_{0i} and u_{1i}, respectively.

Findings

The first set of analysis assessed the degree of within-person variability in our health outcomes. Results from fully unconditional models indicated that 54% of the variability in psychological distress was between people ($\tau_{00} = 7.22$, $z = 19.42$, $p < .001$) and 46% was within people ($\sigma^2 = 6.23$, $z = 55.35$, $p < .001$). In addition, 55% of the variability in physical symptoms was between people ($\tau_{00} = 2.84$, $z = 20.03$, $p < .001$) and 45% was within-people ($\sigma^2 = 2.36$, $z = 55.60$, $p < .001$). Thus these models indicated almost as much within-person daily variation (intraindividual variation) and between-person variation (interindividual variation) in daily indicators of health.

Religious Differences in Physical Reactivity

Religious differences in physical reactivity to stressors are presented in the second column of Table 4.1. Although religious coping (γ_{01}), spirituality (γ_{02}), religious identification (γ_{03}), and church attendance (γ_{04}) were unrelated to the level of physical symptoms, spirituality (γ_{12}), religious identification (γ_{13}), and church attendance (γ_{14}) were each associated with lower physical reactivity to daily stressors. Specifically, people who reported high levels of spirituality, religious identification, and church attendance were less physically reactive to daily stressors compared to people with lower levels of spirituality, religious identification, and church attendance. Estimates of a pseudo-R^2 (Singer & Willett, 2003) were calculated for each model with significant predictors. The spirituality model accounted for 14% of the between-person variability and 7% of the within-person variability in physical symptoms. The religious identification model accounted for 17% of the between-person variability and 6% of the within-person variability in physical symptoms. The church attendance model accounted for 11% of the between-person variability and 6% of the within-person variability in physical symptoms.

Religious Differences in Psychological Reactivity

Religious differences in psychological reactivity are presented in the third column of Table 4.1. Religious coping (γ_{01}), spirituality (γ_{02}), and religious identification (γ_{03}) were unrelated to the average level of psychological distress, but people with higher levels of church attendance reported less psychological distress (γ_{04}). Religious coping (γ_{11}), spirituality (γ_{12}), and religious identification (γ_{13}) were also unrelated to emotional reactivity, but people with higher levels of church attendance were less emotionally reactive to stressors (γ_{14}) compared to people with lower levels of church attendance. The church attendance model accounted

Table 4.1

MULTILEVEL MODEL OF RELIGIOUS EXPERIENCES PREDICTING PHYSICAL AND PSYCHOLOGICAL REACTIVITY TO DAILY STRESSORS

	PHYSICAL SYMPTOMS	PSYCHOLOGICAL DISTRESS
Well-being level, β_0		
Intercept, γ_{00}	1.46*** (.06)	1.16*** (.07)
Coping, γ_{01}	.04 (.03)	−.00 (.03)
Spirituality, γ_{02}	.05 (.03)	.01 (.04)
Religious identification, γ_{03}	.01 (.01)	.00 (.02)
Church attendance, γ_{04}	−.05 (.04)	−.12* (.05)
Reactivity slope, β_1		
Intercept, γ_{10}	.49*** (.05)	1.48*** (.10)
Coping, γ_{11}	−.01 (.02)	−.01 (.05)
Spirituality, γ_{12}	−.07* (.03)	−.07 (.06)
Religious identification, γ_{13}	−.02* (.01)	−.01 (.02)
Church attendance, γ_{14}	−.11** (.04)	−.18* (.08)

Note: Table presents unstandardized estimates (and standard errors).
*p < .05. **p < .01. ***p < .001.

for 44% of the between-person variability and 26% of the within-person variability in psychological distress.

These results illustrate what can be gained by assessing both between- and within-person sources of variability. We found that none of the religion variables were related to overall levels of physical symptoms and that only spirituality was related to psychological distress. A very different picture emerged for stressor reactivity. Church attendance, religious identification, and spirituality each buffered the effects of daily stressors on physical symptoms. Church attendance also buffered the effects of daily stressors on psychological distress.

It is interesting to note that religious coping was not related to well-being level or reactivity to stressors. These findings are consistent with Krause's findings suggesting that the power of religion's influence on health may be in the social ties that come with affiliation to other church members.

CONCLUSION AND FUTURE DIRECTIONS

Studying how people vary in their health behaviors across time is not novel but remains a vital and arguably understudied area of inquiry. Some health behaviors require daily commitment, and multiple competing goals of time and effort can affect these daily activities. In addition to studying how often people engage in these behaviors, studying the patterns of these behaviors, and what predicts these patterns, is an important aim for health psychologists. Understanding what predicts these patterns will allow clinicians to design successful treatment programs. For example, researchers in the area of eating behaviors and alcohol use have studied differences in people with regular habits versus those people characterized by inconsistent, and more dangerous, patterns in their daily lives. Researchers have found, for instance, that inconsistent patterns of eating—assessed by binges—often fluctuate with the stress people experience in their daily lives, as people who report binge eating often do so when they are experiencing stress (Smyth et al., 2007). Training people in positive coping skills and stress inoculation, then, may directly serve to reduce stress, and indirectly serve as an intervention to reduce problematic binge cycles of eating.

Understanding within-person variation in health behaviors will help not only to identify factors encouraging or discouraging health behaviors, but will also offer a new perspective on health promotion. For example, instead of labeling people as those with good or poor health behaviors, a model of within-person variability would view people as having days marked by good or poor health behaviors. Using this conception, people can then learn to identify the trigger points that either enhance or deter certain health behaviors, and researchers can study the types and different reactivities of these triggers with age. Documenting how other health-related behaviors are shaped by daily activities, and how they vary with age, will provide an increased awareness of the best conditions under which people at every point in the life span are capable of achieving health promotion goals.

REFERENCES

Almeida, D. M. (2005). Resilience and vulnerability to daily stressors assessed via diary methods. *Current Directions in Psychological Science, 14,* 64–68.

Almeida, D. M., & Horn, M. C. (2004). Is daily life more stressful during middle adulthood? In O. G. Brim, C. D. Ryff, & R. C. Kessler (Eds.), *How healthy are we?: A national study of well-being at midlife* (pp. 425–451). Chicago: University of Chicago Press.

Almeida, D. M., Wethington, E., & Kessler, R. C. (2002). The daily inventory of stressful events: An investigator-based approach for measuring daily stressors. *Assessment, 9,* 41–55.

Charles, S. T., & Almeida, D. M. (2006). Daily reports of symptoms and negative affect: Not all symptoms are the same. *Psychology and Health, 21,* 1–17.

Charles, S. T., Reynolds, C., & Gatz, M. (2001). Age-related differences and change in positive and negative affect over twenty-five years. *Journal of Personality and Social Psychology, 80,* 136–151.

Del Boca, F. K., Darkes, J., Greenbaum, P. E., & Goldman, M. S. (2004). Up close and personal: Temporal variability in the drinking of individual college students during their first year. *Journal of Consulting and Clinical Psychology, 72,* 155–164.

Hawkins, J. D., Guo, J., Hill, K. G., Battin-Pearson, S., & Abbott, R. D. (2001). Long-term effects of the Seattle social development intervention on school bonding trajectories. *Applied Developmental Science, 5,* 225–236.

Kessler, R. C., Andrews, G., Colpe, L. J., Hiripi, E., Mroczek, D. K., Normand, S. L. T., et al. (2002). Short screening scales to monitor population prevalence and trends in non-specific psychological distress. *Psychological Medicine, 32,* 959–976.

Larsen, R. J., & Kasimatis, M. (1991). Day-to-day physical symptoms: Individual differences in the occurrence, duration, and emotional concomitants of minor daily illnesses. *Journal of Personality, 59,* 387–423.

Leventhal, E. A., Easterling, D., Leventhal, H., & Cameron, L. (1995). Conservation of energy, uncertainty reduction, and swift utilization of medical care among the elderly: II. *Medical Care, 33,* 988–1000.

Leventhal, E. A., Leventhal, H., Schaefer, P., & Easterling, D. (1993). Conservation of energy, uncertainty reduction, and swift utilization of medical care among the elderly. *Journals of Gerontology, Ser. A, 48,* 78–86.

Leventhal, H., Nerenz, D., & Steele, D. (1984). Illness representations and coping with health threats. In A. Baum & J. Singer (Eds.), *A handbook of psychology and health* (Vol. 4, pp. 219–252). Hillsdale, NJ: Erlbaum.

Mallers, M. H., Almeida, D. M., & Neupert, S. D. (2005). Women's daily physical health symptoms and stressful experiences across adulthood. *Psychology and Health, 20,* 389–403.

Meyer, D., Leventhal, H., & Gutmann, M. (1985). Common-sense models of illness: The example of hypertension. *Health Psychology, 4,* 115–135.

Miniño, A. M., Heron, M., Smith, B. L., & Kochanek, K. D. (2006, November 24). *Deaths: Final data for 2004.* Retrieved Month 11, 2006 from http://www.cdc.gov/nchs/products/pubs/pubd/hestats/finaldeaths04/finaldeaths04.htm

Mroczek, D. K., & Kolarz, C. M. (1998). The effect of age on positive and negative affect: A developmental perspective on happiness. *Journal of Personality and Social Psychology, 75,* 1333–1349.

Neupert, S. D., Almeida, D. M., & Charles, S. T. (2007). Age differences in reactivity to daily stressors: The role of personal control. *Journals of Gerontology, Ser. B, 62,* P216–P225.

Prohaska, T. R., Keller, M. L., Leventhal, E. A., & Leventhal, H. (1987). Impact of symptoms and aging attribution on emotions and coping. *Health Psychology, 6,* 495–514.

Rankin, L. A., & Maggs, J. L. (2006). First year college students affect and alcohol use: Paradoxical within- and between-person associations. *Journal of Youth and Adolescence, 35,* 925–937.

Ryff, C. D., Singer, B. H., & Palmersheim, K. A. (2004). Social inequalities in health and well-being: The role of relational and religious protective factors. In O. G. Brim, C. D. Ryff, & R. C. Kessler (Eds.), *How healthy are we?: A national study of well-being at midlife* (pp. 90–123). Chicago: University of Chicago Press.

SAS Institute. (1997). *SAS/STAT software: Changes and enhancements through release 6.12.* Cary, NC: Author.

Singer, J. D., & Willett, J. B. (2003). *Applied longitudinal data analysis: Modeling change and event occurrence.* New York: Oxford University Press.

Smyth, J. M., Wonderlich, S. A., Heron, K. E., Sliwinski, M. J., Crosby, R. D., Mitchel, J. E., et al. (2007). Daily and momentary mood and stress are associated with binge eating and vomiting in bulimia nervosa patients in the natural environment. *Journal of Consulting and Clinical Psychology, 75,* 629–638.

Personality and Cognition

5

From Static to Dynamic: The Ongoing Dialectic About Human Development

NILAM RAM, SYLVIA MORELLI,
CASEY LINDBERG, AND
LAURA L. CARSTENSEN

Each scientific discipline will, in its development, move from more static representations of phenomena to more dynamical ones (West, 1985). The study of behavioral development is no exception. The understanding of cognitive, emotional, and personality development and change has come a long way in the past few decades, moving from relatively static conceptions of individual attributes and debates about their relative stability to more dynamic models of behavioral processes. In turn, the field has advanced in its understanding of the ways that individual development is embedded within cultural contexts (e.g., within-person cross-domain interactive processes and biocultural co-constructive ontogenetic development; Markus & Kitiyama, 1991; Tsai, Knutson, & Fung, 2006). Life span and life course theoretical and methodological frameworks have been key to this shift from static to dynamic (Baltes, Lindenberger, & Staudinger, 2006; Elder, Johnson, & Crosnoe, 2003). The need for

Acknowledgments: The authors gratefully acknowledge the support provided by grant R01-AG08816 from the National Institute on Aging in the preparation of this chapter. Special thanks go to members of the Developmental Systems Group at Pennsylvania State University, the Center for Lifespan Psychology at the Max Plank Institute for Human Development, the Life-Span Development Lab at Stanford University, and Ron Abeles and K. Warner Schaie for helpful comments on earlier versions of this work.

115

articulating and testing hypotheses about a *dialectical interplay* between two *dynamisms*—social structures and individual lives—has demanded innovative approaches from theorists and methodologists, as they have developed new ways of thinking about and modeling the dynamic and complex changes in behavior observed to occur with time and age.

The Social Structures and Aging conferences and book series were, from the outset, conceived as an exploration of these emerging dynamic views (see Riley, 1989). In an early volume, for instance, Abeles and Riley (1987) engaged the dialectic between the aging of individuals and changes in social structure. They reviewed the evidence of how, and through what mechanisms (e.g., family, work environments), changes in social structure (e.g., longevity) influence individual aging processes (e.g., cognitive aging)—and, in turn, how the changes in individual aging influence societal norms and roles and redefine social structures. In this chapter, we explore more generally how ongoing dialectics have pushed researchers into debates and considerations of individuals as dynamic, rather than static, entities. To frame the discussion, we use *complementary pairs* (e.g., person and context; see Kelso & Engstrøm, 2006) to place and organize some of the past and current issues that have characterized the landscape of developmental study. We draw selectively on examples from the fields of personality, emotion, and cognition. Our overarching observation is that the debates and ongoing reconciliations of trait and situation, stability and change, person and context, and socioemotional and cognitive phenomena have positively contributed to and fostered an ongoing transformation and maturation of our discipline—from conceptions of development as static to dynamic (West, 1985). In the sections that follow, we highlight how these complementary pairs have pushed the field by providing new lenses through which the complexities of human behavior can be viewed. We conclude with a note that methodological innovations currently emerging will likely move dynamic perspectives further into the forefront of our scientific discipline.

TRAIT AND SITUATION

The general shift from relatively static to more dynamic inquiry mirrors, and is in some ways an extension of, the trait versus situation debate in psychology. Since early in the 20th century, researchers examined and debated the generality of sampled behaviors (e.g., Allport, 1937; Thorndike, 1906), asking the question, Are individuals behaviorally consistent? Summarizing work in the trait personality arena, Mischel (1968) argued that personality measurements were, given their low correlations with behavioral outcomes, severely limited in their predictive power. Scores of studies in social psychology demonstrated that in a given situation, characteristics of the social and physical context contributed as much, if not more, than personality traits to behavioral outcomes. At the extreme, some contended that personality did not exist. In the ensuing debate about the relevance and primacy of trait or situational characteristics, researchers identified and sought to rectify a number of methodological shortcomings in prior studies (e.g., attenuation, single-item assessment) and examined how novel methodologies might help resolve and/or explain contrasting empirical findings and the conclusions derived from them (e.g., Alker, 1972; Bem, 1972, 1977; Bem & Allen, 1974; Cattell, 1983; Epstein, 1979; Golding, 1975; Nesselroade & Bartsch, 1977; Schaie, Campbell, Meredith, & Rawlings, 1988).

As part of this discourse, in their presentation of the *interactionist* perspective, emphasizing a continuous, multidirectional interaction between person characteristics and situation characteristics, Magnusson and Endler (1977) noted that the "modern interactionist theory of behavior . . . has important consequences for the choice of models and for methods of data collection and data treatment" (p. 409). In particular, an interactional perspective requires information regarding individuals' multidimensional patterns of reactions across situations. A key example is stimulus–response (S–R) inventories, wherein individuals rate their own reactions on a number of scales for each of a number of verbally described situations (e.g., Endler, Hunt, & Rosenstein, 1962). More recently, the multivariate, multisituation (i.e., multioccasion) data provided by S–R-type inventories has been obtained through intensive observation procedures. For example, in a study of social behavior, Shoda, Mischel, and Wright (1994) systematically observed children's behaviors in vivo across a wide variety of interpersonal situations, which occurred in a residential summer camp setting. The intensive data collection provided the raw evidence necessary to evaluate "if . . . then . . . , situation-behavior relations" (p. 676) of the S–R type noted above. Specifically, the repeated hourly measurement of children's behavior across situations (average of 167 hours of observation per child) allowed these researchers to obtain if-then relationships for each child, or in other words, intraindividual, situation-behavior profiles, or *behavioral signatures*. Although these hour-to-hour behavioral signatures differed substantially from child to child, the pattern of relationships was relatively stable from week to week; that is, children exhibited a relatively consistent pattern of situation-behavior responses over time. Such findings can be taken as an indication that situations influence behavior, but in a rather consistent, or traitlike, manner for each person.

Experience sampling paradigms, wherein individuals are measured repeatedly and intensively over a relatively short period of time, have also allowed for further examination and consideration of the interactionist perspective (Bolger, Davis, & Rafaeli, 2003). For instance, Fleeson (2001), in a series of studies examining individuals' behavior across 2–3 weeks of everyday life, found that individuals regularly reported experiencing the full range of personality traits over the course of everyday behavior. Within-person fluctuation of personality states was substantial, with trait-relevant behaviors varying from hour to hour within-person as much or even more than the same behaviors between persons. However, despite individuals' behaviors being inconsistent across situations, the amount and quality of inconsistency (e.g., central tendency, skew, kurtosis of within-person distribution) was stable across time (e.g., week to week) and reliable across persons; that is, behavioral variability itself appears to be a stable and enduring personal characteristic (i.e., a trait). Furthermore, interindividual differences in within-person variability were found, in some domains, to be related to trait personality (e.g., measures of the Big Five). Thus, similar to the observational studies examining behavioral signatures, findings from experience sampling studies provide evidence for both variability and stability of behavior, albeit at different levels of analysis and along different time scales.

The general message conveyed is that by engaging in a dialectic that initially pitted trait and situational characteristics against one another, efforts made in the field to reconcile empirical findings resulted in integrative theoretical perspectives and led to methodological innovations. The debates have pushed and continue to push researchers to question the static nature of individual behavior and to consider if and how individuals function as dynamic beings, that is, people who interact with the situations they encounter in both predictable and fortuitous ways (see, e.g., Bandura, 2006).

As the discussion continues, we see that theoretical accounts of behavior will need to be increasingly precise regarding the particular time scales (e.g., hours, weeks, months, years, etc.) on which behaviors or patterns of behavior are expected to vary and/or be stable. Additionally, as the temporal ordering of intraindividual behavioral variability is considered, new methodologies will be needed that can articulate and test hypotheses regarding if, how, and why individuals tend to exhibit particular temporal signatures and how such temporally ordered patterns of behavior might themselves exhibit stability or change over time.

STABILITY AND CHANGE

Despite the focus on change, the study of development has been viewed as an investigation of early-life phenomena and constrained primarily to the study of infants, children, and adolescents. Reformulating the concept of development as broader than mere growth to one inclusive of the continuities and changes occurring at all ages led to the emergence of a life-span developmental framework that provided a basis for investigating how ontogenesis extends across the entire life course (Baltes et al., 2006). This theoretical merging of the gains occurring during the early phases of life with the seemingly pervasive losses noted in the latter part of life (along with other concurrent theoretical and empirical developments; see, e.g., Elder et al., 2003; Sontag, 1971) has since demanded further reconciliation of when and why development, in both children and adults, is sometimes characterized by stability and sometimes by change (whether gains or losses).

In the personality domain, for example, there has been ongoing argument regarding whether personality characteristics remain stable or change over the life span (Costa & McCrae, 2006; Roberts, Walton, & Viechtbauer, 2006b; Schaie & Parham, 1976; see also Lachman, 1989). Much as in the trait–situation debate, relevant data have provided support for both sides of the argument, some for stability and some for change. In brief, longitudinal and cross-sectional studies simultaneously indicate both relative stability in the rank ordering of individuals on trait measures of personality across time (e.g., relatively high test–retest correlations on the Big Five, e.g., Roberts & DelVecchio, 2000; Schaie, 2005) and substantial change in (group) mean levels of personality with age (e.g., Roberts, Walton, & Viechtbauer, 2006a; Schaie, 2005).

Similarly, in the cognitive domain, arguments have ensued regarding whether aging is characterized by inevitable decline or by stability (see, e.g., Baltes & Schaie, 1976; Horn & Donaldson, 1977). Again, the relevant data can be interpreted as providing support for both sides, with different aspects of cognitive function (e.g., fluid and crystallized abilities) exhibiting different patterns of change with age (Horn & Cattell, 1967). Schaie (2005) and others (e.g., Park et al., 2002), for instance, provided evidence that beginning around age 20, individuals are likely to experience continuous, regular decline in basic cognitive abilities such as perceptual speed inductive reasoning and memory. At the same time, however, verbal ability or knowledge (e.g. vocabulary, synonym and antonym identification) appears to remain stable, or even improve slightly, over the adult life span.

In attempting to make sense of the contradictory evidence, where some data indicate age-related stability and other data indicate age-related change, the life span perspective offered a combined view, or *differential aging* (e.g., Baltes, 1987). From this perspective, rather than pitting stability versus change, both are engaged, and the focus shifts from an either-or question to what characteristics and which persons change *and* what characteristics and which persons remain stable. In this view, individuals are composed of dynamic characteristics that change and remain stable at different rates under different conditions. While intuitively more appealing, such views demand highly sophisticated methodological approaches. Although more work needs to be done, recent studies illustrate some of the ways in which this more dynamic differential aging perspective is being articulated, across domains and across persons.

Schindler, Staudinger, and Nesselroade (2006), for example, were interested in older individuals' motivation to pursue personal goals. Using longitudinal data collected from older adults, they found evidence for differential aging across types of goal engagement. On average, investment in leisure, sexuality, friends, and occupation domains remained stable until age 80, after which it declined precipitously. In contrast, investment in health, cognitive fitness, independence, and family domains remained stable throughout old age. Such results demonstrate how differential aging across constructs is helping to clarify which domains may be considered more or less basic, that is, optional or obligatory investments.

From a similarly dynamic perspective, Rönnlund, Nyberg, Bäckman, and Nilsson (2005) examined differential aging across semantic and episodic memory in a sample of 35- to 80-year-olds. On average, practice-adjusted episodic memory scores remained relatively stable until age 60, then exhibited decline. In contrast, practice-adjusted semantic memory improved through age 60, before also exhibiting decline. The differential pattern of dynamics observed before and after age 60 suggests that various aging processes interact in complex ways, and perhaps in different ways at different parts of the life span. While complicated, such results help to clarify theoretical accounts of the potential processes and causes contributing to memory performance and change (see, e.g., Buchler & Reder, 2007).

In addition to dynamics of change differing across domains, they may also differ across individuals. For example, when examining age-related change in life satisfaction, Mroczek and Spiro (2005) noted inter-individual differences in how some 1,900 men's levels of life satisfaction changed across the 40- to 85-year age span. On average, the prototypical individual's level of life satisfaction was characterized by a slight increase through age 65, followed by a correspondent decrease thereafter (i.e., quadratic curve). Individuals, however, differed significantly in how they changed, with some individuals increasing and/or decreasing more rap-idly than others. These interindividual differences in the trajectory of change were related to the situation or context in which they occurred. In particular, differences were related to levels of individuals' trait ex-traversion and neuroticism, prevalence of memory complaints, and marriage status. In sum, such results highlight that when viewed from a more dynamic perspective, differential changes are prevalent across constructs, across ages, and across persons. More generally, the move to consider and study differential dynamics seems to be providing further insight into the potential causes and consequences of behavior.

Over the past 30 years, research on differential aging has trumped the previous conceptions of exclusive stability or inevitable and uniform growth or decline. The aforementioned studies provide just a few ex-amples of how the move from more static to more dynamic perspectives has advanced our knowledge of differential aging in numerous domains and how it unfolds across the life course. We see that these differential dynamics themselves can provide some of the quasiexperimental para-digms needed for teasing out the causes and consequences of behavior. Continuing inquiry into when and under what conditions constructs or persons change and/or remain stable will, without doubt, further our understanding of how biological, psychological, contextual, social, and other processes interact to produce behavior.

PERSON AND CONTEXT

Almost in parallel to the interactionist resolution of the trait–situation de-bate, developmentalists in the 1970s were reconstituting earlier notions of individual behavior as a function of both person and environment (e.g., Lewin, 1935). The emerging developmental contextual approaches highlighted the ongoing *dynamic interactions* or *transactions* occurring between individuals and their environments (Bronfenbrenner, 1979; Ford & Lerner, 1992; Sameroff & Chandler, 1975). Recent work stemming from this integration of person and context illustrates some of the increasingly dynamic views of behavior that are emerging in the literature.

Tsai and colleagues (2006), for instance, suggested a *dialectic interplay* between cultural and individual phenomena, such that group-level cultural norms (e.g., social structure) and individual-level temperament together influence emotional states. In particular, the interplay suggests that individuals prefer, or would ideally like to feel, those emotions that are valued at the societal level. In line with this hypothesis, young adults from East Asian cultures have been found to disproportionately value positive emotions that are relatively low in arousal, whereas younger adults with American culture have been shown to value positive emotions that are relatively high in arousal. Controlling for individuals' ratings of actual affect, European American undergraduates rated that they would ideally like to feel greater levels of high-arousal positive states (enthusiastic, excited, strong) and lower levels of low-arousal positive states (calm, at rest, relaxed, peaceful) than Asian American undergraduates. Furthermore, these influences seem to be active even early in the life span. For example, Tsai, Louie, Chen, and Uchida (2007) found not only that American children prefer both excited (vs. calm) smiles and exciting activities in storybook content compared to Asian American and Taiwanese children, but also that the top 10 selling storybooks in the United States had greater proportions of excited (vs. calm) expressions and more high-arousal activities (e.g., running) relative to Taiwanese storybooks. As with the more dynamic differential aging views on stability and change, these studies highlight how differences across culture can be useful in identifying how and why persons and contexts interact to affect individual preferences or behavior.

Pushing the idea of interactive dynamics a bit further, developmental contextualist approaches highlight that both persons and contexts are changing over time. Furthermore, the nature or quality of the transactions between these two may also change over time. Taking this notion seriously, researchers have begun examining long-term (i.e., age-related) differences in short-term process. Mroczek, Spiro, Griffin, and Neupert (2006), for example, used daily diary and multilevel modeling methods to describe how stress-related processes occurring at the daily level may change or differ with situational circumstance or age. They found that the *process of neuroticism,* as captured by individuals' short-term day-to-day affective reactivity to daily environmental stress (i.e., the person–context transaction), differs with age. Highly neurotic older adults are not as reactive as their highly neurotic younger counterparts, suggesting that the character of short-term transactions does change over the long term. This research not only spurs new questions regarding how, when, and at what level person–context transactions manifest, but it also highlights how another layer of change must be considered. As increasingly more hypotheses about the temporal course of dynamic processes become the conceptual focus of research on human development, there will be an increasing need for methodologies that can articulate the dynamics of the dynamics.

SOCIOEMOTIONAL AND COGNITIVE PHENOMENA

In the 1980s, Lazarus (1984) and Zajonc (1984) were characterizing the contemporary conceptualizations of emotion and cognition as static, separate processes and debating the primacy of either emotion or cognition. Today, more integrated and dynamic views of emotion and cognition have emerged (Carstensen, Mikels, & Mather, 2006). For instance, from a person-oriented perspective (Magnusson & Stattin, 2006), multiple aspects of function are characterized as functional nodes that interact in concert as a holistic system, in much the same manner that persons and context interact. Said differently, function in any given domain (e.g., cognition) occurs within the context of what is occurring in other domains (e.g., emotion). Over the past 30 years, integrated perspectives on how multiple processes occurring within the same individual influence one another through ongoing and dynamic interactions have gained prominence. The debate has shifted from a view of emotion and cognition as independent and stable processes to one about the mechanisms, reasons, and parameters for the dynamic interaction of socioemotional and cognitive processes.

To illustrate, in studies examining differential responses of the cognitive subsystem in different socioemotional contexts, older adults have been found to perform worse on memory tasks when negative cultural stereotypes about the impact of aging on memory were highlighted. For example, Rahhal, Hasher, and Colcombe (2001) found that instructional manipulations exaggerated age differences in memory performance.

When the memory component of the task was highlighted—using the word *memory* in the instructions—older adults did not perform as well as younger adults. In contrast, when the instructions did not emphasize the memory component of the task, older and younger adults performed at similar levels. Similarly, these researchers found that older adults performed at lower levels in conditions when negative cultural beliefs about the impact of aging on memory were activated, as compared to conditions with minimal or no stereotype threat (Hess, Auman, Colcombe, & Rahhal, 2003). In sum, both studies suggest an ongoing dynamic between cognitive processes (e.g., memory and the ability to use effective strategies) and the socioemotional context (e.g., negative cultural stereotype threat) in which they occur.

Some major theoretical frameworks have also emerged from the debate over the mechanisms, reasons, and parameters for the interaction of socioemotional and cognitive processes. For example, socioemotional selectivity theory suggests that changes in time perspective (i.e., perceived time left in life) lead to shifts in socioemotional goals (Carstensen, 1993, 2006). When time is perceived as limited, individuals focus on more emotional goals (e.g., spending more time with one's family), but when time is viewed as expansive, greater importance is placed on knowledge-related goals (e.g., learning new skills). Empirical evidence generated from socioemotional selectivity theory suggests that socioemotional goals dynamically influence many cognitive processes. Using age and its inherent relationship to time left in life as a proxy for time perspective, age differences in memory and attention—for example, the *positivity effect*—reflect shifts in socioemotional context. The positivity effect is defined by Carstensen et al. (2006) as "a developmental pattern in which a disproportionate preference for negative material in youth shifts across adulthood to disproportionate preference for positive information in later life" (p. 349). While cognitive decline was once thought to be inevitable, the positivity effect demonstrates how socioemotional context selectively influences cognitive processes, more clearly defining the mechanisms, reasons, and parameters for this powerful interaction.

Similarly, dynamic integration theories of affect and cognition (e.g., Labouvie-Vief, 2003; Labouvie-Vief & Medler, 2002) suggest further interplay between socioemotional and cognitive subsystems. Socioemotional functioning (e.g., affect complexity and regulation) is influenced by the quality or amount of cognitive resources available, such that when cognitive resources are high (e.g., younger adulthood), there is sufficient capacity available for complex affective processing and regulation. But when cognitive resources are low (e.g., older adulthood), the complexity of socioemotional processing is necessarily hampered and constrained. For instance, it has been found that the emotions experienced on days when the cognitive subsystem may be overburdened, and reserve resources are low (e.g., high-stress days marked by excessive rumination; see also Linville, 1985), are characterized by less complex structures, as compared to days when cognitive reserves are high (e.g., low-stress days; Zautra, Berkhof, & Nicolson, 2002). Such studies demonstrate how, even within-person, the cognitive context in some way determines or influences socioemotional processes.

The debate over the interaction between socioemotional and cognitive processes spurred theoretical advancement—such as socioemotional selectivity and dynamic integration theories—about specific mechanisms and models. Methodological advancement continues to elucidate these theoretical frameworks and encourage further theoretical advancement. For example, the use of functional magnetic resonance imaging (fMRI) has allowed researchers to investigate the neural systems underlying emotion and cognition. Mather et al. (2004), for example, found that amygdala activation in older adults occurred only in response to viewing positive (as opposed to negative) images. One recent study by Larkin et al. (2007) showed brain activation in older adults when they anticipated gains, but not when they anticipated losses, in contrast to younger adults, who showed brain activation in response to anticipation of both gain and loss. Phelps (2006) argued that neuroimaging research on the amygdala makes a significant contribution to the areas of emotional learning, emotion, and memory; emotion's influence on attention and perception; processing emotion in social stimuli; and changing emotional responses. Social cognitive neuroscience is emerging as a distinct field that seeks to understand relationships among the socioemotional, cognitive, and neural levels of analyses. The methodological advancement of fMRI continues to test the leading edge of theory and more clearly elucidate the interaction between socioemotional and cognitive processes by associating specific neural anatomy with behavior.

Future studies must develop more clearly defined models and theories, using fMRI and integrative methodological approaches to test new ideas. In addition, methodological advancement must inform theory and create hypotheses that make predictions based on neural anatomy and function of emotional and cognitive structures. The debate about the mechanisms, reasons, and parameters for the interaction between socioemotional and cognitive processes must push toward a more accurate, integrated, and specific understanding of these processes.

CONCLUSION

Over the past century, the articulation of theory, and in particular, developmental theory, has made great strides (Lerner, 2006). In this chapter, we examined how some ongoing dialectic tensions have contributed to this transformation. The theoretical merging of traits and situations, stability and change, person and context, and multiple domains within a person has demanded new methods suitable for the examination and organization of the overall structure and sequence of development across the life course. In response to the new empirical needs derived from such theoretical development, powerful multivariate longitudinal conceptions and models have emerged, which can be adapted and used to describe the dynamic complexities of behavioral change (e.g., Box & Jenkins, 1976; Bryk & Raudenbush, 1992; Collins & Horn, 1991; Collins & Sayer, 2001; Schaie et al., 1988). In turn, the innovations in methodological conceptions, measurement, research design, and modeling procedures for studying change have pushed theorists to further refine hypotheses regarding how the processes and mechanisms of development proceed. This ongoing dance between theory and method, wherein sometimes theory leads, and other times method hastens forth and beckons theory to catch up, is one of the hallmarks of the scientific dialectic and certainly has contributed to the reconceptualizations and progression of developmental science from static to dynamic (Wohlwill, 1991).

It may be fair to say that fields advance when dynamic methods are articulated and dynamic theories are tested. In particular, the theoretical complexities of multilevel, multi-time-scale, and interactive dynamisms provide numerous methodological challenges, many of which shall likely require further technical and conceptual innovation. The good news is that many tools exist, and others are emerging, that will be increasingly useful in the study of behavior (see, e.g., Browne & Nesselroade, 2005; Koopmans, 1995; Nayfeh & Balachandran, 1995; Shumway & Stoffer, 2006). As these analytical and statistical modeling tools are incorporated into the psychological literature, we shall be able to unpack and achieve greater understanding of the multiple interactive dynamisms contributing to the complexity of human behavior.

REFERENCES

Abeles, R., & Riley, M. (1987). Longevity, social structure, and cognitive aging. In C. Schooler and K. W. Schaie (Eds.), *Cognitive functioning and social structure over the life course* (pp. 161–175). Norwood, NJ: Ablex.

Alker, H. A. (1972). Is personality situationally specific or intrapsychically consistent? *Journal of Personality, 40,* 1–16.

Allport, G. W. (1937). *Personality: A psychological interpretation.* New York: Holt.

Baltes, P. B. (1987). Theoretical propositions of life-span developmental psychology: On the dynamics between growth and decline. *Developmental Psychology, 23,* 611–626.

Baltes, P. B., Lindenberger, U., & Staudinger, U. M. (2006). Lifespan theory in developmental psychology. In R. M. Lerner (Ed.), *Handbook of child psychology: Vol. 1. Theoretical models of human development* (6th ed., pp. 569–664). New York: John Wiley.

Baltes, P. B., & Schaie, K. W. (1976). On the plasticity of intelligence in adulthood and old age: Where Horn and Donaldson fail. *American Psychologist, 31,* 720–725.

Bandura, A. (2006). Toward a psychology of human agency. *Perspectives on Psychological Science, 1,* 164–180.

Bem, D. J. (1972). Constructing cross-situational consistencies in behavior: Some thoughts on Alker's critique of Mischel. *Journal of Personality, 40,* 17–26.

Bem, D. J. (1977). Predicting more of the people more of the time: Some thoughts on the Allen-Potkay studies of intraindividual variability. *Journal of Personality, 45,* 327–333.

Bem, D. J., & Allen, A. (1974). On predicting some of the people some of the time: The search for cross-situational consistencies in behavior. *Psychological Review, 81,* 506–520.

Bolger, N., Davis, A., & Rafaeli, E. (2003). Diary methods: Capturing life as it is lived. *Annual Review of Psychology, 54,* 579–616.

Box, G. E. P., & Jenkins, G. M. (1976). *Time series analysis: Forecasting and control* (Rev. ed.). San Francisco: Holden-Day.

Bronfenbrenner, U. (1979). *The ecology of human development: Experiments by nature and design.* Cambridge, MA: Harvard University Press.

Browne, M. W., & Nesselroade, J. R. (2005). Representing psychological processes with dynamic factor models: Some promising uses and extensions of ARMA time series models. In A. Maydeu-Olivares & J. J. McArdle (Eds.), *Psychometrics: A festschrift to Roderick P. McDonald* (pp. 415–452). Mahwah, NJ: Erlbaum.

Bryk, A. S., & Raudenbush, S. W. (1992). *Hierarchical linear models: Applications and data analysis methods.* Newbury Park, CA: Sage.

Buchler, N. E. G., & Reder, L. M. (2007). Modeling age-related memory deficits: A two-parameter solution. *Psychology and Aging, 22,* 104–121.

Carstensen, L. L. (1993). Motivation for social contact across the life span: A theory of socioemotional selectivity. In J. E. Jacobs (Ed.), *Nebraska Symposium on Motivation* (pp. 209–254). Lincoln: University of Nebraska Press.

Carstensen, L. L. (2006). The influence of a sense of time on human development. *Science, 312,* 1913–1915.

Carstensen, L. L., Mikels, J. A., & Mather, M. (2006). Aging and the intersection of cognition, motivation and emotion. In J. Birren & K. W. Schaie (Eds.), *Handbook of the psychology of aging* (6th ed., pp. 343–362). San Diego, CA: Academic Press.

Cattell, R. B. (1983). *Structural personality-learning theory: A wholistic multivariate research approach.* New York: Praeger.

Collins, L. M., & Horn, J. L. (1991). *Best methods for the analysis of change.* Washington, DC: American Psychological Association.

Collins, L. M., & Sayer, A. (2001). *New methods for the analysis of change.* Washington, DC: American Psychological Association.

Costa, P. T., Jr., & McCrae, R. R. (2006). Age changes in personality and their origins: Comment on Roberts, Walton, and Viechtbauer (2006). *Psychological Bulletin, 132,* 28–30.

Elder, G. H., Johnson, M. L., & Crosnoe, R. (2003). The emergence and development of life course theory. In J. Mortimer & M. J. Shanahan (Eds.), *Handbook of the life course* (pp. 3–22). New York: Kluwer Academic.

Endler, N. S., Hunt, J. M., & Rosenstein, A. J. (1962). An S-R inventory of anxiousness. *Psychological Monographs, 76,* 1–33.

Epstein, S. (1979). The stability of behavior: I. On predicting most of the people much of the time. *Journal of Personality and Social Psychology, 37,* 1097–1126.

Fleeson, W. (2001). Toward a structure- and process-integrated view of personality: Traits as density distributions of states. *Journal of Personality and Social Psychology, 80,* 1011–1027.

Ford, D. H., & Lerner, R. M. (1992). *Developmental systems theory: An integrative approach.* Newbury Park, CA: Sage.

Golding, S. L. (1975). Flies in the ointment: Methodological problems in the analysis of the percentage of variance due to persons and situations. *Psychological Bulletin, 82,* 278–288.

Hess, T. M., Auman, C., Colcombe, S. J., & Rahhal, T. A. (2003). The impact of stereotype threat on age differences in memory performance. *Journals of Gerontology, Ser. B, 58,* P3–P11.

Horn, J. L., & Cattell, R. B. (1967). Age differences in fluid and crystallized intelligence. *Acta Psychologica, 26,* 107–129.

Horn, J. L., & Donaldson, G. (1977). Faith is not enough: A response to the Baltes-Schaie claim that intelligence does not wane. *American Psychologist, 32,* 369–373.

Kelso, J.A.S., & Engstrøm, D. (2006). *The complementary nature.* Cambridge, MA: MIT Press.

Koopmans, L. H. (1995). *The spectral analysis of time series* (2nd ed.). San Diego, CA: Academic Press.

Labouvie-Vief, G. (2003). Dynamic integration: Affect, cognition, and the self in adulthood. *Current Directions in Psychological Science, 12,* 201–206.

Labouvie-Vief, G., & Medler, M. (2002). Affect optimization and affect complexity: Modes and styles of regulation in adulthood. *Psychology and Aging, 17,* 571–588.

Lachman, M. E. (1989). Personality and aging at the crossroads: Beyond stability versus change. In K. W. Schaie & C. Schooler (Eds.), *Social structure and aging: Psychological processes* (pp. 167–189). Hillsdale, NJ: Erlbaum.

Larkin, G.R.S., Gibbs, S.E.B., Khanna, K., Nielsen, L., Carstensen, L. L., & Knutson, B. (2007). Anticipation of monetary gain but not loss in healthy older adults. *Nature Neuroscience, 10,* 787–791.

Lazarus, R. S. (1984). On the primacy of cognition. *American Psychologist, 39,* 124–129.

Lerner, R. M. (Ed.). (2006). *Handbook of child psychology: Vol. I. Theoretical models of human development* (6th ed.). New York: John Wiley.

Lewin, K. (1935). *A dynamic theory of personality.* New York: McGraw-Hill.

Linville, P. W. (1985). Self-complexity and affective extremity: Don't put all your eggs in one cognitive basket. *Social Cognition, 3*, 94–120.

Magnusson, D., & Endler, N. S. (1977). *Personality at the crossroads: Current issues in interactional psychology.* Hillsdale, NJ: Erlbaum.

Magnusson, D., & Stattin, H. (2006). The person in the environment: Towards a general model for scientific inquiry. In R. M. Lerner (Ed.), *Handbook of child psychology: Vol. 1. Theoretical models of human development* (6th ed., pp. 400–464). New York: John Wiley.

Markus, H., & Kitiyama, S. (1991). Culture and the self: Implications for cognition, emotion, and motivation. *Psychological Review, 98*, 224–253.

Mather, M., Canli, T., English, T., Whitfield, S., Wais, P., Ochsner, K., et al. (2004). Amygdala responses to emotionally valenced stimuli in older and younger adults. *Psychological Science, 15*, 259–263.

Mischel, W. (1968). *Personality and assessment.* New York: John Wiley.

Mroczek, D., & Spiro, A. (2005). Change in life satisfaction during adulthood: Findings from the veterans affairs normative aging study. *Journal of Personality and Social Psychology, 88*, 189–202.

Mroczek, D. K., Spiro, A., Griffin, P. W., & Neupert, S. (2006). Social influences on adult personality, self-regulation and health. In K. W. Schaie & L. Carstensen (Eds.), *Social structures, aging and self-regulation* (pp. 69–83). New York: Springer Publishing.

Nayfeh, A. H., & Balachandran, B. (1995). *Applied nonlinear dynamics.* New York: John Wiley.

Nesselroade, J. R., & Bartsch, T. W. (1977). Multivariate perspectives on the construct validity of the trait-state distinction. In R. B. Cattell & R. M. Dreger (Eds.), *Handbook of modern personality theory* (pp. 221–238). Washington, DC: Hemisphere.

Park, D. C., Lautenschlager, G., Hedden, T., Davidson, N. S., Smith, A. D., & Smith, P. K. (2002). Models of visuospatial and verbal memory across the adult lifespan. *Psychology and Aging, 17*, 299–320.

Phelps, E. A. (2006). Emotion and cognition: Insights from studies of the human amygdala. *Annual Review of Psychology, 57*, 27–53.

Rahhal, T. A., Hasher, L., & Colcombe, S. (2001). Instructional manipulation and age differences in memory: Now you see them, now you don't. *Psychology and Aging, 16*, 697–706.

Riley, M. (1989). Forward: Why this book?. In K. W. Schaie & C. Schooler (Eds.), *Social structure and aging: Psychological processes* (pp. xiii–xv). Hillsdale, NJ: Erlbaum.

Roberts, B. W., & DelVecchio, W. F. (2000). The rank-order consistency of personality traits from childhood to old age: A quantitative review of longitudinal studies. *Psychological Bulletin, 126*, 3–25.

Roberts, B. W., Walton, K. E., & Viechtbauer, W. (2006a). Patterns of mean-level change in personality traits across the life course: A meta-analysis of longitudinal studies. *Psychological Bulletin, 132*, 3–27.

Roberts, B. W., Walton, K. E., & Viechtbauer, W. (2006b). Personality traits change in adulthood: Reply to Costa and McCrae (2006). *Psychological Bulletin, 132*, 29–32.

Rönnlund, M., Nyberg, L., Bäckman, L., & Nilsson, L. G. (2005). Stability, growth, and decline in adult life span development of declarative memory: Cross-sectional and longitudinal data from a population-based study. *Psychology and Aging, 20,* 3–18.

Sameroff, A. J., & Chandler, M. J. (1975). Reproductive risk and the continuum of caretaking casualty. In F. D. Horowitz, E. M. Hetherington, S. Scarr-Salapatek, & G. M. Siegel (Eds.), *Review of child development research* (Vol. 4, pp. 187–244). Chicago: University of Chicago Press.

Schaie, K. W. (2005). *Developmental influences on adult intelligence: The Seattle Longitudinal Study.* New York: Oxford University Press.

Schaie, K. W., Campbell, R. T., Meredith, W., & Rawlings, S. C. (1988). *Methodological issues in aging research.* New York: Springer Publishing.

Schaie, K. W., & Parham, I. A. (1976). Stability of adult personality traits: Fact or fable? *Journal of Personality and Social Psychology, 34,* 146–158.

Schindler, I., Staudinger, U., & Nesselroade, J. (2006). Development and structural dynamics of personal life investment in old age. *Psychology and Aging, 21,* 737–753.

Shoda, Y., Mischel, W., & Wright, J. C. (1994). Intra-individual stability in the organization and patterning of behavior: Incorporating psychological situations into the idiographic analysis of personality. *Journal of Personality and Social Psychology, 67,* 674–687.

Shumway, R. H., & Stoffer, D. S. (2006). *Time series analysis and its applications: With R examples* (2nd ed.). New York: Springer Publishing.

Sontag, L. W. (1971). The history of longitudinal research: Implications for the future. *Child Development, 42,* 987–1002.

Thorndike, E. L. (1906). *Principles of teaching.* New York: Seiler.

Tsai, J. L., Knutson, B., & Fung, H. H. (2006). Cultural variation in affect valuation. *Journal of Personality and Social Psychology, 90,* 288–307.

Tsai, J. L., Louie, J., Chen, E. E., & Uchida, Y. (2007). Learning what feelings to desire: Socialization of ideal affect through children's storybooks. *Personality and Social Psychology Bulletin, 33,* 17–30.

West, B. (1985). *An essay on the importance of being non-linear.* New York: Springer Verlag.

Wohlwill, J. F. (1991). Relations between method and theory in developmental research: A partial-isomorphism view. In P. van Geert & L. P. Mos (Eds.), *Annals of theoretical psychology* (Vol. 7, pp. 91–138). New York: Plenum Press.

Zajonc, R. B. (1984). On the primacy of affect. *American Psychologist, 29,* 117–123.

Zautra, A. J., Berkhof, J., & Nicolson, N. A. (2002). Changes in affect interrelations as a function of stressful events. *Cognition and Emotion, 16,* 309–318.

Those Who Have, Get: Social Structure, Environmental Complexity, Intellectual Functioning, and Self-Directed Orientations in the Elderly

6

CARMI SCHOOLER AND LESLIE J. CAPLAN

There has been a fair amount of contention about whether, as the "use it or lose it" hypothesis implies, older individuals' experience in dealing with intellectually challenging environmental demands can positively affect their intellectual performance (Schooler, 2007). In this chapter, we provide evidence that this is indeed the case, and that these environmental effects are part of a larger pattern of reciprocal effects between intellectually challenging environmental demands and psychological functioning, whose outcome tends to be that "those who have, get"—or, as the original title of this chapter stated, "them that has, gets."

The findings of our National Institute of Mental Health Section on Socioenvironmental Studies (SSES) research program on the relationship between social-structurally determined environmental conditions and psychological functioning frequently indicate that these relationships between environmental demands and psychological functioning tend to be reciprocal. Social-structurally determined environmental conditions affect individuals' psychological functioning; characteristics of individuals' psychological functioning affect their status in their society's social structure. It is the nature of these effects that leads to the title of this chapter. The nature of the reciprocal effects is generally such that with the passage of time (i.e., as people get older), those who start off well—in terms of either their social-structural position or their psychological characteristics—end up relatively even better off both in terms of status and functioning. Those who start off relatively poorly end up even worse. We (and others) have evidence that this general pattern is often the case for a variety of psychological, behavioral, mental health, physical health, and social-structural characteristics, including effective coping mechanisms (Caplan & Schooler, 2007); activities of daily living (Caplan & Schooler, 2003); and socioeconomic status, psychological distress, and health (Mulatu & Schooler, 2002). However, in the present chapter, we will concentrate on the original central concerns of our longitudinal research project: the linkage of two psychological characteristics, intellectual functioning and self-directed orientation, with the environmental characteristics of social-structural position and environmental complexity (Schooler, 1984, 1990b).[1] In the following sections, we will do the following:

1. Set the stage for what follows by presenting a working conceptualization of social structure
2. Briefly describe the SSES research program
3. Describe the reciprocal effects found between occupational self-direction and self-directed orientation and portray the processes through which the relative socioeconomic and psychological advantages that accrue to those who start out in relatively self-directed jobs and/or with relatively self-directed orientations increase over the long term
4. Do the same for occupational self-direction and intellectual flexibility
5. Show that cognitive leisure activity has similar effects on intellectual flexibility as do complex, cognitively demanding work activities
6. Do the same for household work complexity and intellectual flexibility
7. Provide direct evidence for one aspect of the "them that has, gets" view by demonstrating that income differences between individuals manifesting high and low levels of intellectual flexibility

---

[1] According to Schooler (1984, 1990b), the more diverse the stimuli, the greater the number of decisions required , the greater the number of considerations to be taken into account in making these decisions, and the more ill defined and apparently contradictory the contingencies, the more complex the environment.

or self-directed orientation at midlife, respectively, actually increase between these same individuals 20 years later

A WORKING CONCEPTUALIZATION OF SOCIAL STRUCTURE

The working conceptualization of social structure underlying the present chapter is most easily presented through a series of interlocking definitions. These definitions are adaptations of, and extrapolations from, the noted sociologist Robert Merton's (1957) general schema and are well within the mainstream of sociological thought (for an extended discussion and theoretical elaboration of this theoretical framework, see Schooler, 1994).

Status

Status is a position in a social system occupied by designated actors (i.e., individuals or social organizations) that consists of a set of roles that define the incumbents' expected patterns of interrelationships with incumbents of related statuses. Statuses may be *ranked hierarchically* in terms of the interrelated concepts of (a) prestige, (b) unequal distribution of relatively scarce social resources and unequal opportunity for acquiring them, and (c) *power*: the ability to induce others to fulfill one's goals.

When statuses are considered in terms of such a hierarchical perspective, the term *social status* is frequently used. When the emphasis is on Item (b) (i.e., the unequal distribution of resources, etc.), the term *socioeconomic status* (SES) is frequently used.

Social Class

The term *social class* is often used almost interchangeably with the term *social status*. Most sociologists who deal with stratification, however, distinguish between the two. They reserve the use of the term *social class* to reflect the types of societal divisions envisaged by Marx. Thus Kohn and Slomczynski (1990) described social classes as "groups defined in terms of their relationship to ownership and control over the *means of production*, and their control over the labor power of others" (p. 2). The definition is readily expanded to also include ownership and control over the *means of distribution*.

Social Structure

Social structure is the patterned interrelationships among a set of individual and organizational statuses, as defined by the nature of their interacting roles.

Culture

Culture is an historically determined set of denotative (what is), normative (what should be), and stylistic (how done) beliefs, shared by a group of individuals who have undergone a common historical experience and participate in an interrelated set of social structures. In a more expansive form, the definition could include the institutional, instrumental, and material embodiments of these beliefs.

Society or Sociocultural System

Society or a *sociocultural system* is a set of persons and social positions that possesses both a culture and a social structure.

THE SECTION ON SOCIOENVIRONMENTAL STUDIES LONGITUDINAL STUDY

The attempt to specify how the social-structurally determined environmental conditions of modern societies affect psychological functioning was an underlying aim of the project on the psychological effects of occupational conditions conceived by Kohn and Schooler (1969) in the early 1960s. Among the study's major goals was the test of the hypothesis that social status differences, both in individuals' cognitive functioning and in their orientations toward themselves and others, are a function of the nature and conditions of their work.

Method

Sample

The original sample of 3,101 men interviewed in 1964 was representative of all men in the United States employed in civilian occupations. In a 1974 follow-up, a representative subsample of those men ($n = 687$) then under 65 years old was reinterviewed, and their wives ($n = 555$)

and children (n = 352) were interviewed for the first time. In 1994, the SSES carried out a 20-year follow-up survey on the surviving adults interviewed in 1974. We located 95% of the 1974 sample and interviewed about 80% of those eligible (N = 706; 351 men, 355 women).

Measures of Occupational Characteristics

To delineate the exact linkages between individuals' conditions of work and their psychological characteristics, specific occupations were not compared; rather, a job was characterized by a series of dimensions. One of the most critical of these dimensions was *occupational self-direction*. High occupational self-direction is characterized by substantively complex work, low levels of routinization, and relatively loose supervision. Substantive complexity of work (i.e., work that in its very substance requires thought and independent judgment) was, both theoretically and empirically, the keystone concept in regard to occupational self-direction. Indices for the latent concept of substantive complexity were derived from detailed open- and closed-ended questions about participants' work with things, data (or ideas), and people. These questions provide the basis for seven ratings: appraisals of the complexity of each respondent's reported work with things, with data, and with people based on the *Dictionary of Occupational Titles* (U.S. Department of Labor, 1965) as well as the respondents' estimates of the amount of time they spent working at each type of activity and an overall measure of work complexity.

Measures of Psychological Characteristics

The two aspects of psychological functioning central to our present concerns are self-directed orientation and intellectual flexibility. Key to self-directed orientation is "the feeling that locus of control is and should be within oneself" (Schooler, 1972, p. 300) and "the belief that one has the personal capacity to take responsibility for one's actions and that society is so constituted as to make self-direction possible" (Kohn & Schooler, 1983, p. 146). An individual who is high in self-directed orientation is low in authoritarian conservatism and fatalism and high in personally responsible standards of morality. Such an individual holds self-direction and autonomy in high regard and places relatively low value on unthinking conformity.

Intellectual flexibility may be considered the ability to consider objects or questions from multiple perspectives. Its measures were originally assumed to reflect people's "actual intellectual functioning in a non-work situation that seemed to elicit considerable intellectual effort from nearly all the respondents" (Kohn & Schooler, 1983, p. 112). These measures included scores on the Embedded Figures test, an interviewer's rating of a respondent's intelligence, coding of responses to a question requesting arguments for and against allowing cigarette commercials on television, coding of responses to a question asking the factors to be considered in choosing the location for a hamburger stand, and number of times the respondent agreed with agree–disagree questions (see Kohn & Schooler, 1983, for more details).

Measures of Socioeconomic Status

The interview also included three items used as indicators in a measurement model of SES: educational level, family income, and occupational prestige (Hollingshead & Redlich, 1958).

Analyses

The goal of our analyses is to come to a substantively meaningful estimate of how much of a given correlation between an environmental condition and a psychological characteristic is due to (a) the effect of that environmental condition on that psychological characteristic and (b) the degree to which the psychological characteristic affects the likelihood the individual will be subjected to that environmental condition. To do so, our general analytic approach is to use reciprocal effects structural equation modeling (SEM).[2]

---

[2] We identify these nonrecursive models by estimating the reciprocal effects only "concurrently" and by not simultaneously testing for cross-lagged effects. The exclusion of these cross-lagged effects provides instruments to identify the model. This approach follows that of Kohn and Schooler (1983, chap. 6) and Schooler, Mulatu, and Oates (1999; for general discussions, see Heise, 1975, and Kohn & Slomczynski, 1990). For a recent example using this general approach on another body of data to examine the reciprocal effects of occupational self-direction and intellectual functioning, see Hauser and Roan (2007). The consequence of this modeling procedure is that for each pair of variables involved in a reciprocal relationship, the observed concurrent effect of one variable on the other is actually the sum of the true contemporaneous effect and the omitted cross-lagged effect. Thus, when we test a model that only examines "concurrent" effects, without modeling lagged effects, we can reasonably assume that the effects we find significant are real, although we cannot assess how much of the effect is actually contemporaneous and how much is actually lagged. What is certain is that any significant reciprocal paths between our measures of the complexity of paid work and cognitive functioning represent the *total* effect of each type of measure on the other over the two time periods.

OCCUPATIONAL SELF-DIRECTION AND SELF-DIRECTED ORIENTATION

Our analyses of the interrelationships between occupational self-direction and self-directed orientation (Schooler, Mulatu, & Oates, 2004) are based on those individuals in our sample who were working for pay in both 1974 and 1994 ($n = 244$).[3] In this reciprocal effects SEM analysis, occupational self-direction was allowed to affect self-directed orientation, and vice versa. Both 1974 characteristics were positively correlated with SES 1974 (for occupational self-direction, $r = .83$, $p < .001$; for self-directed orientation, $r = .68$, $p < .001$).

Both occupational self-direction and self-directed orientation were modeled as second-order factors. The model of self-directed orientation included three first-order latent factors: authoritarian conservatism, personally responsible morality, and fatalism (see Table 6.1). The model for occupational self-direction also included three first-order latent factors: substantive complexity, closeness of supervision, and routinization of work (see Table 6.2). Figure 6.1 presents the loadings of these first-order factors on their respective second-order factors (Schooler et al., 2004). It also presents the results of a model evaluating the reciprocal effects between occupational self-direction and self-directed orientation. The model was a multigroup model, in which the two groups were defined by a median split on age (younger group = 41–57 years; older group = 58–83 years).

The results demonstrate the existence of at least moderate-sized positive reciprocal effects between occupational self-direction and self-directed orientation: high degrees of one lead to high degrees of the other (see Figure 6.1). There is no significant difference between older and younger groups in the magnitude of these effects. These results provide further support for the hypothesis that cognitively demanding complex environments increase the value an individual places on self-direction and autonomy (Schooler, 1990a). In turn, those values affect the complexity of one's environment. The finding that there is no reliable difference between the older and younger segments of our sample in the magnitude of the reciprocal effects provides support for the hypothesis that the magnitude of these psychological effects

---

[3] The results described in this section are taken in somewhat modified form from Schooler, Mulatu, and Oates (2004).

Table 6.1

STANDARDIZED LOADINGS OF THE INDICATORS OF FIRST-ORDER LATENT VARIABLES FROM A SECOND-ORDER MODEL OF SELF-DIRECTED ORIENTATION: AUTHORITARIAN CONSERVATISM, PERSONALLY RESPONSIBLE MORALITY, AND FATALISM

	1974	1994–1995
Authoritarian conservativism		
The most important thing to teach children is obedience to parents	.75*	.68*
Young people shouldn't be allowed to read books likely to confuse them	.56*	.50*
In this complicated world, the only way to know what to do is rely on leaders	.63**	.47**
No decent man can respect a woman who has had premarital sex	.64**	.56**
Any good leader should be strict with people under him to gain their respect	.57**	.50**
Personally responsible morality		
It is all right to do anything you want if you stay out of trouble	–.69**	–.61**
If something works, it doesn't matter whether it is right or wrong	–.59**	–.48**
It is OK to go around the law as long as you don't break it	–.48**	–.43**
It is all right to do whatever the law allows	–.23**	–.28**
Fatalism		
Never faults self when things go wrong	.54**	.57**
Hardly blames self for one's own problems	.76**	.59**
Things that happen are out of personal control	.73**	.65**

Note: From "Effects of Occupational Self-Direction on the Intellectual Functioning and Self-Directed Orientations of Older Workers: Findings and Implications for Individuals and Societies," by C. Schooler, M. S. Mulatu, and G. Oates, 2004, *American Journal of Sociology, 110*, p. 181.
$*p < .05; **p < .01.$

Table 6.2

STANDARDIZED LOADINGS OF THE INDICATORS OF FIRST-ORDER LATENT VARIABLES FROM A SECOND-ORDER MODEL OF OCCUPATIONAL SELF-DIRECTION: SUBSTANTIVE COMPLEXITY, CLOSENESS OF SUPERVISION, AND ROUTINIZATION OF WORK

	1974	1994–1995
Substantive Complexity		
1. Complexity of work with data	.68**	.77**
2. Complexity of work with people	.60**	.60**
3. Hours of work with data	.43**	.26**
4. Hours of work with people	.37**	.25**
5. Overall complexity of work	.72**	.74**
Closeness of supervision		
1. Freedom to disagree with supervisor	−.67**	−.75**
2. Self-rated assessment of the closeness of supervision	.78**	.76**
3. Supervisor tells respondent what to do	.77**	.75**
4. Importance of doing what one is told	.89**	.91**
Routinization of work		
1. Routineness of work	1.00	1.00

Note. From "Effects of Occupational Self-Direction on the Intellectual Functioning and Self-Directed Orientations of Older Workers: Findings and Implications for Individuals and Societies," by C. Schooler, M. S. Mulatu, and G. Oates, 2004, *American Journal of Sociology,* 110, p. 178.
**$p < .01$.

of work, which generalize well beyond the workplace, are unaffected by age.

These results are relevant to our original hypothesis: that social status differences, both in individuals' cognitive functioning and in their orientations toward themselves and others, are a function of the nature and conditions of their work. Those in higher social status positions and

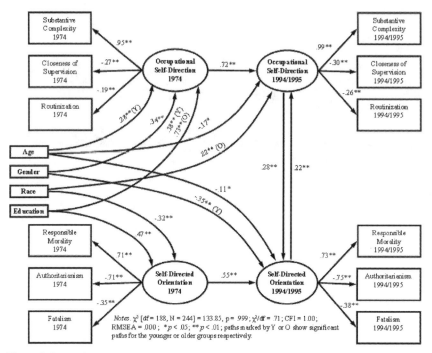

Figure 6.1 Multigroup reciprocal effects model of occupational self-direction and self-directed orientation.

From "Effects of Occupational Self-Direction on the Intellectual Functioning and Self-Directed Orientations of Older Workers: Findings and Implications for Individuals and Societies," by C. Schooler, M. S. Mulatu, and G. Oates, 2004, *American Journal of Sociology, 110,* p. 185.

from relatively higher social status backgrounds tend to have higher levels of self-directed orientations. Our findings suggest the existence of a loop: Having such self-directed orientations, in turn, contributes to the likelihood that people will obtain relatively high-status, self-directed jobs (Kohn & Schooler, 1983). This outcome provides clear support for Stinchcombe's (1990) view that "skills acquired by workers . . . on the job are often a function of unequal opportunities flowing to these workers because of their race and social class" (p. 357). Thus, through the perpetuation of this loop throughout their careers, people who early in life hold jobs likely to be linked to having self-directed orientations (e.g., high-status jobs) are likely to have careers leading to jobs with increasingly higher social status and income. On the other hand, people who early in life hold jobs linked to having non-self-directed orientations (e.g., low-status jobs) are likely to have careers leading to jobs with lower and lower social status and less and less income.

OCCUPATIONAL SELF-DIRECTION AND INTELLECTUAL FLEXIBILITY

We have similarly investigated the reciprocal effects between occupational self-direction and intellectual flexibility (Schooler et al., 2004), again relying on data from those individuals who worked in both 1974 and 1994.[4] SES 1974 is again highly correlated with the psychological variable in 1974 (for intellectual flexibility, $r = .76$, $p < .001$). Figure 6.2 shows the loadings of the indices of our latent intellectual flexibility factor; it also shows that intellectual flexibility correlates highly ($r = .87$) with a latent factor (standard cognitive functioning) based on more standard psychometric measures of cognitive/intellectual functioning.

Like the preceding model, this model was a multigroup model, in which the two groups were defined by a median split on age. The results indicated once again that there are significant reciprocal effects between environmental and psychological variables: occupational self-

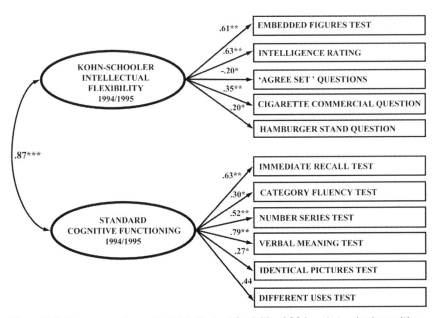

Figure 6.2 Measurement model of intellectual flexibility 1994 and standard cognitive functioning.

---

[4] The findings described in this section are also taken from Schooler, Mulatu, and Oates (2004).

direction and intellectual flexibility have positive effects on one another (see Figure 6.3). Since there is no significant difference between the effects of occupational self-direction on our older compared to our younger respondents, the findings indicate that within the age range of our sample (41–83 years), the effects of occupational self-direction on intellectual flexibility are at least as strong for older as for younger adults. Indeed, earlier findings about the greater effects of substantively complex work on intellectual functioning in older and younger adults (Schooler, Mulatu, & Oates, 1999) suggest that, if anything, the intellectual functioning of older adults may be more positively affected by cognitively demanding environmental conditions than is that of younger adults.

In terms of career trajectories, the positive reciprocal relationship between occupational self-direction and intellectual flexibility, like the similar relationship between occupational self-direction and self-directed orientation, means that those who start their careers with

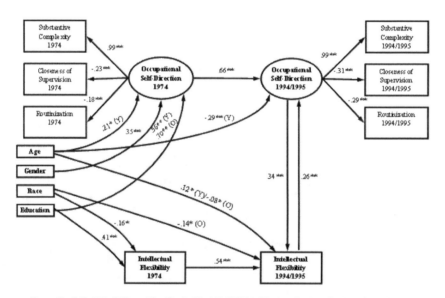

Notes. χ² [df = 83, N = 244] = 75.83, p = .699; χ/df = .91; CFI = 1.00; RMSEA = .000 ; *p < .05; **p < .01; paths marked by Y or O show significant paths for the younger or older groups respectively.

Figure 6.3 Multigroup reciprocal effects model of occupational self-direction and intellectual flexibility.

From "Effects of Occupational Self-Direction on the Intellectual Functioning and Self-Directed Orientations of Older Workers: Findings and Implications for Individuals and Societies," by C. Schooler, M. S. Mulatu, and G. Oates, 2004, *American Journal of Sociology, 110*, p. 187.

relatively low levels of intellectual functioning are doubly disadvantaged: In general, the cognitive effects of their jobs tend to decrease their cognitive functioning even further. Lower social status workers are particularly likely to be caught in a negative loop. The relatively low-status, non-self-directed jobs that they are likely to get, in part because of their relatively low levels of cognitive functioning (Farkas, England, Vicknair, & Kilbourne, 1997), are likely to lead to yet lower levels of intellectual functioning, which in turn further decrease the likelihood of their obtaining higher status jobs, thus leading to a downward career spiral. The reverse is true for those who start out functioning relatively well intellectually—their work careers are relatively more likely to spiral upward.

More generally, being in a self-directed job fosters both intellectual functioning and self-directed orientations (both of which lead to more self-directed, generally higher status, better paying jobs). Consequently, preexisting socioeconomic differences are intensified. This intensification occurs to the extent that workers are selected (or self-select) for self-directed jobs on the basis of intellectual functioning, self-directed values, or social characteristics (such as social status) linked to these psychological characteristics.

THE RECIPROCAL EFFECTS BETWEEN COGNITIVE LEISURE ACTIVITY AND INTELLECTUAL FLEXIBILITY AND THEIR SOCIOECONOMIC AND PSYCHOLOGICAL CONSEQUENCES

A potential difficulty of the two analyses discussed previously is that they include only respondents who were working for pay.[5] In an attempt to investigate reciprocal effects between intellectual functioning and cognitive environmental demands for more of our respondents, we investigated an alternative environmental condition—the cognitive demandingness of leisure time activities—using the same data set (Schooler & Mulatu, 2001). In this sample ($N = 635$), SES 1974 was highly correlated with the cognitive demandingness of 1974 leisure time activities ($r = .78, p < .001$).

---

[5] The results described in this section are based on those of Schooler and Mulatu (2001).

We constructed a reciprocal effects model conceptually similar to those described previously, this time involving the complexity of leisure time activities and intellectual flexibility. This model was also a multigroup model; however, this time, the two groups consisted of individuals who were working for pay and those who were not. Figure 6.4 shows the indices of our latent factor assessing the cognitive demands of the individuals' leisure time activities and their loadings on that factor. As before, we obtained significant positive reciprocal effects between intellectual flexibility and cognitive leisure activity (see Figure 6.5). We also obtained a significant positive path from SES to intellectual flexibility among both those working and those not working. These reciprocal effects occur even when the effects of health, exercise, and work status are controlled. Thus, in a reciprocal relationship analogous to that found for substantively complex work and intellectual functioning, carrying out cognitively demanding leisure time activities raises the level of intellectual functioning; in turn, higher levels of intellectual functioning lead to more cognitively demanding leisure time activities. The pattern of findings indicates not only that intellectual flexibility leads to an increase in cognitive leisure activity, but also that SES directly affects intellectual flexibility. Therefore high SES indirectly increases the likelihood that individuals will engage in more cognitive leisure activity and, in doing so, also increases the likelihood their level of intellectual functioning will be further increased. As we have previously seen, there are also reciprocal paths between intellectual functioning and self-directed, generally higher

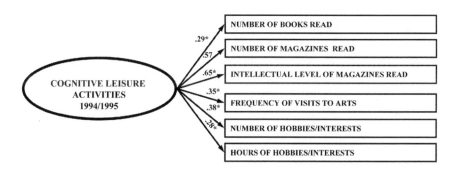

* p < .001

Figure 6.4 Measurement model of cognitive leisure time activities.

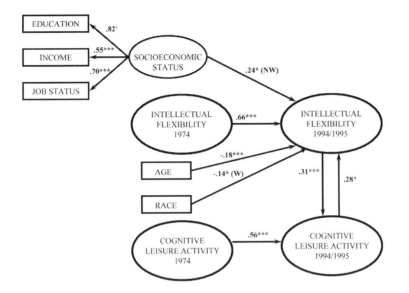

Paths with W indicate that the parameters were estimated to be significant for the working group only; paths with NW indicate that the parameters were estimated for the nonworking group only. χ^2 (612, N = 635) = 938.10, p < .001; RMSEA = .04, CFI = .93. † = reference value whose p-value cannot be computed; * p < .05, *** p < .001

Figure 6.5 Longitudinal (1974–1994/1995) reciprocal effects model of cognitive leisure activity and intellectual flexibility for working and nonworking participants.

From "The Reciprocal Effects of Leisure Time Activities and Intellectual Functioning in Older People: A Longitudinal Analysis," by C. Schooler, and M. S. Mulatu, 2001, *Psychology and Aging, 16*, p. 473.

status paid work. Thus the pattern of interrelationships among cognitive leisure time activities, intellectual functioning, and self-directed and higher status work indicates that carrying out complex leisure time activities is yet another mechanism that leads to increased differentiation across the life course between those who start out relatively privileged and those who do not.

THE RECIPROCAL EFFECTS BETWEEN HOUSEHOLD WORK COMPLEXITY AND INTELLECTUAL FLEXIBILITY AND THEIR SOCIOECONOMIC AND PSYCHOLOGICAL CONSEQUENCES

In this analysis, we investigated another nonoccupational source of environmental complexity and cognitive demand: the nature of household work.[6] To test for the psychological effects of household work complexity, we developed models of household work complexity conceptually similar to those that we developed for paid work and leisure time activities. Given known gender differences between men's and women's work in the home, we used different indicators for men and women when developing measurement models (see Figures 6.6 and 6.7), and separate SEM models were constructed for men and for women. Our analyses indicated that doing complex household work had a positive effect on the intellectual functioning of both men and women. The reciprocal path, from intellectual flexibility to household work complexity, was marginally significant for women ($.05 < p < .10$; see Figure 6.8) and clearly not significant for men. In addition, for women, status indicators (1974 education and occupational prestige) were related to intellectual functioning, although not to complexity of household work. Nevertheless, we still have tentative evidence of the loop of reciprocal effects between the psychological variable intellectual flexibility (itself affected by social sta-

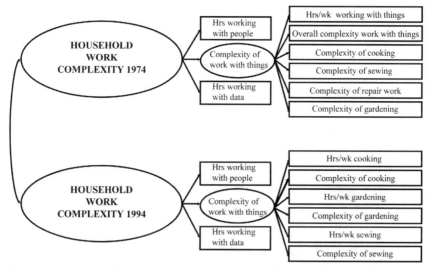

Figure 6.6 Measurement model of household work complexity for women.

Based on "Household Work Complexity, Intellectual Functioning, and Self-Esteem in Men and Women," by L. J. Caplan and C. Schooler, 2006, *Journal of Marriage and Family, 68.*

---

[6] The results described here are based on the work of Caplan and Schooler (2006).

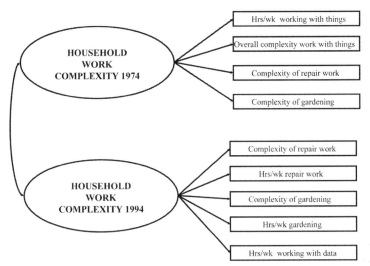

Figure 6.7 Measurement model of household work complexity for men.

Based on "Household Work Complexity, Intellectual Functioning, and Self-Esteem in Men and Women," by L. J. Caplan and C. Schooler, 2006, *Journal of Marriage and Family,* 68.

tus) and household work complexity. Thus women who are at an initial intellectual advantage would see this advantage increase over time due to their performance of relatively complex household work. However, we have no clear evidence that this is the case for men.

SPIRALING SOCIOECONOMIC EFFECTS OF INITIAL PSYCHOLOGICAL DIFFERENCES

All the evidence discussed until this point makes a strong theoretical case for the proposition that initial differences in SES between the psychologically advantaged (e.g., those people with relatively high levels of intellectual functioning or self-directed values) and disadvantaged (e.g., those people with relatively low levels of intellectual functioning or self-directed values) should increase over time. To test this hypothesis, we conducted two new sets of analyses.

In the first set, we used median splits to divide our sample into two halves, on the basis of either 1974 intellectual flexibility or 1974 self-directed orientation. We then conducted two analyses of vari-

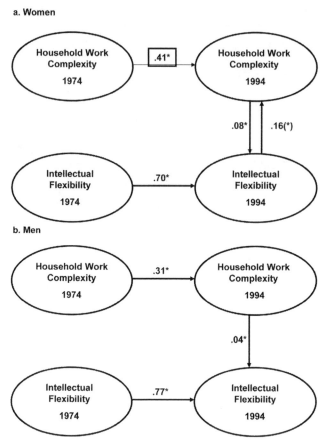

Figure 6.8 Longitudinal (1974–1994/1995) reciprocal effects model of household work complexity and intellectual flexibility for women and men.

From "Household Work Complexity, Intellectual Functioning, and Self-Esteem in Men and Women," by L. J. Caplan and C. Schooler, 2006, *Journal of Marriage and Family, 68,* p. 893.

ance to compare family incomes in 1974 to family incomes in 1994 (in estimated 1974 dollars), using logarithmic transformations of family income to normalize the distributions. In each analysis, time (1974, 1994) was the within-subject variable, and the psychological characteristic (either 1974 intellectual flexibility or 1974 self-directed orientation) was the between-subject variable. The interactions between time and each of the 1974 psychological characteristics were significant: Although income generally decreased over time throughout the sample, the decrease was less for individuals who were either initially high in intellectual flexibility, $F(1, 638) = 38.66$, $p < .001$, or high in self-directed orientation, $F(1, 638) = 9.65$, $p < .01$ (see Figures 6.9 and 6.10).

In the second set of analyses, we used a different measure of SES. We created a latent variable, 1994 financial status, whose indicators were family income, total assets, and whether the individual owned his or her own home. We calculated a 1994 financial status factor score for each individual. We then used analysis of covariance to examine the effects of 1974 intellectual flexibility (based on median split) on 1994 financial status, while controlling for 1974 family income. Individuals who had been higher in intellectual flexibility in 1974 had higher financial status 20 years later than those who had been lower in intellectual flexibility, $F(1, 675) = 76.71$, $p < .01$ (see Table 6.3a). We also conducted a parallel analysis, comparing the 1994 financial status of people who were either high or low in 1974 self-directed orientation (based on median split), again controlling for family income in 1974. As in the intellectual flexibility results, individuals who had been

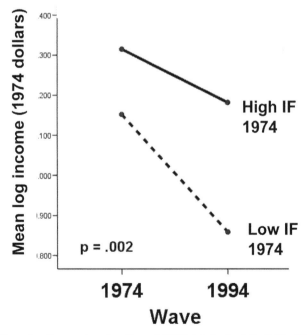

Figure 6.9 Mean log (income) as function of 1974 intellectual flexibility (IF).

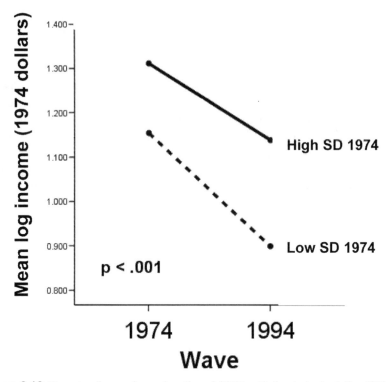

Figure 6.10 Mean log (income) as a function of 1974 self-directed orientation (SD).

higher in self-directed orientation in 1974 had higher financial status in 1994 than those who had been lower in self-directed orientation, $F(1, 675) = 27.62$, $p < .01$ (see Table 6.3b). These spiraling effects of initial psychological advantage, as demonstrated by the increasing over-time financial advantage of people with higher initial levels of intellectual flexibility or self-directed orientation, provide strong empirical support for the theoretically based proposal that the reciprocal effects between psychological advantages and status-based advantages lead to increasing disparities over time.

CONCLUSIONS

Much of the literature on the effects of SES leads to the hypothesis that SES is part of a web of interconnected sociological and psychological phenomena. Our results lend support to this hypothesis: They

Table 6.3A

MEAN FINANCIAL STATUS 1994 FACTOR SCORES AS A FUNCTION OF 1974 INTELLECTUAL FLEXIBILITY AND SELF-DIRECTEDNESS OF ORIENTATION (NET OF 1974 FAMILY INCOME): INTELLECTUAL FLEXIBILITY

	HIGH INTELLECTUAL FLEXIBILITY 1974	LOW INTELLECTUAL FLEXIBILITY 1974	DIFFERENCE
1994 financial status	.810	–.765	1.575**

**p < .01.

Table 6.3B

MEAN FINANCIAL STATUS 1994 FACTOR SCORES AS A FUNCTION OF 1974 INTELLECTUAL FLEXIBILITY AND SELF-DIRECTEDNESS OF ORIENTATION (NET OF 1974 FAMILY INCOME): SELF-DIRECTEDNESS OF ORIENTATION

	HIGH SELF-DIRECTION 1974	LOW SELF-DIRECTION 1974	DIFFERENCE
1994 financial status	.506	–.469	.975**

**p < .01.

reveal that over a lifetime, the continuous occurrence of reciprocal effects between intellectually challenging environmental demands and psychological functioning can lead to greater disparities between the "haves" and "have-nots." They demonstrate that early psychological advantages lead to later socioeconomic advantage; conversely, their pattern strongly suggests that early socioeconomic advantages lead to later psychological advantages.

In more general terms, we have examined the causal interrelationships among phenomena at the social-structural and psychological levels. Our examination has focused on how these interrelationships affect the cognitive complexity of people's environments and, by doing so, predict disparities in well-being over the life course. We believe that in focusing on these reciprocal effects between social-structurally influenced environmental conditions and psychological functioning in later stages of the life course, our chapter exemplifies the principles that have guided the Penn State Conference Program on Social Structures and Aging over the last 20 years.

REFERENCES

Caplan, L. J., & Schooler, C. (2003). The roles of fatalism, self confidence and intellectual resources in the disablement process in older adults. *Psychology and Aging, 18,* 551–561.

Caplan, L. J., & Schooler, C. (2006). Household work complexity, intellectual functioning, and self-esteem in men and women. *Journal of Marriage and Family, 68,* 883–900.

Caplan, L. J., & Schooler, C. (2007). Socioeconomic status and financial coping strategies: The mediating role of perceived control. *Social Psychology Quarterly, 70,* 63–78.

Farkas, G., England, P., Vicknair, K., & Kilbourne, B. S. (1997). Cognitive skill, skill demands of jobs, and earnings among young European American, African American, and Mexican American workers. *Social Forces, 74,* 913–938.

Hauser, R., & Roan, C. (2007). *Work complexity and cognitive functioning at midlife: Cross-validating the Kohn–Schooler hypothesis.* Paper presented at the annual meeting of the American Sociological Association, New York.

Heise, D. R. (1975). *Causal analysis.* New York: John Wiley.

Hollingshead, A., & Redlich, F. C. (1958). *Social class and mental illness: A community study.* New York: John Wiley.

Kohn, M. L., & Schooler, C. (1969). Class, occupation, and orientation. *American Sociological Review, 34,* 659–678.

Kohn, M. L., & Schooler, C. (1983). *Work and personality: An inquiry into the impact of social stratification.* Norwood, NJ: Ablex.

Kohn, M. L., & Slomczynski, K. M. (1990). *Social structure and self-direction: A comparative analysis of the United States and Poland.* Oxford, England: Basil Blackwell.

Merton, R. K. (1957). *Social theory and social structure.* New York: Free Press.

Mulatu, M. S., & Schooler, C. (2002). Causal connections between SES and health: Reciprocal effects and mediating mechanisms. *Journal of Health and Social Behavior, 43,* 22–41.

Schooler, C. (1972). Social antecedents of adult psychological functioning. *American Journal of Sociology, 78,* 299–322.

Schooler, C. (1984). Psychological effects of complex environments during the life span: A review and theory. *Intelligence, 8,* 259–281.

Schooler, C. (1990a). Individualism and the historical and social-structural determinants of people's concerns over self-directedness and efficacy. In J. Rodin, C. Schooler, & K. W. Schaie (Eds.), *Self-directedness: Cause and effects throughout the life course* (pp. 19–49). Hillsdale, NJ: Erlbaum.

Schooler, C. (1990b). Psychosocial factors and effective cognitive functioning through the life span. In J. E. Birren & K. W. Schaie (Eds.), *Handbook of the psychology of aging* (pp. 347–358). Orlando, FL: Academic Press.

Schooler, C. (1994). A working conceptualization of social structure: Mertonian roots and psychological and sociocultural relationships. *Social Psychology Quarterly, 57,* 262–273.

Schooler, C. (2007). Use it—and keep it, longer, probably: A reply to Salthouse (2006). *Perspectives on Psychological Science, 2,* 24–29.

Schooler, C., & Mulatu, M. S. (2001). The reciprocal effects of leisure time activities and intellectual functioning in older people: A longitudinal analysis. *Psychology and Aging, 16,* 466–482.

Schooler, C., Mulatu, M. S., & Oates, G. (1999). The continuing effects of substantively complex work on the intellectual functioning of older workers. *Psychology and Aging, 14,* 483–506.

Schooler, C., Mulatu, M. S., & Oates, G. (2004). Effects of occupational self-direction on the intellectual functioning and self-directed orientations of older workers: Findings and implications for individuals and societies. *American Journal of Sociology, 110,* 161–197.

Stinchcombe, A. L. (1990). *Information and organizations.* Berkeley: University of California Press.

U.S. Department of Labor. (1965). *Dictionary of occupational titles.* Washington, DC: U.S. Government Printing Office.

Commentary: Personality, Emotion, and Cognition

FREDDA BLANCHARD-FIELDS

There is a substantial literature on cognitive changes that take place with advancing age. Historically, cognitive processes were typically studied separately from both emotional processes and personality characteristics. In this sense, they were largely viewed as logically distinct areas of research. This is not surprising given that in the past, cognitive research, especially in aging research, was largely seen as of primary importance. The dominance of cognitive aging research in isolation of emotion and personality is evidenced by past research concerned with the possibility that cognitive performance may be confounded by age differences in arousal or affect (e.g., a concern with performance-inhibiting emotional states such as test anxiety), as opposed to reflecting a function of age changes in basic cognitive processes (see Botwinick, 1984; Kausler, 1990). The classic studies by Eisdorfer and colleagues (see, e.g., Eisdorfer, 1968) argued, for example, that age differences in paired associate learning could be an artifact of overarousal of older persons in test situations. In these studies, the primary questions about cognition and emotion were being asked by researchers primarily interested in age-related changes in basic cognitive processes. Emotion and personality tended to be treated as completely separate (although equal) domains of psychological construct, each studied by aging researcher experts in the respective areas. From the point of view of gerontologists interested in cognitive processes, emotional and personality constructs were really little more than nuisance factors to be controlled to better assess age changes in cognition.

Thus there is a mainstay of aging research in each of these three domains. For example, historically, emotion research reflected such areas as the degree to which emotional intensity dampened with increasing age (Diener, Sandvik, & Larsen, 1985), age differences in the subjective experience of emotions (Levenson, Carstensen, Friesen, & Ekman 1991), or changes in autonomic arousal in conjunction with emotional experience (Levenson et al., 1991). Personality researchers were primarily interested in charting the developmental trajectory of personality in terms of stability or change (e.g., McCrea & Costa, 1994). More recently, socioemotional selectivity theory came into the forefront; however, the initial focus was more prominently on motivational shifts in time perspective and the resulting press toward emotionally gratifying social relationships in older adulthood (Carstensen, 1998). Finally, evidence of treating these constructs as separate but equal is highlighted in the examination of their separate developmental trajectories. Thus, although there is a wealth of evidence showing cognitive decline with advancing age, emotion shows a positive developmental trajectory; in other words, emotion appears to be spared from the age-related decline most evident in the cognitive aging literature (Carstensen, Pasupathi, Mayr, & Nesselroade, 2000; Charles & Carstensen, 2004; Kunzmann & Grühn, 2005). It is only recently that the interface between emotion and cognition has become of great interest to aging researchers.

Around the same time, cognitive psychologists began to openly question whether emotion can be separated from cognition, either theoretically or empirically (Bower, 1991; Clore, Schwarz, & Conway, 1994; Forgas, 1995). Rather than argue about issues such as whether emotional responses can be formed without cognition, or whether emotions require prior cognitive appraisal, researchers have focused on the interactions between emotional states and cognitive processes. Today, aging researchers have also stressed the reciprocal relationship between emotion and cognition in the laboratory and in everyday life (see Carstensen, Mikels, & Mather, 2006, for a review). As eloquently stated by Ram, Morelli, Lindberg, and Carstensen (this volume), "the debate has shifted from a view of emotion and cognition as independent and stable processes to one about the mechanisms, reasons, and parameters for the dynamic interaction of socioemotional and cognitive processes" (p. 123). The same can be said about personality processes. Research on personality and cognition has moved from separate but equal nonoverlapping domains to examining the reciprocal interface between the two (Sliwinski, Smyth, Hofer, & Stawski, 2006). This is nicely illustrated by Schooler and Caplan (this volume), for example, in their analysis of the reciprocal relationships between intellectual flexibility and self-directed orientation.

Similar to the Ram et al. and Schooler and Caplan chapters, the remaining discussion will focus on views that cognition, personality, and emotion are reciprocally related in a complex manner that varies widely across individuals and situations. Emotional states and personality characteristics influence cognitive processes (i.e., memory, decision making, social judgments, learning), but cognitions also influence emotions and the manifestation of personality (i.e., mood induction, cognitive appraisal).

EMOTION AND COGNITION

The adult development and aging literature has grown considerably in the past 7 years in its focus on the changing nature of emotion–cognition relationships with advancing age. The importance of this area has manifested itself in rapidly increasing research and theories on the interplay of cognition and emotion from an adult developmental perspective (e.g., socioemotional selectivity theory, dynamic integration theory); an increase in handbook and overview chapters (e.g., Birren & Schaie, 2006); and increases in grant proposals, scientific presentations, and recent publications such as the special section on cognition and emotion in *Psychology and Aging* (Blanchard-Fields, 2005). Emotion is no longer thought of exclusively as a confounding variable; it now commands attention in the cognitive aging and neuroscience literature.

The chapter by Ram and colleagues nicely outlines some of the major theoretical frameworks that have emerged from the recent focus on adult development and the reciprocal relationship between emotional and cognitive processes. The primary question asked is how shifts in goals and motivations change the way older adults process information. For example, as stated in the Ram et al. chapter, socioemotional selectivity theory (SST) has recently stepped up to the plate by explicitly developing a theoretical stance on the changing relationship between emotion and cognition in older adulthood (Carstensen & Mikels, 2005). Carstensen and colleagues (2006) posit a positivity effect in which older adults show a processing priority for positive information over negative information, leading, for example, to an accurate recall of positive information. This preference is linked to changing temporal horizons, with increasing age motivating the older adults to selectively focus on positive information when processing materials in their environments. What is of particular importance in the Ram et al. chapter is that they show that these socioemotional goals dynamically influence cognitive processes. On one hand, the socioemotional context changes for older adults (shifting temporal horizons) and selectively influences cognitive processes. However, it is also important to consider the reciprocity of this relationship. Thus the dynamic integration theory of affect and cognition (Labouvie-Vief, 2003) demonstrates how existing cognitive resources in older adults influence emotional experience and expression. As indicated in the Ram et al. chapter, the quality of cognitive resources available is critical for complex affective processing and regulation. By embracing both of these theoretical perspectives, the reciprocal interaction between emotion and cognition is nicely illustrated.

PERSONALITY AND COGNITION

Such a reciprocal interaction is aptly demonstrated in the Schooler and Caplan chapter examining cognitively complex environments and intellectual functioning. For example, among many interacting relationships, these authors explicitly demonstrate the reciprocal interaction between phenomena such as the degree to which cognitive demands in leisure time activities influence intellectual functioning and how levels of intellectual functioning lead to more or less cognitively demanding leisure time activities. Placing this relationship into an adult developmental context, they find that the importance of this reciprocal relationship may even be greater for older adults. They conclude that this interactive relationship can have a spiraling effect in that initial differences in status, whether socioecomonic or level of intellectual functioning, may create an increasing disparity between the advantaged and disadvantaged. In other words, early psychological advantages lead to later socioeconomic advantages, and conversely, early socioeconomic disadvantages lead to later psychological disadvantages. Thus, in contrast to the literature on emotion and cognition relationships, Schooler and Caplan reveal a negative by-product of personality–cognition interactions: the problem of a disadvantaged start. This leads to important considerations regarding when personality and emotion interactions with cognition provide a facilitative effect and when they produce a maladaptive effect.

ADAPTIVE VALUE OF AGE-RELATED CHANGES IN EMOTION, PERSONALITY, AND COGNITION RELATIONSHIPS

In each of these chapters, it is of critical importance to address the question of how these approaches inform adaptive functioning in the older adult. Let us take the case of emotion–cognition relationships. Focusing on the positive may operate in service of heightening emotional well-being in older adulthood and facilitate the integrity of close relationships, whereas avoiding negative information may have the adaptive effect of reducing one's exposure to negative experiences. More specifically, overarousal and fragmentation in experiencing negative emotions can be particularly detrimental to older adults, who have lower tolerance for high negative arousal levels (Consedine, Magai, & Bonanno, 2002). However, processing and attending to pertinent negative material may be essential to making decisions (Rozin & Royzman, 2001). Overall, it appears that personality and emotions facilitate cognition when they create a supportive context, and they create impediments when they create arousal and interference.

Empirical evidence supports this viewpoint. In the context of processing emotions, the distinctiveness of emotions has been shown to reduce false memories in older adults (Kensinger & Corkin, 2004; May, Rahhal, Berry, & Leighton, 2005), enhance recall and the processing of complex material (Carstensen & Mikels, 2005; Carstensen et al., 2006), and highlight important information to attend to when making decisions (Löckenhoff & Carstensen, 2004). By focusing on the positive to the exclusion of the negative, older adults may be able to create a positive and nontoxic environment that will not strain their limited cognitive as well as physiological resources.

Empirical evidence also demonstrates when emotions impede information processing. For example, processing in older adults is at a disadvantage when cognitive tasks place high demands on executive control processes (Mather & Knight, 2005; Wurm, Labouvie-Vief, Aycock, Rebucal, & Koch, 2004) and create situations of high arousal (Kensinger & Corkin, 2004; Wurm et al., 2004). Cognitive functioning is adversely affected in decision making when older adults focus only on positive information. In this case, their decision making can lead them to overlook important criteria for making a quality decision (Löckenhoff & Carstensen, 2004). Overall, it will be important to understand under what conditions it is important for older adults to attend to negative stimuli; in other words, when is deploying attention to positive information and diverting it away from negative information more adaptive, and when is it maladaptive?

Drawing from the Schooler and Caplan chapter, the problem of a disadvantaged start and its vicious cycle in the reciprocal relationship between, for example, cognitively complex environments and intellectual functioning generates a number of questions related to the adaptive functioning of older adults. Can we tailor activities to provide for a more facilitating complex context to promote older adult functioning to preempt the increasing disparity between the advantaged and disadvantaged? Do complex environments have different meanings for older adults with differing personality characteristics such as those who are high versus low in neuroticism or high versus low in extraversion? Overall, Schooler and Caplan have elegantly demonstrated the reciprocal relationship between social structure variables and various aspects of functioning. The next step is to translate this research into intervention applications that perturbate malfunctioning reciprocal relationships such as those found in the disadvantaged start.

CHALLENGES AND FUTURE DIRECTIONS

Placing behavior in a social, emotional, and biological context has broadened the investigation of adult developmental theories from a narrow focus on unidimensional mechanisms to the consideration of multiple determinants of behavioral change. For example, changes in processing of information are not simply a function of biological decline, but instead are also influenced by social context, personality, motivation, and emotions, among others. As a result, we can observe a proliferation of research examining the nature of the emotion–cognition and personality–cognition interfaces in the aging mind.

As methodologies for time sampling are becoming more accessible and reliable, the interactions between emotion and personality and cognition can be more explicitly examined in and generalized to an everyday life context. Furthermore, it will be necessary to address the long-term consequences to truly assess its adaptive value. In conjunction with these approaches, advances in statistical procedure analyzing intraindividual variability and the coupling of psychological constructs will allow for an on-line assessment of the coupling between emotion and/or personality and cognition. Finally, as indicated in the Ram et al. chapter, current advances in neuroscientific methods will allow us to explore how these interactions are reflected in structural and functional changes in the brain.

CONCLUSIONS

Overall, the chapters by Ram and colleagues and Schooler and Caplan have reinforced the importance of examining personality and emotion as they interact with cognition. The proliferation of new and more advanced methods and technologies is providing important tools to examine and advance the research in these areas. However, it is also important not to lose sight of the adaptive significance of the interplay between emotion, personality, and cognition. For example, age-related motivational shifts in goal orientations and processing preferences have strong implications for designing effective environments for older adults. For example, the fact that older adults have less difficulty processing emotional information, while at the same time, they focus less on negative information, needs to be taken into consideration when designing learning materials, instructional materials, medical information, and so on. Evidence suggests that facilitative social contexts promote optimal functioning on the part of older adults. The groundbreaking findings related to health interventions influencing cognition suggest that promoting a healthy lifestyle can facilitate adaptive functioning in the elderly. The search for aspects of the aging process that have adaptive value for developing adults may be advanced with more studies examining the interface between cognition, personality, and emotion.

REFERENCES

Birren, J. E., & Schaie, K. W. (Eds.). (2006). *Handbook of the psychology of aging* (6th ed.). San Diego, CA: Elsevier.

Blanchard-Fields, F. (2005). Introduction to the Special Section on Emotion—Cognition interactions and the aging mind. *Psychology and Aging, 20,* 539–541.

Botwinick, J. (1984). *Aging and behavior.* New York: Springer Publishing.

Bower, G. H. (1991). Mood congruity of social judgments. In J. P. Forgas (Ed.), *Emotion and social judgments* (pp. 31–53). Elmsford, NY: Pergamon Press.

Carstensen, L. L. (1998). A life-span approach to social motivation. In J. Heckhausen & C. Dweck (Eds.), *Motivation and self-regulation across the life span* (pp. 341–364). New York: Cambridge University Press.

Carstensen, L. L., & Mikels, J. A. (2005). At the intersection of emotion and cognition: Aging and the positivity effect. *Current Directions in Psychological Science, 14,* 117–121.

Carstensen, L. L., Mikels, J. A., & Mather, M. (2006). Aging and the intersection of cognition, motivation, and emotion. In J. E. Birren & K. W. Schaie (Eds.), *Handbook of the psychology of aging* (6th ed., pp. 343–362). San Diego, CA: Elsevier.

Carstensen, L. L., Pasupathi, M., Mayr, U., & Nesselroade, J. R. (2000). Emotional experience in everyday life across the adult life span. *Journal of Personality and Social Psychology, 79,* 644–655.

Charles, S. T., & Carstensen, L. L. (2004). A life-span view of emotional functioning in adulthood and old age. In P. T. Costa & I. C. Siegler (Eds.), *Advances in cell aging and gerontology: Vol. 15. Recent advances in psychology and aging* (pp. 133–162). Amsterdam: Elsevier.

Clore, G. L., Schwarz, N., & Conway, M. (1994). Affective causes and consequences of social information processing. In R. S. Wyer & T. K. Srull (Eds.), *Handbook of social cognition* (Vol. 1, 2nd ed., pp. 323–419). Hillsdale, NJ: Erlbaum.

Consedine, N. S., Magai, C., & Bonanno, G. A. (2002). Moderators of the emotion inhibition-health relationship: A review and research agenda. *Review of General Psychology, 6,* 204–228.

Diener, E., Sandvik, E., & Larsen, R. J. (1985). Age and sex differences for emotional intensity. *Developmental Psychology, 21,* 542–546.

Eisdorfer, C. (1968). Arousal and performance: Experiments in verbal learning and a tentative theory. In G. Talland (Ed.), *Human behavior and aging: Recent advances in research and theory* (pp. 189–216). New York: Academic Press.

Forgas, J. P. (1995). Mood and judgment: The affect infusion model (AIM). *Psychological Bulletin, 117,* 39–66.

Kausler, D. (1990). Motivation, human aging, and cognitive performance. In J. E. Birren & K. W. Schaie (Eds.), *Handbook of the psychology of aging* (3rd ed., pp. 171–182). New York: Academic Press.

Kensinger, E. A., & Corkin, S. (2004). The effects of emotional content and aging on false memories. *Cognitive, Affective and Behavioral Neuroscience, 4,* 1–9.

Kunzmann, U., & Grühn, D. (2005). Age differences in emotional reactivity: The sample case of sadness. *Psychology and Aging, 20,* 47–59.

Labouvie-Vief, G. (2003). Dynamic integration: Affect, cognition, and the self in adulthood. *Current Directions in Psychological Science, 12,* 201–206.

Levenson, R. W., Carstensen, L. L., Friesen, W. V., & Ekman, P. (1991). Emotion, physiology, and expression in old age. *Psychology and Aging, 6,* 28–35.

Löckenhoff, C. E., & Carstensen, L. L. (2004). Socioemotional selectivity theory, aging, and health: The increasingly delicate balance between regulating emotions and making tough choices. *Journal of Personality, 72,* 1395–1424.

Mather, M., & Knight, M. (2005). Goal-directed memory: The role of cognitive control in older adults' emotional memory. *Psychology and Aging, 20,* 554–570.

May, C. P., Rahhal, T., Berry, E. M., & Leighton, E. A. (2005). Aging, source memory, and emotion. *Psychology and Aging, 20,* 571–578.

McCrae, R. R., & Costa, P. T. (1994). The stability of personality: Observation and evaluations. *Current Directions in Psychological Sciences, 3,* 173–175.

Rozin, P., & Royzman, E. B. (2001). Negativity bias, negativity dominance, and contagion. *Personality and Social Psychology Review, 5,* 296–320.

Sliwinski, M. J., Smyth, J. M., Hofer, S. M., & Stawski, R. S. (2006). Intraindividual coupling of daily stress and cognition. *Psychology and Aging, 21,* 545–557.

Wurm, L. H., Labouvie-Vief, G., Aycock, J., Rebucal, K. A., & Koch, H. E. (2004). Performance in auditory and visual emotional stroop tasks: A comparison of older and younger adults. *Psychology and Aging, 19,* 523–535.

Technology and the Workplace

Technology as Multiplier Effect for an Aging Workforce

8

NEIL CHARNESS

Technological innovations have been important catalysts for changes in social structures, particularly in recent decades. However, other important trends have paralleled technology diffusion, particularly changes in wealth and education. Such trends influence and are influenced by the development of social structures. The role of such trends is discussed from the perspective of present and future prospects for our aging workforce.

This discussion is motivated by the missive to look at some of the accomplishments and omissions in a few of the recent volumes from within the 20-year Social Structures and Aging series. Overviewing accomplishments is rather easy—there is clearly a wealth of ideas within the series that has served as a wonderful resource to researchers and practitioners over the years—but trying to identify omissions, particularly for the case of relatively recent volumes, has forced me to dig into other fields of social science, such as economics and demography, to provide what Wahl and Mollenkopf (2003) termed the *macro perspective level of analysis* in their chapter in one of the more recent volumes.

Acknowledgments: This research was supported by NIA 1 PO1 AG17211-07 to the Center for Research and Education on Aging and Technology Enhancement (CREATE) and by SSHRC to Workforce Ageing in the New Economy (WANE). I thank Jill Quadagno, Tiffany Jastrzembski, Roy Roring, Katinka Dijkstra, and Wendy Rogers for helpful comments on earlier drafts.

167

As background for assessing technology's impact on our aging workforce, I will selectively review economic and social trends that have been shaping our current social structures, including a few that I think have been insufficiently appreciated. Then I will overview a few of the prior themes in the series that pertain to work and technology and try to assess where we stand today. Finally, I will speculate on the near future for technology and our aging workforce.

THE BIG TWO: AGING AND TECHNOLOGY

Many disciplines have noted two major societal changes that have occurred in the past century or so. The first revolution we have witnessed is the striking aging of our population and the associated gender disparity in life span favoring women. We have also experienced a technological revolution, the speed of which has accelerated with the invention of the microprocessor by Intel in 1971.

Both topics have received detailed attention in two of the volumes in the series that I will address, namely *Impact of Work on Older Adults* (Schaie & Schooler, 1998) and *Impact of Technology on Successful Aging* (Charness & Schaie, 2003). Population aging has been the underlying current running through the series as a whole. Technology was explicitly dealt with in the 2003 volume.

Schaie and Schooler (1998) dealt with a series of issues around the aging workforce. Among the major accomplishments in that volume, in my view, was getting some perspective from economics, a social science that seems to attract little attention from mainstream psychologists and sociologists. For better or for worse, economics has the attention of policy makers in a way that sociology and psychology do not, particularly because economics directly addresses the financial impacts of policy decisions. (Governments are constrained by a different big two: trust and tax revenue. The former is reasonably stable in democracies, and the latter is variable, but necessary.) I also noticed the presence of economic viewpoints in the most recent Social Structures and Aging volume (Schaie & Carstensen, 2006). The Charness and Schaie (2003) volume dealt in depth with implications of technology for our aging population, a field of inquiry that has been termed *gerontechnology* by Harrington and Harrington (2000), or sometimes *gerotechnology* (Burdick & Kwon, 2004), though the former term should probably be preferred (Charness, 2004).

TECHNOLOGY: INVENTION VERSUS ADOPTION

Although the term *structural lag* was coined by Matilda White Riley to discuss the lag between changes in attributes of the population, such as longevity, and changes in social structures, such as workplaces, lag is a frequently occurring feature of many human endeavors such as the creation and widespread dissemination of new technologies (e.g., Charness & Czaja, 2005). Examples can be seen in Table 8.1.

I picked just a few technology-related inventions and some important precursors to inventions. Scientists are usually the first to uncover the important principles of operation for natural phenomena that others later capitalize on to invent consumer products. There is a very long lag between time of patenting for an invention and its widespread adoption in the case of the older cohorts of inventions. The best example is the facsimile (fax) machine, patented in the first half of the 19th century, with its widespread adoption only occurring in the second half of the 20th century. Compare that 100+-year gestation period to the roughly 10-year time to widespread diffusion and adoption of http protocol and the Web browser. Lag is clearly decreasing for the younger cohort of inventions. Such speedup is probably attributable to many causes such as the improved infrastructure for distribution that has evolved (e.g., telegraph lines were used for telephone transmissions; telephone lines and cable TV coax cables provide Internet access) and particularly increases in wealth, discussed later.

REFLECTIONS ON AGE AND WORK: WHAT HAS CHANGED SINCE 1998?

Pension Changes and Retirement

In their chapter, Schooler, Caplan, and Oates (1998) noted the massive changes in the prior century in age of retirement from work. About two-thirds of 65-year-old men worked in 1900, when small firms and farms dominated the employment landscape. By 1980, fewer than 20% worked past age 65. The authors concluded that the normative age for retirement from work was now firmly 65 years of age. As Burtless (2006) noted, there are really retirement peaks at both ages 62 and 65. At the time of the 1998 chapter, Schooler, Caplan, and Oates noted the move toward age neutrality in pensions, which might have discouraged the trend toward earlier retirement.

Table 8.1

TECHNOLOGICAL INVENTION AND DATE OF INVENTION

INVENTION	DATE (INVENTOR)
Electric telegraph	1837 (Morse)
Facsimile machine	1843 (Bain)
Telephone	1876 (Bell)
Television	1884 (Nipkow); in 1926, Baird demonstrated the TV system
Microwaves produced	1886 (Hertz)
International wireless telegraphy	1901 (Marconi)
Videophone	1930 (AT&T)
Mobile telephone	1946 (radiotelephone by AT&T)
Transistor	1947 (Bardeen, Brattain, and Shockley)
Earth satellite	1957 (Glushko and Korolyov)
Laser	1960 (Maiman)
Consumer microwave oven	1967 (Amana)
Microprocessor invented	1971 (Intel)
Personal computer	1974, MITS Altair kit; 1976, Apple I; 1977, Apple II (Jobs and Wozniak); 1981, IBM PC
Internet	1983, TCP/IP network; 1969, ARPANET
World Wide Web	1989, http protocol (Berners-Lee at CERN); 1992, text-based browser

Note: From Encyclopedia Britannica online, academic edition (http://search.eb.com/).

In fact, there had been an important shift under way in private pension types: Defined benefit plans had given way to defined contribution ones (see Figure 8.1). Defined benefit plans in the United States, in combination with social security, tax, and benefit policies, tend to encourage employees to retire on time because for every year worked past entitlement age (e.g., age 65), the employee can lose real income from this lifetime benefit (Butrica, Johnson, Smith, & Steuerle, 2006). Defined contribution plans continue to accrue real value with each year worked and, given vagaries in market fluctuations for investments, tend to keep individuals working longer to ensure that they have adequate funds for retirement because that form of retirement income is not guaranteed.

Concurrent with this shift have been changes in social security policy in the United States, encouraging a later retirement for baby boom generations beyond the earlier full benefit date of 65 years of age. In the future, full social security benefits will occur only at age 67 for those born after 1960. Just as the introduction of social security shifted preference

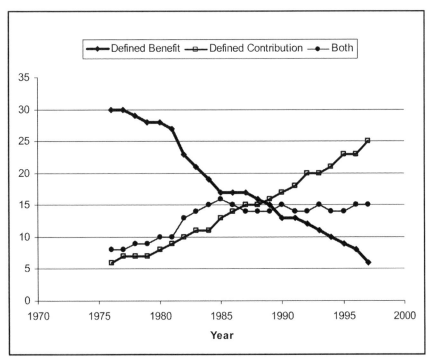

Figure 8.1 Percentage of U.S. workers by type of retirement plan. Data are from the Pension and Welfare Benefits Administration.

to earlier retirement (e.g., Burtless, 2006), later social security pension entitlement age coupled with shifting private pension types will likely contribute to a declining rate of early retirement, and perhaps even to its reversal given lengthening life expectancy coupled with improving health status. So a potentially important trend for the future of the workforce appears to be later retirement and a potential for older workers to stay in paid employment longer, if economic penalties for staying in the labor force, or for returning postretirement, are reduced. A potential counterbalancing force, though, could be the trend of increasing individual (and family) wealth, which might lead upper-income people to retire earlier.

Farr, Tesluk, and Klein (1998) commented on the rapidly aging workforce, citing a projection that by 2010, the median age of the workforce would rise to 40. I recently calculated that we likely reached that figure in 2006, some 4 years ahead of that projection. In a July 2006 release, the Bureau of Labor Statistics cited a median age of 41 projected for 2008. Although some have been concerned at the macroeconomic level about the potential productivity declines that an aging workforce might engender (e.g., Eberstadt, 2006), it is worth recalling that in 1962, the median age of the labor force was 40.5 (Bureau of Labor Statistics, 2006). Furthermore, as meta-analyses have shown at the micro (worker productivity) level on a number of occasions, there seems to be little relationship between age and productivity (McEvoy & Cascio, 1989; Sturman, 2004; Waldman & Avolio, 1986).[1] However, given that we survived an older workforce back in 1962 with a far less productive or wealthy society (see subsequent discussion), we should not be overly concerned about the impact of a graying labor force in the next decade or so, with a few caveats.

The first caveat is that if a greater proportion of older workers are persuaded to stay in labor markets or to reenter them, we run a risk of depressing wages for them and the rest of the labor force, which can lead to a negative feedback loop in times of high unemployment (Weller, 2006). The second caveat is that I am moderately concerned about the ability of older workers to adapt to a fast-paced, fast-changing labor market, given the very robust age-related slowing in learning rate that older adults typically experience (e.g., Charness, Kelley, Bosman, & Mottram, 2001; Salthouse, 1996).

---

[1] One important feature that is needed, though, to link macro- with microlevel analyses is an agreed on definition of *productivity*. Macroeconomic studies typically factor in wages, whereas micropsychological studies look at worker output or job performance ratings and ignore wage levels.

However, it is also evident that having the right training techniques is essential to effective interventions with older workers. Research on training older and younger adults on representative white-collar tasks has shown that older adults can learn to do computer-based tasks, though often not as proficiently at the end of training as younger adults (e.g., Czaja & Sharit, 1993, 1998). There is an indication that emphasizing direct, hands-on procedural training in place of conceptual training results in differential benefit for older compared to younger adults in tasks such as learning to use an ATM or Internet searching (Mead & Fisk, 1998; Mead, Spaulding, Sit, Meyer, & Walker, 1997). Ability to adapt and learn new skills is becoming increasingly important in today's volatile job market.

Volatility of Labor Markets and Career Options

It is pretty clear that as societal incentives change, so, too, do corresponding behaviors such as choice of time to retire (Burtless, 2006). However, we are probably in a more volatile labor market situation than ever before because of the global competition for jobs. Bernanke (2006), chairman of the Federal Reserve Bank in the United States, recently noted the accelerating pace of globalization of economic activity. Perhaps as a result of broader competitive pressures, employers are shifting more of the risk of producing retirement income from their firms to their employees. (This shift of risk from firms to individuals is even more worrisome in the case of health care benefits in the United States because reasonably priced basic health insurance is typically only available from employers.) Firms also are more able than ever before to find ways to reduce labor costs because of the shift in the United States away from unionization (which tends to tilt salary bargaining power toward employees) and the increasing availability of skilled labor in developing nations.

Technology has a lot to do with the option to outsource labor because computers and communication channels permit more and more people to engage in work at a distance: telework. This may actually be a positive trend because telework may be particularly suited to older workers' needs and abilities (Charness, Czaja, & Sharit, 2007). We are perhaps entering an era where the mix of job types is shifting closer to what Sørenson (1998) called the *spot market* situation for labor (vs. job competition or promotion system jobs), where jobs are less secure, and many potential workers compete actively for them. As Bernanke (1996) warned, though, governments have the added responsibility to ensure that the benefits of globalization are spread to all segments of the population and that those workers losing jobs to international competition are given an opportunity to retrain. As is evident in meta-analyses conducted a decade apart on attitudes toward older workers and older adults, generally, older workers are (still) perceived as less suitable for learning or training (Finkelstein, Burke, & Raju, 1995; Kite, Stockdale, Whitley, & Johnson, 2005). Thus the willingness of management to offer retraining to older workers and the willingness of older workers to take up such infrequent offers remain in doubt (Farr et al., 1998).

Similarly, organizational structures at work for large-scale employers are probably continuing to change in the direction of leaner production, with flatter hierarchies and more of a shift toward workers being expected to build their own careers, rather than having the employer support that activity (e.g., Ekerdt, 2006).

Work–Family Boundaries

Another recent change, not necessarily for the better, is the ever more permeable boundary between work life and home life, particularly because of mobile telecommunication devices such as the cell phone (or the Blackberry, which provides constant access to e-mail) and the home computer attached to the Internet. The ability of technology to bridge distance is one facet of what I am calling the multiplicative effects of technology on our labor force.

Those who can take advantage of technological innovations, whether employer or worker, can carry out production activities more efficiently, including at a distance from the nominal company headquarters. However, in a multinational (Canada, United States, European Union, Australia) Workforce Aging in the New Economy project focusing on the information technology (IT) industry, we heard interview complaints, mainly from younger workers, about constantly being on call for company projects. However, older workers express more conflict on a questionnaire item that asks about the intersection between work life and other parts of life: "To what extent do you agree or disagree with each of the following statements?—My working hours interfere with my family responsibilities." Here workers over the age of 40 (n = 213) are significantly more likely to express agreement or strong agreement with this statement than those under 40 (n = 266): 29.6% versus 20.3%. Negotiating the work–family boundary is probably becoming more difficult for all age groups as firms seek to compete in an increasingly global market and demand more from their employees.

WHAT HAS NOT CHANGED SINCE 1998: RECIPROCAL INFLUENCES ON SOCIAL STRUCTURES

As Matilda Riley (1998) pointed out, aging occurs within social structures. Different cohorts age differently and in turn effect change in social structures. However, there is usually a significant lag to changes in social structures needed to accommodate the latest aging cohorts in terms of opportunities for work, leisure, and education. We might also expect that over time, there is going to be little change in such reciprocal influences given the natural tensions between people and their institutional structures.

For instance, as Hoyer (1998) pointed out in his commentary chapter, the decision to leave the workforce at the individual level may be a response to a myriad of (microculture) individual and (macro) social influences. However, retirement from work depends a great deal on financial features, bringing me to the most important change across time that few social scientists bother to consider: The rise in personal wealth through income.

A SPECTACULAR SOCIAL TREND: INCOME WEALTH THROUGH PRODUCTIVITY GAINS

In the United States, per capita gross domestic product follows an exponentially increasing function (only briefly interrupted by wars or recessions), as seen in Figure 8.2. Undoubtedly, this growth has been driven by factors such as capital investment (equipment, education, and training) on the part of individuals, industry, and government as well as by concurrent technological innovation.

The rise, particularly post–World War II, is very steep. It is worth noting that per capita income is not now just at historical highs in the United States. In fact, the United States ranked third in 2005, behind Luxembourg and Norway. However, it is also worth contemplating that many less developed countries today have less income per capita than did the United States in the 1890s. Of the roughly 180 countries for which per capita income figures are available, about 80 fall into this category (http://en.wikipedia.org/wiki/List_of_countries_by_GDP_%28PPP%29_per_capita).

Did this productivity gain in the United States translate to income for families? Figure 8.3 shows that until fairly recently, those gains accrued to families in exponential form as well.

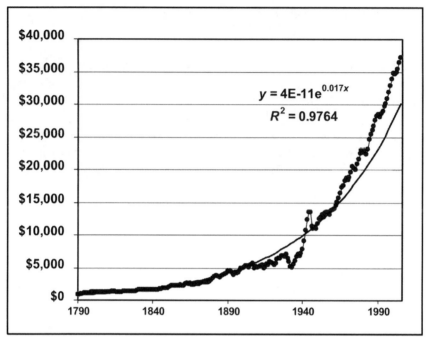

Figure 8.2 Changes in U.S. per capita GDP measured in year 2004 dollars. Data are from "The Annual Real and Nominal GDP for the United States, 1790–Present," by Louis D. Johnston and Samuel H. Williamson, October 2005, Economic History Services, retrieved June 30, 2006, from http://www.measuringworth.com/usgdp/

The values in Figure 8.3 are given in constant (real) dollars, adjusted for inflation over that time period. The rise in median family income, from approximately $3,000 in 1947 to approximately $54,000 in 2004, is striking, though some of that increase is probably attributable to the sharp rise in women moving into the paid labor force in the 1970s. Another likely factor in recent decline is a change in the mix of family types, with more single-income family units (e.g., single mothers).

Although it almost goes without saying, evolutionary influences on the human genome have not resulted in large-scale changes in genotypes or corresponding phenotypes since 1900 that could be responsible for our massive increases in societal wealth. As Schaie (1994) noted for the Seattle Longitudinal Study, different birth cohorts do seem to vary in basic psychological ability levels. It is not clear whether cohort differences, such as the trend for better performance on cognitive ability

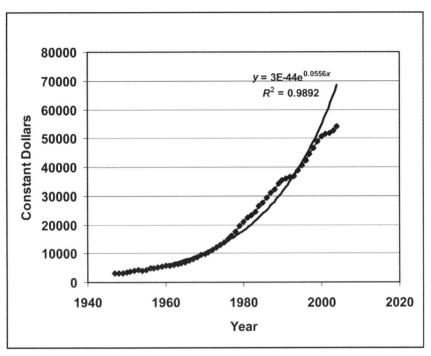

Figure 8.3 U.S. family median income by year in constant 2004 dollars. Data are from U.S. Census Bureau, Current Population Survey, Annual Social and Economic Supplements; Historical Income Tables: Families. http://www.census.gov/hhes/www/income/histinc/f08ar.html

tests across generations (e.g., the Flynn effect; Dickens & Flynn, 2001), have been partly responsible for the rising productivity of the workforce, as seen in Figure 8.3. Whatever the source, that rise has been exceptional.

One consequence of these huge changes in both productivity and income is that people who are reasonably successful in saving for retirement may choose to retire from paid work because they can literally afford to stop working and maintain a reasonable standard of living. Even those of us enjoying the privileged position of university researchers probably recognize that many people do not enjoy their jobs. The development of a government-sponsored social security system (only affordable because of the relative wealth in the country) stimulated the initial trend toward earlier and earlier retirement. Finally, increases in family wealth permit a more rapid diffusion and adoption of new technology by individuals and households.

MULTIPLIER EFFECTS FOR TECHNOLOGY ON PRODUCTIVITY

There was a long period in which people were unable to detect a productivity gain for massive investments in technology such as computer systems, best illustrated by a quote that is typically attributed to Nobel Prize economist Robert Solow in 1987: "We see computers everywhere but not in the productivity statistics." Eventually, it became clear that general productivity gains were related to technology investment (e.g., Organisation for Economic Co-operation and Development, 2003), and mechanisms for tracing the impact of investment in research and development on industry productivity are becoming better developed (e.g., Wilson, 2002).

My personal speculation is that there is always a significant lag between technology introduction and effective use because people are limited in acquiring requisite skills to use the technology efficiently by their relatively slow learning rate (Simon, 1974), coupled with the necessity to balance effort between learning and producing goods and services within their jobs. It takes considerable time, hundreds to thousands of hours, to build up a skill to a high level of expertise (Ericsson, Charness, Feltovich, & Hoffman, 2006). Academics are relatively privileged to occupy jobs that provide the luxury (pretenure faculty would say the necessity) of taking time off to learn new things as part of their job descriptions.

One index of the importance of the computer and electronics sector to the economy as a whole can be seen in Figure 8.4, created from productivity data supplied by the Bureau of Labor Statistics.

It is little wonder that prices for computers have plummeted over the years considering the spectacular increases in productivity that this industry has enjoyed relative to other sectors. Computers do enable increases in efficiency, particularly in the communications field. Carrying on correspondence with multiple people (mass mailings) used to mean generating a base letter followed by serial printing of letter after letter, followed by inserting each in an envelope and dumping them in a mail distribution system. Today, after composition of the text message, access to an e-mail alias list enables practically simultaneous distribution and nearly instant delivery of the message. Alas, such synergies can be used for good or evil, and, as most e-mail readers today will recognize, spammers have taken unfair advantage of this efficient distribution channel. But given the exponential growth that the United States has enjoyed in income since 1900, long before computers made their appearance, other factors than computerization should be credited for our increasing wealth. This brings me to another undervalued social influence: education.

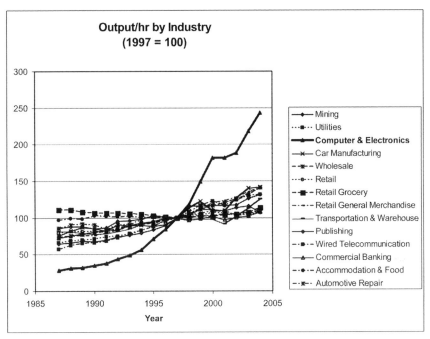

Figure 8.4 Changes in productivity (output/hr) by industry sector (1985–2005). Data are scaled to 100 for the year 1997.

Source: Retrieved August 2006 from http://data.bls.gov/PDQ/servlet/SurveyOutputServlet.

INCREASING EDUCATIONAL ATTAINMENT

The ever-increasing levels of education in the labor force is a critical social trend, as seen in Figure 8.5.

However, research has yet to untangle whether it is the case that education makes you smarter (hence more valuable as a worker) or whether there are other factors that make people smart (hence more likely to progress further in educational systems and do better at jobs). Nonetheless, it is striking to see how, in a little over 60 years, high school completion rates have risen from 25% to 85%, and college completion rates now border on 30%, compared to 5% earlier. The much maligned educational system in the United States must be doing something right. There is the caveat about how much knowledge and skill today's high school or college graduate has relative to yesterday's graduate. And one might keep in mind the concept that a primary function of educational attainment is to serve as a *signaling system* (Spence,

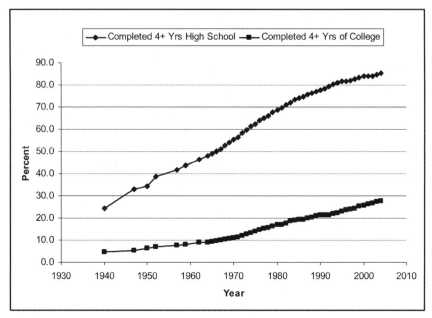

Figure 8.5 Educational attainment for those aged 25 years and over, 1940–2004. Data are from "U.S. Census Bureau Educational Attainment," retrieved August 20, 2006, from http://www.census.gov/population/www/socdemo/educ-attn.html

1974) that enables productive people to stand out from the crowd in hiring decisions.

A very important consequence of higher educational attainment is the likelihood that future training and retraining within the working years will go more smoothly for an ever-increasing proportion of the working population. We are likely to experience a positive *Matthew effect*, where the rich are likely to get richer in knowledge and skills. One of the strongest predictors of success in learning a new software package, independent of learner age, is breadth of experience with software packages (Charness et al., 2001).

Another potential spin-off from higher education levels and more challenging occupational niches is better cognition during the working years and in old age (see Schooler and Caplan, this volume). Recent research has shown the importance of education (and occupation) as protective factors for maladies such as dementia (e.g., as reviewed in Charness, 2006). Despite this rosy picture, there are still important cohort differences in education and in breadth of experience with technology.

THE TECHNOLOGY GAP FOR OLDER COHORTS

Cohorts that are more recent arrivals in the workplace apparently acquired skill with computer technology more easily. In an earlier volume in this series, Czaja and Lee (2003) pointed out that older adults, at that time, were lagging their younger counterparts in use of computers and the Internet. If we examine Figure 8.6, showing a cross-sectional picture of computer use over a 6-year interval (Pew Foundation, http://www. pewinternet.org/datasets.asp/), we can see that even in 2006, less than 40% of U.S. adults aged 65 years and older used a computer. Even those cohorts still within nominal working age, 50- to 64-year-olds, significantly lagged younger aged cohorts. So we can add the age gap in technology use as one feature that has remained constant since the 2003 book. However, education is also a powerful predictor of computer use (National Telecommunications and Information Administration, n.d.). Here, too, older cohorts are likely to be disadvantaged in that they have had fewer years of formal education.

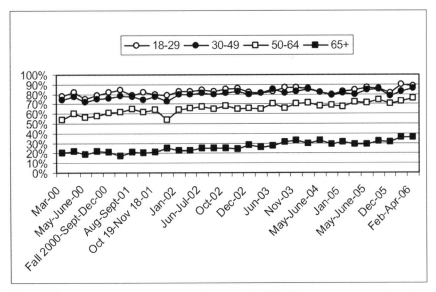

Figure 8.6 Computer use by age group. Response to Q5: "Do you use a computer at your workplace, at school, at home, or anywhere else on at least an occasional basis?" Data are from the Pew Internet and American Life Tracking Survey, March 2000 to February–April 2006, retrieved September 15, 2006, from http://www.pewinternet. org/datasets.asp/

Both education and income (which tend to be highly correlated), two factors discussed above, are important mediators of these cohort differences in Internet access. A Kaiser Family Foundation study (Rideout, Neuman, Kitchman, & Brodie, 2005) noted that education and income are both important predictors of ever having gone online within the 65+ population, as seen in Figure 8.7.

However, as Liu and Park (2003) noted, the baby boom cohorts will likely have reasonable levels of computer literacy when they approach old age, so the problem of age-related gaps in computer and Internet use may decline over time. However, new tools will continue to be introduced, and the cohort gap in the facility with which such tools will be utilized may not narrow. Given that computers are potential multipliers for productivity, it seems likely that older cohorts are and will be disadvantaged in the workplace to the extent that their jobs could be enhanced by greater efficiency at using computer technology.

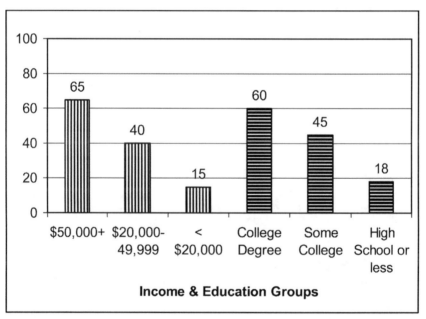

Figure 8.7 Percent U.S. seniors (65+ years) reporting that they had ever gone online by income and education levels. Data are from "E-Health and the elderly: How seniors use the Internet for health information: Key findings from a national survey of older adults," by V. Rideout, T. Neuman, M. Kitchman, and M. Brodie, 2005, Kaiser Family Foundation, retrieved September 22, 2006, from http://www.kff.org/entmedia/upload/e-Health-and-the-Elderly-How-Seniors-Use-the-Internet-for-Health-Information-Key-Findings-From-a-National-Survey-of-Older-Americans-Survey-Report.pdf

An important question to address is why older cohorts are less likely to use computer systems. Among the likely culprits are differences between cohorts in access, motivation, and learning ability, coupled with differential usability of technical systems (Charness, 2003). The latter may be a critical factor. A salient example is the continuing presence of badly designed Web sites, despite good guidelines and effective techniques for doing usability testing (e.g., Morrell, Dailey, & Rousseau, 2003). Ironically, whereas technology is diffusing faster than ever, adoption of best practices still appears to have a significant lag.

OTHER RECENT ADVANCES: THE RISE OF SMART HOMES AND ROBOTICS

Wahl and Mollenkopf (2003) made the argument that it would not be necessary to review developments in intelligent housing or robotics, though those fields were advancing. Since that time, there has continued to be significant progress in both fields, but particularly in the area of smart homes, a major focus of the Georgia Institute of Technology component of the Center for Research and Education on Aging and Technology Enhancement (CREATE) project (e.g., Mynatt, Melenhorst, Fisk, & Rogers, 2004). A high-technology chronic care institution has become well established in Oregon (Oatfield Estates, http://www.elite-care.com/oatfield.html). At the deployment end of robotics, it is worth noting that there are apparently more than 1.5 million robotic vacuum cleaners in U.S. households (Kelleher, 2005), though that number represents less than 2% penetration. But because technology has been diffusing more rapidly over time, we can expect to see robotic appliances reaching significant numbers in the near future.

CONCERNS GOING FORWARD

Although we are aging better than ever before from a morbidity and disability perspective (e.g., Manton, Stallard, & Corder, 1995), there are normative age-related declines in aspects of perception, cognition, and psychomotor ability that affect large numbers of older adults even within the usual working years (e.g., Schieber, 2003). As many people have commented, and as was the focus of the 2003 Social Structures and Aging volume, appropriate sensitivity to those changes should lead people to design technology artifacts that can be used effectively and comfortably by older users.

However, as Fozard (2003) noted in his commentary chapter, the same recommendations about improving design for older adults have been made numerous times by numerous authors. Yet we see too little attention to recommendations. So what can we do to improve the chances that well-understood design principles will be implemented? Chapters like this one in yet another Social Structures and Aging volume are probably not the solution. It seems to me that guidelines may at some point need to become regulations; legislative remedies can be an important agent for change in social structures.

Several examples come to mind from U.S. law. Extending rights to impaired individuals was first tackled through the Americans With Disabilities Act of 1990 (http://www.usdoj.gov/crt/ada/adahom1.htm). Another example is Section 508 of the Rehabilitation Act (http://www.section508.gov/), dealing specifically with technology design issues. It holds sway in the public sector and with those private sector groups that want to do business with the federal government. Of course, in the area of work, the Age Discrimination in Employment Act of 1967 was passed to protect aging workers (age 40+; http://www.eeoc.gov/policy/adea.html).

However, the current antiregulation attitude in Washington, D.C., makes the prospect of new regulations unlikely in the near future in the United States. It should be kept in mind that the United States is probably unique as a nation in its individualistic approach to social change. It seems to prefer that informal, low-level social structures (self-help groups, charitable organizations) take the lead in social innovation, rather than relying on formal structures such as municipal, state, and federal governments.

Of course, competitive pressures will eventually force manufacturers and designers to heed the needs (and wants) of the large and relatively wealthy baby boom cohorts. *Eventually* may be too long a time to serve the needs for many older adults, unfortunately, particularly those in lower income groups.

Aging is associated with general slowing in information processing rates (e.g., Salthouse, 1996). Such slowing might be expected to reduce learning rates in older adults, for instance, for job-related information. It does, though that slowing effect is mediated (e.g., Charness et al., 2001) by the knowledge base that older workers have already acquired their accumulated stock of knowledge (see earlier discussion for age productivity meta-analyses). Nonetheless, particularly in a social context of rapid change in work environments (lean production, just-in-time production), slowing is going to make older workers less valuable to their employers, unless those workers have compensatory knowledge (e.g., about production, management of resources). Life in the workplace is undoubtedly going to become harder for the older worker over time.

So, what social structures can be called on to buttress the opportunities for older workers? First, we have to consider contextual factors that influence willingness to offer employment. The state of the business cycle (current match between labor supply and demand) is still likely to be more critical than demographic factors, such as the smaller cohorts following the baby boom generation, when it comes to employment trends (e.g., Cappelli, 2003). When economies expand, demand for workers increases. When there are contractions (recessions), demand slackens. During the boom period before the IT investment bubble burst in 2000, low-skilled younger workers and older workers alike benefited from the need for labor.

We also have to consider the willingness of older workers to seek employment. When older workers have adequate resources to live comfortably without working, many will opt for leisure over work. Social incentives and disincentives for work (such as presence of social security pensions, defined contribution vs. defined benefit pension plans, tax policy) affect resources and retirement timing. Finally, we need to consider the willingness of aging workers to keep their skills current (through training and retraining). One of the striking findings in the Bray and Howard (1983) longitudinal study of managers at AT&T was the difference in the lifestyle trajectories, and corresponding attitudes, of those who moved up the management ladder from those who stalled at lower levels. Willingness to expend effort in a work environment to acquire new skills seems to be a complex function of individual (micro) and organizational (macro) social structures. It is here that a combination of industrial–organizational psychology research paired with human factors research may play an important role in fashioning effective interventions with older workers.

TECHNOLOGY AS MULTIPLIER FACTOR FOR SOCIAL STRUCTURES

With all the bad news about how technological innovation has been instrumental in facilitating greater intrusiveness of work life into home life, in making labor markets more volatile, and also in forcing employers to shift pension and health care risk to workers, one might be tempted to adopt a Luddite attitude to such innovation. However, we also need to note the positive sides of technology (aside from the way it has enriched incomes). For those with disabilities, technology has provided assistive devices that can promote independence and forestall institutionalization (e.g., Mann, 2003). Technology has made possible improved communication in family life. As my wife and I have discovered, desktop video-conferencing is not the same thing as being there for grandparents and grandchildren, but it certainly helps to maintain and enrich ties. Rituals can develop around videoconferencing that bind geographically separated generations together in a more satisfying way than did weekly long distance phone calls in my generation, or as did letters in my parents' and grandparents' generations.

So, as Riley (1998) stated so aptly in her commentary chapter, we need to pay closer attention to agents of change, not just ego, the older worker, but also those who influence the way in which ego behaves, namely, the alters. Technology, by almost anyone's definition, has taken on the role of agent, and not just in the form of science fiction's autonomous robot. My colleagues at Georgia Tech now like to discuss the Georgia Tech aware home (Mynatt et al., 2004; Rogers & Fisk, 2003) as taking on the role of technology coach, certainly an agentic role. Putting intelligence in technology agents is a very active area of research that is continuing to progress, albeit slowly. We are still a long way from the Jetsons' helpful robotic maid Rosie, or even the evil computer HAL from *2001: A Space Odyssey*. Nonetheless, products such as Roomba™ and Scooba™, the robotic vacuum cleaner and robotic floor scrubber, do provide a glimpse into how technology products can facilitate the cleaning of a house, one of the less enjoyable instrumental activities of daily living (IADL). It is surprising how many IADLs can now be facilitated by today's technology (Charness, 2005).

Technology has also opened up employment opportunities for less mobile older adults in the form of telework. The loss of driving privileges need no longer equate to the loss of the opportunity for meaningful work. Similarly, advances in telemedicine and telehealth, potentially embeddable within smart homes, may also obviate the need for frequent visits to a physician's office, as health becomes more fragile in old age. Although the price of such technology, both in terms of monetary cost and learning cost, is likely still too high for the average retired adult, productivity gains in this industry are making technology more affordable with each passing year, though the slowing learning rate within an aging population is also making technology products more difficult to learn to use. Judicious use of human factor guidelines and principles (e.g., Fisk, Rogers, Charness, Czaja, & Sharit, 2004) may tip the balance in favor of the aging worker and consumer.

In summary, technology is a potent multiplier factor for those aging workers who can take advantage of it. It can expand options for those who can master its use, or it can constrict them for those left behind. Hence the future holds both risks and rewards that are predicated on successful incorporation of technology into our lives. Will the necessary social structures be there to support its incorporation? Although there is always a significant lag between aging populations and their social structures, as Riley pointed out so many years ago, I am cautiously hopeful that the lag can be shortened. Increased education, better health, greater wealth, and advancing technology provide ideal conditions to begin to shorten this lag and provide new opportunities for our aging workforce and aging population.

NEW RESEARCH DIRECTIONS

Although the prior Social Structures and Aging volumes have created an impressive foundation for research, there are some new directions that can be considered. First, we need a better sense of how technology diffuses generally, and more specifically, how it diffuses to older adults. Assessing the role of individual difference variables for technology adoption seems to be an important avenue, given that studies have already shown that psychological ones, such as fluid and crystallized intelligence (e.g., Czaja et al., 2006), and socioeconomic ones, such as education and income (Rideout et al., 2005), play important roles. Multiple-cohort longitudinal studies would seem to be an effective way to proceed here.

Another important issue that is still poorly understood is, What are the best methods for training older workers? One meta-analysis showed that older adults benefit less from training than younger adults (Kubeck, Delp, Haslett, & McDaniel, 1996). This is predictable from general slowing in learning with age. Still, a large range of training techniques do work successfully within an older worker group, as seen in the meta-analysis by Callahan, Kiker, and Cross (2003). However, the critical question is really, Are there techniques that promote differential gain for older workers relative to younger workers? As mentioned earlier, Mead and colleagues (Mead & Fisk, 1998; Mead et al., 1997) have shown that procedural training seems to result in differential benefit relative to conceptual training. However, much more work needs to be conducted to identify the controlling variables for successful training at the micropsychological process level. But an important part of the process will involve identifying organizational and attitudinal barriers to training, given some persistent stereotypical beliefs about older worker capabilities by management. Training in most job settings rarely takes place in a pristine, lablike environment with minimal personal context.

There continue to be a large number of questions to be answered about retirement processes. They include financial ones such as how to encourage people to invest wisely to ensure adequate retirement income (and probably more importantly, adequate health care coverage in the United States). Another concerns how to avoid penalizing individuals financially when they wish to work past nominal retirement age. As well, we need to know more about how personal factors play into the decision to retire.

Finally, from the point of view of design of technology to help older workers and older adults generally, we need to find more efficient methods of design. Although guidelines have been published (e.g., Fisk et al., 2004), in many cases, they are too general to help with low-level design decisions (e.g., for cell phone menu structure). Pooling existing experimental studies to come up with older adult information processing parameters for simulation techniques, such as goals, operators, methods, selection rules (GOMS) modeling (Jastrzembski & Charness, 2007), is a promising avenue to pursue.

REFERENCES

Bernanke, B. S. (2006, August 25). *Global economic integration: What's new and what's not?* Paper presented at the Federal Reserve Bank of Kansas City's 30th annual economic symposium, Jackson Hole, WY. Retrieved 8/25/2006 from http://www.federal reserve.gov/newsevents/speech/Bernanke20060825a.htm

Bray, D. W., & Howard, A. (1983). The AT&T longitudinal studies of managers. In K. W. Schaie (Ed.), *Longitudinal studies of adult psychological development* (pp. 112–146). New York: Guilford Press.

Burdick, D. C., & Kwon, S. (Eds.). (2004). *Gerotechnology: Research and practice in technology and aging—A textbook and reference for multiple disciplines* (pp. 42–53). New York: Springer Publishing.

Bureau of Labor Statistics. (2006, July). *Working in the 21st century*. Retrieved February 16, 2008, from http://www.bls.gov/opub/working/page2b.htm

Burtless, G. (2006). Social norms, rules of thumb, and retirement: Evidence for rationality in retirement planning. In K. W. Schaie & L. Carstensen (Eds.), *Social structures, aging, and self-regulation* (pp. 123–160). New York: Springer Publishing.

Butrica, B. A., Johnson, R. W., Smith, K. E., & Steuerle, C. E. (2006). The implicit tax on work at older ages. *National Tax Journal, 64,* 211–234.

Callahan, J. S., Kiker, D. S., & Cross, T. (2003). Does method matter? A meta-analysis of the effects of training method on older learner training performance. *Journal of Management, 29,* 663–680.

Cappelli, P. (2003). Will there really be a labor shortage? *Organizational Dynamics, 32,* 221–233.

Charness, N. (2003). Access, motivation, ability, design, and training: Necessary conditions for older adult success with technology. In N. Charness & K. W. Schaie (Eds.), *Impact of technology on successful aging* (pp. 15–27). New York: Springer Publishing.

Charness, N. (2004). Coining new words: Old (Greek) wine in new bottles? (Reply). *Gerontechnology, 3,* 52–53.

Charness, N. (2005). Age, technology, and culture: Gerontopia or dystopia? *Public Policy and Aging Report, 15,* 20–23.

Charness, N. (2006). The influence of work and occupation on brain development. In P. B. Baltes, F. Rösler, & P. Reuter-Lorenz (Eds.), *Lifespan development and the brain: The perspective of biocultural co-constructivism* (pp. 306–325). New York: Cambridge University Press.

Charness, N., & Czaja, S. J. (2005). Adaptation to new technologies (7.13). In M. L. Johnson (Gen. Ed.), *Cambridge handbook on age and ageing* (pp. 662–669). Cambridge, England: Cambridge University Press.

Charness, N., Czaja, S. J., & Sharit, J. (2007). Age and technology for work. In K. S. Schulz & G. A. Adams (Eds.), *Aging and work in the 21st century* (pp. 225–249). Mahwah, NJ: Erlbaum.

Charness, N., Kelley, C. L., Bosman, E. A., & Mottram, M. (2001). Word processing training and retraining: Effects of adult age, experience, and interface. *Psychology and Aging, 16,* 110–127.

Charness, N., & Schaie, K. W. (Eds.). (2003). *Impact of technology on successful aging.* New York: Springer Publishing.

Czaja, S. J., Charness, N., Fisk, A. D., Hertzog, C., Nair, S. N., Rogers, W. A., et al. (2006). Factors predicting the use of technology: Findings from the Center for Research and Education on Aging and Technology Enhancement (CREATE). *Psychology and Aging, 21,* 333–352.

Czaja, S. J., & Lee, C. C. (2003). The impact of the Internet on older adults. In N. Charness & K. W. Schaie (Eds.), *Impact of technology on successful aging* (pp. 113–133). New York: Springer Publishing.

Czaja, S. J., & Sharit, J. (1993). Age differences in the performance of computer-based work. *Psychology and Aging, 8,* 59–67.

Czaja, S. J., & Sharit, J. (1998). Ability-performance relationships as a function of age and task experience for a data entry task. *Journal of Experimental Psychology: Applied, 4,* 332–351.

Dickens, T., & Flynn, J. R. (2001). Heritability estimates versus large environmental effects: The IQ paradox resolved. *Psychological Review, 108,* 346–369.

Eberstadt, N. (2006). Growing old the hard way: China, Russia, India. *Policy Review, 136*. Retrieved September 15, 2006, from http://www.policyreview.org/136/eberstadt.html

Ekerdt, D. (2006). *No career for you: Is that a good or bad thing?* Paper presented at the Pennsylvania State University conference on social structures and aging individuals: continuing challenges, University Park, PA.

Ericsson, K. A., Charness, N., Feltovich, P., & Hoffman, R. (Eds.). (2006). *Cambridge handbook of expertise and expert performance.* Cambridge, England: Cambridge University Press.

Farr, J. L., Tesluk, P. E., & Klein, S. R. (1998). Organizational structure of the workplace and the older worker. In K. W. Schaie & C. Schooler (Eds.), *Impact of work on older adults* (pp. 143–185). New York: Springer Publishing.

Finkelstein, L. M., Burke, M. J., & Raju, N. S. (1995). Age discrimination in simulated employment contexts: An integrative analysis. *Journal of Applied Psychology, 80,* 652–663.

Fisk, A. D., Rogers, W. A., Charness, N., Czaja, S. J., & Sharit, J. (2004). *Designing for older adults: Principles and creative human factors approaches.* Boca Raton, FL: CRC Press.

Fozard, J. (2003). Commentary: Using technology to lower the perceptual and cognitive hurdles of aging. In N. Charness & K. W. Schaie (Eds.), *Impact of technology on successful aging* (pp. 100–112). New York: Springer Publishing.

Harrington, T. L., & Harrington, M. K. (2000). *Gerontechnology: Why and how.* Maastricht, Netherlands: Shaker.

Hoyer, W. J. (1998). Commentary: The older individual in a rapidly changing work context: Developmental and cognitive issues. In K. W. Schaie & C. Schooler (Eds.), *Impact of work on older adults* (pp. 28–44). New York: Springer Publishing.

Jastrzembski, T. S., & Charness, N. (2007). The Model Human Processor and the older adult: Parameter estimation and validation within a mobile phone task. *Journal of Experimental Psychology: Applied, 13,* 224–248.

Kelleher, K. (2005, November 11). *iRobot sweeping hearts and minds.* Retrieved September 7, 2006, from http://www.thestreet.com/tech/kevinkelleher/10252502.html

Kite, M. E., Stockdale, G. D., Whitley, B. E., Jr., & Johnson, B. T. (2005). Attitudes toward younger and older adults: An updated meta-analytic review. *Journal of Social Issues, 61,* 241–266.

Kubeck, J. E., Delp, N. D., Haslett, T. K., & McDaniel, M. A. (1996). Does job-related training performance decline with age? *Psychology and Aging, 11,* 92–107.

Liu, L. L., & Park, D. C. (2003). Technology and the promise of independent living for adults: A cognitive perspective. In N. Charness & K. W. Schaie (Eds.), *Impact of technology on successful aging* (pp. 262–289). New York: Springer Publishing.

Mann, W. C. (2003). Assistive technology. In N. Charness & K. W. Schaie (Eds.), *Impact of technology on successful aging* (pp. 177–187). New York: Springer Publishing.

Manton, K. G., Stallard, E., & Corder, L. (1995). Changes in morbidity and chronic disability in the U.S. elderly population: Evidence from the 1982, 1984, and 1989 National Long Term Care Surveys. *Journal of Gerontology: Social Sciences, 50,* S194–S204.

McEvoy, G. M., & Cascio, W. F. (1989). Cumulative evidence of the relationship between employee age and job performance. *Journal of Applied Psychology, 74,* 11–17.

Mead, S., & Fisk, A. D. (1998). Measuring skill acquisition and retention with an ATM simulator: The need for age-specific training. *Human Factors, 40,* 516–523.

Mead, S. E., Spaulding, V. A., Sit, R. A., Meyer, B., & Walker, N. (1997). Effects of age and training on World Wide Web navigation strategies. In *Proceedings of the Human Factors and Ergonomics Society 41st Annual Meeting* (pp. 152–156). Santa Monica, CA: Human Factors and Ergonomics Society.

Morrell, R. W., Dailey, S. R., & Rousseau, G. K. (2003). Applying research: The NIHSeniorHealth.gov project. In N. Charness & K. W. Schaie (Eds.), *Impact of technology on successful aging* (pp. 134–161). New York: Springer Publishing.

Mynatt, E. D., Melenhorst, A. S., Fisk, A. D., & Rogers, W. A. (2004). Aware technologies for aging in place: Understanding user needs and attitudes. *IEEE Pervasive Computing, 3,* 36–41.

National Telecommunications and Information Administration. (n.d.). *Falling through the NET II: New data on the digital divide, 1998.* Retrieved May 5, 1999, from http://www.ntia.doc.gov/ntiahome/net2/falling.html

Organisation for Economic Co-operation and Development. (2003). *ICT and economic growth: Evidence from OECD countries, industries and firms.* Paris: Author.

Rideout, V., Neuman, T., Kitchman, M., & Brodie, M. (2005). *E-Health and the elderly: How seniors use the Internet for health information: Key findings from a national survey of older adults.* Retrieved September 22, 2006, from Kaiser Family Foundation Web site: http://www.kff.org/entmedia/upload/e-Health-and-the-Elderly-How-Seniors-Use-the-Internet-for-Health-Information-Key-Findings-From-a-National-Survey-of-Older-Americans-Survey-Report.pdf

Riley, M. W. (1998). Commentary: Psychology, sociology, and research on aging. In K. W. Schaie & C. Schooler (Eds.), *Impact of work on older adults* (pp. 20–27). New York: Springer Publishing.

Rogers, W. A., & Fisk, A. D. (2003). Technology design, usability, and aging: Human factors techniques and considerations. In N. Charness & K. W. Schaie (Eds.), *Impact of technology on successful aging* (pp. 1–14). New York: Springer Publishing.

Salthouse, T. A. (1996). The processing-speed theory of adult age differences in cognition. *Psychological Review, 103,* 403–428.

Schaie, K. W. (1994). The course of adult intellectual development. *American Psychologist, 49,* 304–313.

Schaie, K. W., & Carstensen, L. (Eds.). (2006). *Social structures, aging, and self-regulation.* New York: Springer Publishing.

Schaie, K. W., & Schooler, C. (Eds.). (1998). *Impact of work on older adults.* New York: Springer Publishing.

Schieber, F. (2003). Human factors and aging: Identifying and compensating for age-related deficits in sensory and cognitive function. In N. Charness & K. W. Schaie (Eds.), *Impact of technology on successful aging* (pp. 42–84). New York: Springer Publishing.

Schooler, C., Caplan, L., & Oates, G. (1998). Aging and work: An overview. In K. W. Schaie & C. Schooler (Eds.), *Impact of work on older adults* (pp. 1–19). New York: Springer Publishing.

Simon, H. A. (1974). How big is a chunk? *Science, 183,* 482–488.

Sørenson, A. B. (1998). Career trajectories and the older worker. In K. W. Schaie & C. Schooler (Eds.), *Impact of work on older adults* (pp. 207–234). New York: Springer Publishing.

Spence, M. A. (1974). Job market signaling. *Quarterly Journal of Economics, 87,* 355–374.

Sturman, M. C. (2004). Searching for the inverted u-shaped relationship between time and performance: Meta-analyses of the experience/performance, tenure/performance, and age/performance relationships. *Journal of Management, 29,* 609–640.

Wahl, H.-W., & Mollenkopf, H. (2003). Impact of everyday technology in the home environment on older adults' quality of life. In N. Charness & K. W. Schaie (Eds.), *Impact of technology on successful aging* (pp. 215–241). New York: Springer Publishing.

Waldman, D. A., & Avolio, B. J. (1986). A meta-analysis of age differences in job performance. *Journal of Applied Psychology, 71,* 33–38.

Weller, C. E. (2006). Gambling with retirement: Market risk implications for social security privatization. *Review of Radical Political Economics, 38,* 334–344.

Wilson, D. J. (2002). Is embodied technological change the result of upstream R&D? Industry-level evidence. *Review of Economic Dynamics, 5,* 342–362.

9

No Career for You: Is That a Good or Bad Thing?

DAVID J. EKERDT

For 55 years, from the ages of 19 to 74, Jim Glynn worked for the same employer, the Kansas City Livestock Exchange. At this site in the West Bottoms of the Kansas and Missouri Rivers, live cattle from the Great Plains were funneled into meat-processing plants to provision the tables of 20th century America. The Kansas City facility, second only to Chicago's in size, was served by 16 railroads in its heyday. Each workday, Jim arose in his city neighborhood, put on his boots, took his whip, and drove down to the stockyards to herd cattle. As a yard foreman, he worked outdoors and directed the unloading of railcars and trucks, sending livestock down a maze of alleys into pens for auction or sale. If you ate meat any time between 1920 and 1975, the odds are good that Jim Glynn saw your meal trot by. But by the time he retired, the stockyard's business had already dropped off, and it closed in 1991.

Up the hill in more elegant environs, Jim's sister Bernadine Glynn began work at Harzfeld's in Petticoat Lane, the premier salon for women's famous-label couture in Kansas City. Her career with this concern would last over 50 years. She was initially a seamstress, then a fashion buyer, and eventually head of alterations at the shop, selecting clothes and advising on style and fit for Harzfeld's select clientele. In the course of her career, she could point to women in the society pages and proudly identify the ones she had "dressed." Harzfeld's underwent ownership changes beginning in the 1970s, and it closed in 1984. Bernadine was asked to stay on when the store's business migrated to Bonwit Teller, but she declined to remain for another ownership change 7 years later, retiring in 1991 at the age of 80.

Steady employment lasting for decades at a single job in a single place now seems a dated practice, like urban stockyards and ladies' dress salons.

In this chapter, I will visit and develop a theme from Volume 10 of the Social Structures and Aging series, titled *The Impact of Work on Older Adults*, edited by K. Warner Schaie and Carmi Schooler, which appeared midway through the two-decade series. The theme emerged directly in two of that volume's six presentations and their associated commentaries: the chapter by Farr, Tesluk, and Klein (1998) about work environments for older workers and the chapter by Sørenson (1998) about labor markets and the careers of older workers. Because the conference was focused on the changing nature of work, the theme was also a back-story for most of the volume's other articles. My own contribution to that conference (Ekerdt, 1998) described how organizational structures shape individual expectations about the future, a notion that is also consistent with the matter to be discussed here.

The theme that was more or less explicit in Volume 10 was the erosion of long-term work careers—how stable, predictable employment was growing less available to current workers and oncoming cohorts. The text that crystallized the idea for me was the following passage, cited by Marshall (1998), from a focus group interview, during which a human resources manager at a large insurance firm said,

> The word career has been stricken literally from all Human Resources Development material. So after 23 years with a company, what do you have? You're not allowed to have a career any more because your job is, you know, could be eliminated tomorrow. . . . Career is taboo, you can't even say the word when you're discussing it with someone, you cannot talk career; you cannot have the word career in documentation because there are no careers here anymore; and that's been very clearly spelled out to everyone. (p. 199)

Marshall's (1998) informant and the other authors in Volume 10 were referring to a trend that had been underway in the American economy for about 20 years. This chapter begins by bringing the story up-to-date: how organizational restructuring has changed employment relationships, job stability, and job security. Next is a consideration of how work careers matter for individual lives. What does it afford one to possess, or expect to possess, a stable location in the social structure? Is there a positive way to regard the more episodic work careers of today? The chapter concludes with a note of concern about the consequences when work is less secure.

At the outset, it is important to clarify the term *career*. It literally means "the course over which a thing runs." *Career* is a common term in life course research, loosely interchangeable with the idea of a pathway or trajectory, all of which denote a sequence of experiences or roles. These component segments have durations, with special attention paid to the transitions between segments. The career sequence may also have identifiable occasions of entry and exit (Elder, Johnson, & Crosnoe, 2004). One can be said to have a family career, or a consumer career, or an illness career. Careerlike series of experience are the timbers and joists of the life course perspective. One other point of usage is that the career (or trajectory or pathway) can be seen alternately as the experience of the individual—a biography, if you will—or as a feature of social structure, a recognizable pattern to be followed.

Career is most conventionally used to describe a sequence of work or employment experience, and that is the domain addressed here. There is a prescriptive and a neutral way to talk about work careers (Spilerman, 1977). In the prescriptive sense, a *career* is an orderly progression through positions of increasing responsibility or rewards, typically occurring within a firm that offers a career ladder and chances for promotion as part of a so-called internal labor market (Rosenfeld, 1992). This narrow usage of the term omits many kinds of employment opportunity and experience, and so there is a more neutral way to talk about work careers as including all sorts of job histories, ones with and without unilineal progression and ones that may unfold across organizational and industrial boundaries.

Relaxing the assumption that a work career must consist of progressive promotions, there is a further useful contrast to be made between *career* and *career line*. Following Spilerman (1977), a *career* is an individual's job history. A *career line* is an empirical regularity in the labor market, a sequence of jobs in which there is a high probability of movement from one position to another. Thus the worker has a career by occupying an institutionalized career line. The distinction is relevant here because what the authors of Volume 10 saw was the reduced availability of career lines.

Among other things—and it is possible to examine many aspects of careers, such as how they are gained, how they end, what direction or form they take—the feature of interest here is the way that they afford the workers the expectation of ongoing employment: steady work, job stability, security. The contract between employer and employee might be explicit or implicit on this point, but workers with career-line jobs count on continuity. The expectation of ongoing employment is likewise shared with others in the jobholder's social network, and so the enduring nature of the employment relationship is a kind of symbolic life course—an outlook about the way that life will go (Dannefer & Uhlenberg, 1999).

As already noted, the prescriptive view of career lines as role sequences within a single organization is somewhat narrow. Yet career lines of this type are the most conceivable. These are typically so-called standard work arrangements, which Kalleberg (2000) characterized as work done on a full-time basis that continues indefinitely and is performed at the employer's place of business under the employer's control. But it is also possible to have a career of steady predictable employment in nonstandard jobs, a category that includes part-time and contract work, and also self-employment. Workers in some occupations have knowledge and skills that are in high demand, which afford them control over their conditions of work. This human capital can be carried from organization to organization, even industry to industry (Kalleberg, 2003). One thinks of an occupation such as nursing in this regard. A career as a nurse can and often does cross many different settings (Robinson, Murrells, & Marsland, 1997).

Whether in standard or nonstandard work arrangements, the reduced availability of stable employment in the U.S. economy is seen to have begun in the 1970s. The authors of Volume 10, as they concentrated on the way that work structures affect individual lives, were observing a trend under way for 20 years. A decade later, the ebbing of long-term security has not reversed.

ORGANIZATIONAL RESTRUCTURING

A century ago, it would have been unremarkable for one's working years to be marked by intermittent or part-time work, punctuated by spells of unemployment. Today, this is called *contingent work*, so named because the employment is not expected to continue (Polivka & Nardone, 1989). But what was already in motion a century ago was the rise of steady work (Jacoby, 2004; Uchitelle, 2006). Industrial capitalism had begun to institute labor practices that would mobilize workers for mass production, especially in the period after World War II. Large hierarchical organizations extended good wages and job security in return for labor's acceptance of employer control. Regimes of stability and routinization became the norm for blue- and white-collar work (R. Hall, 1982). Of course, certain segments of the American population never had a shot at these career jobs with their living wages, long-term employment contracts, paid vacations, pensions, and company-provided health insurance. It must also be said that workers and critics pushed back against routinization, conformity, and the gaze of the efficiency expert. Bureaucracy, by turns, could oppress workers, but it also protected them (Sennett, 2006).

And then, in the 1970s, the organization of work began to change. The story has several skeins (Harrison & Bluestone, 1988; Mishel, Bernstein & Schmitt, 2001; Schor, 1991). Foreign competition challenged U.S. hegemony in production and manufacturing, aided now by the demise of fixed exchange rates for major currencies. Oil embargoes slowed economic growth and raised unemployment. New economic thinking favored market forces over government solutions and led to the deregulation of entire industries and weaker labor laws. So-called impatient capital bullied organizations into cost-cutting (Harrison, 1994). Spates of acquisitions, divestitures, and mergers spread the specter of layoffs now to the ranks of white-collar workers. New kinds of communication and information technologies allowed firms to decentralize functions, while maintaining effective control over production and service processes.

What resulted were workplaces designed strategically to be more responsive to changing conditions and demands. They were marked by flexibility of two kinds (Smith, 1997). *Functional flexibility*, in theory, asked employees to become more involved in task design, decision making, and training and hence more engaged in securing organizational outcomes. The other kind, *numerical flexibility*, had organizations committing themselves to a smaller core workforce, while externalizing (outsourcing) more tasks among contingent, part-time, and contract workers (Kalleberg, 2000). As this occurred—the increasing segmentation of the workforce into those with core versus peripheral (internal vs. external) employment—the verb *downsize* came into common parlance. It was originally applied in the mid-1970s to describe the redesign of automobiles but soon came to describe the refashioning of the company or business itself, and has eventually become a euphemism for dismissals and layoffs.

Thinking in terms of pyramidal bureaucracy, the reorganized work structure is flatter (delayered) in the sense that it has fewer levels of hierarchy. And it is narrower, with workers—human resources—regarded like other resources and materials, to be acquired or shed as conditions dictate (Farr et al., 1998). Yet the reengineered firm still needs to produce goods and services, still needs to respond to customers, but it does so using more contingent and nonstandard work arrangements (Cappelli, 2003). These tend to be lower quality jobs that come with lower wages and fewer benefits such as health insurance and pensions. Kalleberg, Reskin, and Hudson (2000) find that such so-called bad job characteristics also correlate with their occupants' perceptions of job insecurity. (These authors also note, in fairness, that some kinds of contract work and self-employment can approximate the profile of the standard, full-time job.)

Workers not subject to flexible staffing, those who retained a place in the core workforce of the firm, are the ostensible winners of organizational restructuring, insulated from competition for their jobs within internal labor markets (Sørenson, 1998). Yet they may confront a less determinate career ladder, the task-shifting demands of functional flexibility, the scrutiny of performance-based job evaluation, and ongoing anxiety about the next round of restructuring. And the growing ranks of contingent workers should be a lesson to anyone that, as Marshall's (1998) personnel manager said, "your job could be eliminated tomorrow."

The General Social Survey (Davis & Smith, 1992) has carried a question since 1973 that has asked successive cross sections of U.S. adults whether at any time during the last 10 years, they had had a spell of unemployment that lasted as long as a month. Table 9.1 summarizes reports about exposure to monthlong unemployment at decade intervals for survey respondents who were currently working full-time. For workers in their 30s, there was an increase of 10 percentage points between the mid-1970s and mid-1980s in the proportion claiming to have had monthlong unemployment, a level of displacement experience that has not fallen back and continues to be reported up to the present. Workers in their 40s, more entrenched in the labor force, would be expected to have seen less displacement than workers in their 30s—and they did. But the secular pattern is similar: Unemployment events increased in the first decade of the period to a level that has been consistently reported since the mid-1980s. Nowadays, approximately 30% to 40% of adult full-time workers have had an experience of discontinuous employment, and these rates are one-third to one-half again higher than had been claimed 30 years ago.

Table 9.1

PERCENTAGE OF PERSONS CURRENTLY WORKING FULL-TIME RESPONDING YES TO THE QUESTION, "AT ANY TIME DURING THE LAST 10 YEARS, HAVE YOU BEEN UNEMPLOYED AND LOOKING FOR WORK FOR AS LONG AS A MONTH?"

SURVEY YEARS	AGE 30–39	AGE 40–49
1973–1974	30.3 (300)[a]	19.8 (272)
1983–1984	39.8 (437)	28.6 (276)
1993–1994	39.0 (551)	30.2 (441)
2002 and 2004	38.5 (257)	29.3 (246)

Note: Author's calculations from the General Social Survey Cumulative File (http://www. icpsr.umich.edu/cocoon/ICPSR/STUDY/04697.xml)
[a]Marginal *n* in parentheses.

Documentation of the reduced availability of career lines is not unambiguous. Smith's (1997) review concluded that while the evidence for a secular decrease in job stability is tenuous, the perception is firm that job security is on the decline. As a prominent example, in March 1996, *The New York Times* carried a multipart series on the topic titled "The Downsizing of America." It portrayed a "searing climate of insecurity" ("Downsizing and Its Discontents," 1996) among the nation's workers at all levels and ranks. Economic studies of the employment relationship, however, do not show the sharp break with historical patterns that has been implied in media and anecdotal reports. Instead, time series that describe worker–employer attachments suggest a more modest change. Average job tenures have fallen, more so among men than women, and more so among those with less education (Farber, 1995; Gross, 2006). Stevens (2005) examined the longest jobs ever held by men (ages 58–62) who were nearing the end of their careers, and her findings showed men's tenures shifting to shorter durations since 1980. Among such men surveyed in 1980 (who had work careers over the 1940s through 1970s), the median longest job had been 24 years. Among men surveyed in 2002 (work careers from the 1960s through 1990s, including the period of organizational restructuring), the median longest job was 21 years. For men with less than a high school education, the longest job went from a median of 23 to 17 years. Research reports have shown an increase in the proportion of the workforce that works part-time but prefers full-time work (Stratton, 1996; Tilly, 1996) and in the extent of employment in temporary services (Kalleberg, 2000). Surveys of firms suggested to Kalleberg (2003) that "between one third and one half of U.S. establishments have adopted some form of core-periphery labor utilization strategy" (p. 158).

Whether these developments herald a profound change in the employment relationship is a matter of argument, and various reviews have attempted to grapple with the apparent disparity between rhetoric and reality. Neumark (2000) held that "the bonds [between workers and firms] may have weakened, but they have not broken" (p. 1). Jacoby (2003) concluded that "these are changes of degree, not of kind" (p. 179).

One approach to the controversy draws a distinction between job stability as objectively measured (tenure, job loss, separations) and workers' subjective expressions of job security. Workers' anxiety about job loss, even among those who keep their jobs, and especially among the managerial class, may be driving public perceptions of change. For example, Schmidt (1999) studied workers' beliefs about job security between 1977 and 1996 and found them to be more pessimistic in the 1990s compared to the 1980s. Levels of concern about job loss had converged between blue-collar and (formerly insulated) white-collar workers. Cappelli (2003) emphasized that a stable job is not necessarily a secure one. Aggregate data on tenures can be misleading because some workers never had a long-duration job to lose. Although the economy still provides good jobs, their security has been undermined, according to Cappelli, by the volatility of product markets, which makes firms fragile; by the increasing practice of outside hiring; and by risk shifting from employer to employees, that is, declining coverage for health insurance and pensions. In all, objective and subjective data point to a change in the employment relationship since the 1970s, but how great a change remains in dispute.

Two further points are worth making. First, secular change in job stability and security have also been investigated abroad (Böckerman, 2004). Comparisons to American experience, however, are difficult because the United States, unlike European countries, has the special legal custom of *at-will employment*, where employer and employee are more free to terminate employment at any time (Muhl, 2001). Second, organizational restructuring is only one reason for short tenures and multiple-job careers. A lot of job mobility is voluntary, more so in tight labor markets, when workers hope to improve their circumstances. And part-time and temporary jobs are not necessarily unwanted. People's own choices and agency as well as social structure may keep them from steady work.

THE AFFORDANCES OF A CAREER

If the possibility of having a career-line job is receding, what might be the life course implications of this development? I next turn to outline how a career matters to the job holder and his or her social circle. If you have the presumption of indefinite employment, what do you have? I will address this question for individual lives *away* from the domain of work, though the job-specific dimensions of career experience have been a worthy area of study, including how people manage work continuity, execute the expectations of a career line, behave in the workplace, and relate to peers and supervisors (Sullivan, 1999). I suggest six lifestyle features that a career-line job may afford, though these things can and do happen in the absence of career-type employment. My contention is that steady work makes them more surely occur.

First and fundamentally, a career yields a stream of income. Not only are there reliable wages from season to season, but there is also the outlook for wage increases. In fact, people seek out career lines precisely for the advancement prospects that are scheduled into them (Spilerman, 1977). Extended tenure and/or continuous income are also the guarantors of a stronger pension position, be it for Social Security retirement benefits, the traditional defined-benefit pension, or a defined-contribution plan. Pensions, in turn, become the future stream of income that is the necessary condition for retirement. One stream begets another in a process of cumulative advantage (Dannefer, 2003).

Continuous income permits people to entertain longer horizons in their financial affairs. They can embark on extended projects of consumption or saving. Career income makes consumer debt more feasible, allowing people to borrow for immediately unaffordable items such as houses, education, and automobiles, while assuming a reasonable risk that the debt can be paid. Predictable paychecks allow people to meet insurance contracts on life and property, protecting themselves against loss. The paid vacations that can come with career jobs make leisure consumption predictable and schedulable. As for savings, a course of income reduces the need for liquidity and large amounts of cash on hand, freeing money to be tied up in longer term arrangements with more favorable rates of return.

Second, careers put a consistent footing under family life. One career stabilizes a marriage; two careers are better. The expectation of continuous employment facilitates the creation of a household, its provisioning, and its maintenance; sets a standard of living; and insulates it from the shock of financial shortfalls. Just as there is self-selection to career lines, so, too, in mating, there is self-selection to partners with career prospects. One spouse with a career backs the other one up should he or she become unemployed or want to suspend employment, experiment with jobs, or pursue an education. And should the marriage dissolve, reliable employment would provide the career holder with financial autonomy for the split.

Steady work makes more conceivable one of the most serious extended projects of the life course: raising children. Therefore we should expect careers to have a positive effect on family formation and to govern its timing. At the same time, once parenthood is launched, dual-career households would be more likely to limit the number of children. Parents with long-term employment can be a role model for children, helping socialize them to the value of deferred gratification, commitment, and moderation—an ethic that fits children for educational attainment. Adults with careers also lend their spouses and family members a stable status in the wider community. The child that can say, "I'm the one whose mother is . . ." or "I'm the one whose father works at . . ." has a socially handy way to matter, fit, be named, and be remembered. The parental career that anchors and stabilizes the family is ultimately an important mechanism for the intergenerational transmission of advantage.

Whereas careers may be a boon for marital and family life, they do not benefit every relationship and responsibility, as, for example, when their demands compete with family roles. Women's work careers, in particular, have been seen to reduce the availability of adult children for caregiving to older relatives.

Third, a work career requires a regime for the body. The simple act of daily presenting oneself at a workplace, ready for the functions of the job, calls out patterns of behavior that generally tend to preserve well-being. I say this while acknowledging that there is plenty of dangerous, stressful, and fatiguing work—albeit steady—that can do a body harm. At the least, the need to show up every day limits the more self-abusive practices. But more, the discipline of daily work probably raises the likelihood of better hygiene regarding personal cleanliness, sleep, diet, exercise, recreational drugs, self-medication, driver safety, and sexual practices. The extent to which routine work contributes to moderation can be easily imagined by the frequency of the evening-ending announcement, "I've got to get up for work in the morning." To manage a consistent appearance of being ready and able, workers may need to train or groom themselves in certain ways, to keep themselves together. On occasion, the need to show work commitment and fitness may be a motivation to rebound from illness. Practices of self-care and preservation are aided by steady income from a career and the health insurance benefits that such jobs are likely to carry for the purchase of products and services and for access to health care and fitness facilities.

Fourth, long-term jobs invite geographic stability (with the notable exception of career sequences that require frequent place moves). Strong employment prospects help secure better terms for a home mortgage. With property ownership and continuity in place comes commitment to the community and its implications for economic life, schools, churches, civic organizations, and customs. Place affiliation then may discourage job seeking elsewhere. Community roots deepen further when they come to be valued by one's own children as they make their life choices. When the next generation stays, it reinforces the prospects for mobilizing emotional and instrumental support within the family. Altogether, the advantages of residential settledness are particularly apparent when it is disrupted, for example, by the departure of the industry from a one-industry town.

Fifth, careers weave people into social networks. In his commentary in Volume 10, Juster (1998) pointed out that the returns from ongoing work are not just monetary, that jobs provide a major source of social contact for life away from the workplace. These relationships afford what Juster calls *flows of utility* in the form of information, material assistance, socialization, affection, leisure enjoyment, and integration into the community. The implication into community institutions that comes with geographic stability, noted earlier, is also an entrée into systems of social relationship that likewise have economic and cultural value.

Sixth, a work career is a stream of identity. Belonging at work is a basis for self-definition in a number of ways. One can credit oneself as reliable and steadfast, perhaps to the principle of work, perhaps to coworkers, or even to the employer. One may credit oneself as a capable and confident performer in an occupational role—as a stockyard foreman or a fashion buyer. One may credit oneself as an instrument for the ends of the work enterprise—a contributor. These identities are portable away from the job, ideas of one's self against which other identities can lean: spouse, parent, consumer, neighbor, friend, member, citizen. With an ongoing way to locate oneself in some field of human affairs, it is possible then to have a self-story, a narrative that makes sense of the flow of experience. According to Sennett (1998), "narratives are more than simple chronicles of events; they give shape to the forward movement of time, suggesting reasons why things happen, showing their consequences" (p. 30). This sustained interpretive resource becomes yet another basis for feeling subjectively secure.

To recapitulate, the affordances of reliable work organize life in a durable way and, in so doing, reinforce one another. Two things must be emphasized at this point. First, this life course pattern does not happen automatically. It requires suitable role performance over time at work, at home, and in the community. There are many ways in which the entire project can come off the rails. Career lines underpin an opportunity structure for lives away from work but do not guarantee it. Second, it would be wrong to conclude that workers who lack career-line jobs have chaotic lives. They, too, can earn income year in and year out, keep themselves together, form and maintain households, settle down in a place, have social support, and fix on ways to define themselves. My contention is that career-challenged adults pursue the tasks of the life course with less certainty of fulfillment than if reliable work steadied the project.

RESILIENCE AND INDIVIDUAL RESPONSIBILITY

If an era of more episodic employment has arrived—or returned, taking the longer historical view—is there a positive way to frame the matter? Indeed, the wave of corporate restructuring has spawned an ample supply of advice about how to cope.

In a labor market with fewer career lines, just as in one with more career lines, the structure leads individuals to develop or accentuate certain capacities. Sørenson (1998) noted in Volume 10 that so-called internal workforce arrangements insulate employees from competition for their jobs. The flexible organization model, on the other hand, exposes more individuals to outside labor markets. Unprotected by a bureaucratic regime, their wages depend more directly on individual productivity and performance. To sustain or improve their incomes, they must be ready to move to another job (if not first moved out). Work histories characteristically fill out with multiple jobs and lateral moves. One significant implication of this model for aging workers is that wages are not likely to grow beyond middle age (Belous, 1990).

To swim in these choppier waters, career management specialists advise adults to a lifetime habit of adaptability, rather than organizational conformity. The pieces by Farr et al. (1998) and by Howard (1998) in Volume 10 conveyed this counsel. Workers should embrace reinvention, renewal, and self-direction, developing the meta-skill of learning how to learn. As individuals shoulder the responsibility for career management, they benefit themselves with a protean, or malleable, career. Early in the era of organizational restructuring, D. T. Hall (1976) defined the *protean career* as "a process which the person, not the organization, is managing. It consists of all the person's varied experiences in education, training, work in several organizations, changes in occupational field, and so forth" (p. 106). This is more than simply piecing together a series of jobs. One builds, as personal needs demand, a portfolio of skills by apprenticing to and mastering a situation, and then starting the cycle again (D. T. Hall & Mirvis, 1995). In the protean career, employment is tied less to maturity, experience, and fit with the organization and more to the fitness that one can maintain over time. This means constantly seeking ways to put oneself in line to be taken up by the restless, ever-tacking employer who is in the market for contract or contingent workers. It means more networking. When migration from position to position is the norm, then there is no shame in termination; it can be valued for the reskilling opportunity that it presents. Self-regard and identity flow not from organizational roles and their requirements, but from the intrinsic satisfactions of having mastered challenges and shown initiative.

Employees, even core employees, can be guided to this way of thinking, in the first place, by disabusing them of any notion that their job is guaranteed. Marshall's (1998) informant cited previously had thus been leveled with: "Career is taboo, you can't even say the word." Firms, moreover, are encouraged to motivate workers toward self-development and continuous learning. One way is to expose them to diverse assignments and experiences (via functional flexibility) so that learning how comes to be second nature. When the job ends, as it will, the individual will possess a wider array of knowledge and skills to carry to the next situation, with less embarrassment about having to do so. Rather than being at the mercy of employers, workers can maintain a sense of control if they anticipate and prepare for the inevitable turn of events. In this way, the proactive individual is an analogue of the flexible firm itself—both surviving by being nimble, risk taking, and responsive to change.

The extent to which the episodic career is preferable to a routinized one, about this one can get a good argument (Micklethwait & Wooldridge, 1996; Uchitelle, 2006). Frequent job mobility results in more lateral moves, wage plateaus, and fewer benefits. Instead of generating self-regard for having shown initiative and responsibility, people may be vulnerable to self-blame (Ehrenreich, 2005). Some point out, however, that flexible work arrangements can benefit older workers, providing the part-time and bridge jobs that older workers may seek (Quinn, 1999). Because bureaucracies and seniority systems typically discount experience, flexible organizations could offer senior workers real challenge and responsibility—without the ageism (Farr et al., 1998). And a more fluid labor market could be beneficial to all ages, freeing up positions in which long-tenured workers had hunkered down.

The career management advisors are either apologists for flexible employment schemes (this is the way it should be) or pragmatists (this is how it is—deal with it). In thinking about episodic employment and its desirability, it is also interesting to recall the work of another participant in Volume 10, Matilda White Riley.

Riley, Kahn, and Foner (1994) discussed life course patterns of work engagement in their volume on age and structural lag. As the argument goes, social structures have lagged behind the reality of increased longevity. In particular, people at young and old ends of the age spectrum still have limited role opportunities: the young segregated within educational roles and the old relegated to leisure. The adults in between mainly work, and this comprises a picture of an age-differentiated, three-box life (Riley & Riley, 1994). Imagine, instead, an age-integrated social structure that spreads education, work, and leisure more evenly across the life course. The young would partake of the grown-up affair of work, and the old would sharpen their minds on education. Riley and Riley (1994) also argued the benefits of flexible structures for the middle-aged, who could intersperse work with education and leisure, experiment with new jobs, and use these work absences to accommodate family roles. However, time freed from work, even by part-time jobs, has a cost: "To be sure, reducing the hours of paid work can entail reductions in income and loss of benefits" (p. 27). Somehow, though, this cycling in and out will make work matter less as a basis for judging one's worth:

> Working part-time or starting over in new careers, since they typically mean accepting periods of reduced income or loss of benefits, now tend to be regarded as signs of failure—but not so under age-integrated conditions.

Flexible structures place less value on economic competition and comparative achievement and more on responsibilities and other rewards—affection from family and friends, respect from the community, esteem for contributions to science and the arts, recognition for personal fulfillment. (p. 30)

Riley and Riley (1994) clearly esteem the flexible life course over the rigid (male) life course that has people employed for decades at a stretch. Their optimism notwithstanding, these authors seem to assume that the coming and going from work roles will all be voluntary, matters of individual agency. And there is an assumption that the work organizations can readily be reentered. We are, in fact, seeing a version of the age-integrated work career with intermittent time off, retraining, and reskilling, but in many cases, it is not the individual, but the structure, that has scheduled the sabbatical. Reinvention and second acts are much admired as life course turns, but what we have at present with downsizings, layoffs, and displacements is structural liberation as a consequence of people being set adrift.

CONCLUSION

The U.S. economy still offers career-line jobs, but there are fewer of them, and they are less secure than a generation ago. Recent figures on the duration of jobs (Bureau of Labor Statistics, 2006) described the experience of young adults (born 1957–1964) up through 2004, a group that continued to have large numbers of short-duration jobs as they approached middle age. Among all jobs started by persons aged 31–35, only 18% were ongoing (same employer) 5 years later. Among all jobs started between ages 36 and 40, only 28% were ongoing 5 years later. (There was scant difference in the job durations of men and women.) The 30s are the decade of life when adults establish themselves as spouses, parents, householders, and participants generally in the institutions of society. Here begin the trajectories for middle age and later life, and only a minority of the cohort reported here were able to gain the anchor of long-term employment once in their 30s.

There are things to be said for steady work, and they can be summarized by observing that long-term employment lets people plan and helps things cumulate: wealth, relationships, identity, and values. At the same time, routine can trap and dull human development and possibility. So, on one hand, let us acknowledge the benefits of a more improvisational life course. In new flexible work systems, individuals have the opportunity, through initiative and self-development, to locate the work arrangements that best suit their needs, especially the demands of family life. And who knows? Their enterprise and experimentation may land a long-term job. On the other hand, the entrepreneurial, self-managed career is continually on the lookout for the next chance, a circumstance that truncates the possibility of sustained relationships.

There is a smaller prospect today for work careers such as were held by Jim and Bernadine Glynn, brother and sister, whose courses of life coincided with the mid-20th-century opportunity for lifetime jobs. If I had a wish for cohorts entering the labor force now, I would wish first that they had such a chance for such roles, but also the agency to reject a continuous, one-job career in favor of an age-integrated life course that weaves in time out for leisure and education.

The authors of Volume 10 pondered the impact of work structures on individual lives. I have earlier cited Richard Sennett's (1998) attention to *narrative*, the self-story that functions over time as an interpretive resource. When work institutions no longer provide a sustained frame for this, when instability is the new normal, when employees learn the values of detachment and superficial cooperation, how, asks Sennett, do individual lives attempt coherence?

> How can long-term purposes be pursued in a short-term society? How can durable social relations be sustained? How can a human being develop a narrative of identity and life history in a society composed of episodes and fragments? (p. 26)

The concern is not only for the coherence of individual lives, but also for community, which requires loyalty and commitment. If work matters less for our life project of understanding what we mean and how we matter and where we belong, then something else will have to matter more—perhaps family, perhaps religion, or political ideology, or consumerism. Identity, in the end, will be ribbed by something.

REFERENCES

Belous, R. S. (1990). Flexible employment: The employer's point of view. In P. B. Doeringer (Ed.), *Bridges to retirement: Older workers in a changing labor market* (pp. 111–129). Ithaca, NY: ILR Press.

Böckerman, P. (2004). Perception of job instability in Europe. *Social Indicators Research, 67,* 283–314.

Bureau of Labor Statistics. (2006). *Number of jobs held, labor market activity, and earnings growth among the youngest baby boomers: Results from a longitudinal survey.* Retrieved February 1, 2007, from http://www.bls.gov/nls/nlsy79r19.pdf

Cappelli, P. (2003). Career jobs are dead. In O. S. Mitchell, D. S. Blitzstein, M. Gordon, & J. F. Mazo (Eds.), *Benefits for the workplace of the future* (pp. 203–225). Philadelphia: University of Pennsylvania Press.

Dannefer, D. (2003). Cumulative advantage/disadvantage and the life course: Cross-fertilizing age and social science theory. *Journals of Gerontology, Ser. A, 53,* S327–S337.

Dannefer, D., & Uhlenberg, P. (1999). Paths of the life course: A typology. In V. L. Bengtson & K. W. Schaie (Eds.), *Handbook of theories of aging* (pp. 306–326). New York: Springer Publishing.

Davis, J. A., & Smith, T. W. (1992). *The NORC General Social Survey: A user's guide.* Thousand Oaks, CA: Sage.

"Downsizing and its discontents." (1996). *New York Times,* March 10.

Ehrenreich, B. (2005). *Bait and switch: The (futile) pursuit of the American dream.* New York: Metropolitan Books.

Ekerdt, D. J. (1998). Workplace norms for the timing of retirement. In K. W. Schaie & C. Schooler (Eds.), *Impact of work on older adults* (pp. 101–123). New York: Springer Publishing.

Elder, G. H., Jr., Johnson, M. K., & Crosnoe, R. (2004). The emergence and development of life course theory. In J. T. Mortimer & M. J. Shanahan (Eds.), *Handbook of the life course* (pp. 3–19). New York: Springer Publishing.

Farber, H. S. (1995). *Are lifetime jobs disappearing? Job duration in the United States: 1973–1993* (Working Paper No. 5014). Cambridge, MA: National Bureau of Economic Research.

Farr, J. L., Tesluk, P. W., & Klein, S. R. (1998). Organizational structure of the workplace and the older worker. In K. W. Schaie & C. Schooler (Eds.), *Impact of work on older adults* (pp. 143–185). New York: Springer Publishing.

Gross, D. (2006, September 10). Behind that sense of job insecurity. *The New York Times,* Sect. 3, p. 4.

Hall, D. T. (1976). *Careers in organizations.* Glenview, IL: Scott, Foresman.

Hall, D. T., & Mirvis, P. H. (1995). Careers as lifelong learning. In A. Howard (Ed.), *The changing nature of work* (pp. 322–361). San Francisco: Jossey-Bass.

Hall, R. (1982). The importance of lifetime jobs in the U.S. economy. *American Economic Review, 72,* 716–724.

Harrison, B. (1994). *Lean and mean: The changing landscape of corporate power in the age of flexibility.* New York: Basic Books.

Harrison, B., & Bluestone, B. (1988). *The great U-turn: Corporate restructuring and the polarizing of America.* New York: Basic Books.

Howard, A. (1998). Commentary: New careers and older workers. In K. W. Schaie & C. Schooler (Eds.), *Impact of work on older adults* (pp. 235–245). New York: Springer Publishing.

Jacoby, S. M. (2003). Are career jobs headed for extinction? In O. S. Mitchell, D. S. Blitzstein, M. Gordon, & J. F. Mazo (Eds.), *Benefits for the workplace of the future* (pp. 178–202). Philadelphia: University of Pennsylvania Press.

Jacoby, S. M. (2004). *Employing bureaucracy: Managers, unions, and the transformation of work in the 20th century* (Rev. ed.). Mahwah, NJ: Erlbaum.

Juster, F. T. (1998). Commentary: Career trajectories and the older worker. In K. W. Schaie & C. Schooler (Eds.), *Impact of work on older adults* (pp. 246–251). New York: Springer Publishing.

Kalleberg, A. L. (2000). Nonstandard employment relations: Part-time, temporary, and contract work. *Annual Review of Sociology, 26,* 341–365.

Kalleberg, A. L. (2003). Flexible firms and labor market segmentation: Effects of workplace restructuring on jobs and workers. *Work and Occupations, 30,* 154–175.

Kalleberg, A. L., Reskin, B. F., & Hudson, K. (2000). Bad jobs in America: Standard and nonstandard employment relations and job quality in the United States. *American Sociological Review, 65,* 256–278.

Marshall, V. W. (1998). Commentary: The older worker and organizational restructuring: Beyond systems theory. In K. W. Schaie & C. Schooler (Eds.), *Impact of work on older adults* (pp. 195–206). New York: Springer Publishing.

Micklethwait, J., & Wooldridge, A. (1996). *The witch doctors: Making sense of the management gurus.* New York: Times Books.

Mishel, L., Bernstein, J., & Schmitt, J. (2001). *The state of working America.* Ithaca, NY: Cornell University Press.

Muhl, C. J. (2001). The employment-at-will doctrine: Three major exceptions. *Monthly Labor Review, 12,* 3–11.

Neumark, D. (2000). Change in job stability and job security: A collective effort to untangle, reconcile, and interpret the evidence. In D. Neumark (Ed.), *On the job: Is long-term employment a thing of the past?* (pp. 1–31). New York: Russell Sage Foundation.

Polivka, A. E., & Nardone, T. (1989). On the definition of "contingent work." *Monthly Labor Review, 112,* 9–16.

Quinn, J. F. (1999). *Retirement patterns and bridge jobs in the 1990s* (Issue Brief No. 206). Washington, DC: Employee Benefit Research Institute.

Riley, M. W., Kahn, R. L., & Foner, A. (Eds.). (1994). *Age and structural lag: Society's failure to provide meaningful opportunities in work, family, and leisure.* New York: Wiley Interscience.

Riley, M. W., & Riley, J. W., Jr. (1994). Structural lag: Past and future. In M. W. Riley, R. L. Kahn, & A. Foner (Eds.), *Age and structural lag: Society's failure to provide meaningful opportunities in work, family, and leisure* (pp. 15–36). New York: Wiley Interscience.

Robinson, S., Murrells, T., & Marsland, L. (1997). Constructing career pathways in nursing: Some issues for research and policy. *Journal of Advanced Nursing, 25,* 602–614.

Rosenfeld, R. A. (1992). Job mobility and career processes. *Annual Review of Sociology, 18,* 39–61.

Schmidt, S. R. (1999). Long-run trends in workers' beliefs about their own job security: Evidence from the General Social Survey. *Journal of Labor Economics, 17,* S127–S141.

Schor, J. B. (1991). *The overworked American.* New York: Basic Books.

Sennett, R. (1998). *The corrosion of character: The personal consequences of work in the new capitalism.* New York: W. W. Norton.

Sennett, R. (2006). *The culture of the new capitalism.* New Haven, CT: Yale University Press.

Smith, V. (1997). New forms of work organization. *Annual Review of Sociology, 23,* 315–339.

Sørenson, A. B. (1998). Career trajectories and the older worker. In K. W. Schaie & C. Schooler (Eds.), *Impact of work on older adults* (pp. 207–234). New York: Springer Publishing.

Spilerman, S. (1977). Careers, labor market structure, and socioeconomic achievement. *American Journal of Sociology, 83,* 551–593.

Stevens, A. H. (2005). *The more things change the more they stay the same: Trends in long-term employment in the United States, 1969–2002* (Working Paper No. 11878). Cambridge, MA: National Bureau of Economic Research.

Stratton, L. S. (1996). Are "involuntary" part-time workers indeed involuntary? *Industrial Labor Relations Review, 49,* 522–536.

Sullivan, S. E. (1999). The changing nature of careers: A review and research agenda. *Journal of Management, 25,* 457–484.

Tilly, C. (1996). *Half a job: Bad and good part-time jobs in a changing labor market.* Philadelphia: Temple University Press.

Uchitelle, L. (2006). *The disposable American: Layoffs and their consequences.* New York: Alfred A. Knopf.

Commentary: New Employment Structures—Varieties of Impact on Aging Workers

10

JAMES L. FARR AND ALEXANDER R. SCHWALL

Almost everything about the nature of work has been changing in dramatic ways over the past several decades, as many authors have noted (e.g., Charness, this volume; Ekerdt, this volume; Howard, 1995; Schaie & Schooler, 1998). Continued change is almost a sure bet, and organizational scholars (e.g., Lawler, 2007) argue that organizations must both develop cultures that embrace change and align their financial, technological, and human resource systems and procedures to encourage innovation and adaptability. We focus here on selected implications of work-related change for aging workers, based on themes that emerged from our reading of the chapters by Charness and Ekerdt.

The first broad theme that we use to organize our thoughts is that primary responsibility for many aspects of work life continues to shift from the employing organization to the individual employee. The second is that changes in organizational and socioeconomic structures, made possible by enhanced technology, represent both opportunities for and threats to employee career success. Third, individual differences in the capacities needed to take advantage of career opportunities and to deflect career threats result in highly varied sets of outcomes for employees. These three themes have clear links to each other, and our discussion reflects these interconnections. We emphasize their implications for today's older workers and offer a few speculations regarding future older workers.

CAREERS AND CAREER LINES

Perhaps no work-related factor is more affected by the confluence of individual responsibility, technological and structural change, and employee capacities than career planning and management. Following Ekerdt, we define a *career* as the job history of an individual and a *career line* as a sequence of jobs in the labor market, in which the empirical probability of moving from one job to the next one in the sequence is high. Ekerdt notes that career lines are fewer today than previously as organizations have downsized, become flatter (fewer hierarchical levels), outsourced more functions to other firms, and utilized more temporary and contract (fixed-term) workers, and as technological introductions have resulted in frequent and short-lived changes in employee skill requirements. Less stability and predictability in skill requirements have reduced the extent to which organizations provide employee training and development at company expense and on company time. Employees must now be concerned with and responsible for their personal employability, that is, their attainment of required job skills for current and future jobs.

Ekerdt notes that both traditional career lines and *episodic* careers (characterized by less predictability, increased organizational transitions, and more self-direction) have potential advantages and disadvantages for the employee. We consider next some of the ways in which these career types can play out for older workers.

Implications for Older Workers

Ekerdt states that changes in the nature of work require both organizations and individuals to be more flexible and adaptive and further emphasizes that it is increasingly necessary for individuals to engage in career self-management to maneuver the "choppier waters" (p. 205) of the changing career. Various other authors have suggested that *protean careers* and *boundaryless careers* may be suitable strategies to stay successfully at sea, that is, to react to the less secure and more demanding requirements of today's labor market (Hall & Mirvis, 1995; O'Mahony & Bechky, 2006).

Protean and boundaryless careers are partially overlapping and have often been used interchangeably (Hall, Briscoe, & Kram, 1997). Briscoe and Hall (2006) recently attempted to clarify their similarities and differences. According to Briscoe and Hall, a protean career is characterized by two central features. First, protean careers are value driven. The employee's values and goals drive the career and provide guidance, not goals and objectives set by the organization. Second, protean careers are self-directed. The individual successfully enacting a protean career has the ability to flexibly and adaptively react to changes in work- and career-related demands. Briscoe and Hall emphasized that the protean career is primarily defined by the orientation or mind-set that a person has, not the precise shape of the career. Success in a protean career is primarily subjective in nature, measured by the individual's standards and goals, not those defined by the organization, such as rank, pay, or promotions. A protean career is not defined by a set of prescribed behaviors (Briscoe & Hall, 2006), but by an attitude toward the career that assists freedom, self-direction, and choices based on personal values.

Briscoe and Hall (2006) noted that the definition of a boundaryless career emphasizes physical and/or psychological physical mobility or change (cf. Arthur, Khapova, & Wilderom, 2005; Arthur & Rousseau, 1996). *Physical mobility* typically refers to changing organizations or changing geographic location. *Psychological mobility* refers to subjective phenomena such as self-identity, perceptions of work–family role relationships, and self-evaluations of career and work success. Thus, although most research on the boundaryless career has focused on individuals who change employers or make major occupational shifts within the same (usually large) organization, the boundaryless career encompasses more than job mobility. For example, an individual's career may be considered psychologically boundaryless when one's work-related identity is defined by individuals and organizations outside the employer (e.g., university faculty who look to their disciplinary peers for reputation and acclaim) or when an employee self-defines career success as achieving sufficient work-related flexibility to accommodate family needs (e.g., the employee can decide to work at home when a child is ill).

As noted previously, the concepts of protean and boundaryless careers have often been used synonymously in the research and applied literature. Both concepts explicitly or implicitly embrace the assumption that the modern career requires an employee who actively seeks careers and relevant skills, but who also transcends traditional boundaries such as organizational membership and career paths procured by the employer. However, neither the protean nor boundaryless career research literatures can provide clear answers to whether either form of career can accommodate older employees and meet work-related needs that are particular to an aging workforce. We do attempt to provide some partial answers by looking more closely at protean and boundaryless career research from the perspective of the older worker. Ekerdt asks, "No career for you—is that a good or a bad thing?" We agree that there is no easy answer to this question, and we suggest that the choppy waters may even be rougher than often assumed.

Like Ekerdt, we will use the general term *episodic career* in the remainder of this chapter to refer broadly to nontraditional or non-career-line careers. Ekerdt notes that nontraditional careers frequently consist of sequences or episodes of employment that may entail different employers, different occupations, and/or different skill sets. These nontraditional careers are characterized by less predictability, increased organizational transitions, and more self-direction, but may not always fit well the more specific definitions of protean or boundaryless careers. When a particular research study or conceptual paper is based more closely on protean or boundaryless career definitions, we will use the appropriate term for increased precision.

Episodic Careers and Older Workers' Skills and Competencies

Most employed persons want to succeed at their work, or at least do not want to fail. The motivations for desiring adequate or better performance are many and varied across persons, but work represents an important component of identity and is a frequent basis for social comparisons. An episodic career filled with new work demands requiring a constantly changing mix of skills and knowledge may be an exhilarating challenge for some employees, especially those who are striving to prove their worth in the world of work. Older workers who believe in their ability to learn and adapt may also be strongly motivated to show that they can learn new tricks. For other older workers, the new tasks and required skills are not opportunities, but threats to well-being, job performance, and employment security.

We believe that to understand the effects of the episodic career, it is necessary to specify how job demands are changing and how quickly skill sets become obsolete. At a conceptual level, jobs can be located on a continuum that reaches from a high rate of obsolescence to a low rate of obsolescence. At the low end, for example, is an academic position, in which knowledge and expertise accumulate and benefit the individual as he or she can draw from a larger literature to inform his or her research (Karp, 1986). At the other end is a job with a high rate of obsolescence, for example, the job of information technology (IT) professionals, who constantly have to update to fight obsolescence (Dubin, 1990). If older employees are working in occupations with low rates of obsolescence, a protean career will lead to a broad portfolio of various applicable and valuable skills, providing the employee a considerable edge in the labor market. In such situations, tenure and age may be equated with experience and marketability. Especially for individuals with high occupational commitment (Lee, Carswell, & Allen, 2000), such accumulative settings may contribute to job satisfaction and high job performance. In contrast, in settings with high rates of knowledge obsolescence, individuals may perceive the constant updating as an uphill battle, in which only current expertise is valuable. In comparison with other employees, the playing field is constantly leveled as existing skills do not provide an advantage. This environment of constant "competence destroying changes" (Ang & Slaughter, 2000, p. 310) may lead to chronic worry and stress for some employees (Tsai, Compeau, & Haggerty, 2007). If competences are continuously destroyed, age and experience do not lead to increases in expertise and competence. We conjecture that older employees may perceive less job satisfaction in such environments. This reaction is reflected in Tsai, Compeau, and Haggerty's description of an older employee in the IT industry: "This particular interviewee had witnessed technology evolution from the punch card era to today's Internet world. After undertaking migrations from one area to another for more than 20 years, this IT professional seemed to feel the limitations in his or her capacity to constantly learn new things, no matter how joyful this activity had been" (p. 399).

As highlighted by the example just provided, much of the concern about older workers within employment settings that require changing skill and knowledge sets is related to the stereotypic view that older workers are less able to learn and less motivated to learn (Maurer, Wrenn, & Weiss, 2003). Maurer et al. (2003) further noted that research has shown that these beliefs are widely held not only by older workers' managers and coworkers, but also by many older workers themselves. Possible consequences of such beliefs include fewer training and development opportunities made available to older workers by their employing organizations and less active seeking of developmental activities by older workers. Research examining organization-funded, on-the-job training and development has generally supported the existence of these consequences (Simpson, Greller, & Stroh, 2002).

However, more recent research by Greller and colleagues (e.g., Greller & Richtermeyer, 2006; Simpson et al., 2002) found different results. In particular, Simpson et al. (2002) found in a national sample that late career workers (aged 50–65) did participate less overall in developmental activities than younger individuals, but that older workers participated more than younger workers in many types of targeted human capital investment activities that develop occupation-based skills, including on-the-job computer-based training. Simpson et al. (2002) noted that most earlier research did not examine as wide a range of or as many specific training activities, and the aggregate measures that were used may have confounded the results obtained.

Simpson et al. (2002) found that older participants generally favored development activities over which they could exercise some control over the timing and place of delivery of program content. Control over the pace of instruction has also been found to be an important and consistent facilitator of older workers' learning in training programs (Callahan, Kiker, & Cross, 2003). Greller and Richtermeyer (2006) found little age-related variation in the amount of perceived support for training and development in a sample of finance and accounting professionals when they examined such support from a broad range of sources (family, coworkers, supervisor, colleagues in other organizations, and friends). An important finding was that sources outside of one's own employing organization were frequently very important both for social support and development, but also in providing information about possible developmental activities and related occupational issues.

The Episodic Career and Psychological Needs

As suggested by Ekerdt, a career may afford more than just a stream of income or financial benefits. Various authors have suggested that individuals work for reasons other than income (Friedman & Havighurst, 1954; Steers & Porter, 1979). A critical question may be if the potentially boundaryless nature of an episodic career provides other critical benefits of work such as social contacts (Sverko & Vizek-Vidovic, 1995). Social contacts have been shown to be important for development, either as mentoring relationships (Kram, 1983) or other forms of relationships (Allen & Finkelstein, 2003; Kram & Isabella, 1985). To the degree that episodic careers lead to severance of social networks, this critical affordance might get lost. Again, following Ekerdt's suggestion, episodic careers may be a double-edged sword. On one hand, a flexible employee, developing a self-managed and multifaceted career, may develop large social networks that span various departments and organizations that may allow the individual to serve as a boundary spanner (Richter, West, Van Dick, & Dawson, 2006). However, following an episodic career may come at the cost of having to leave one's immediate social support (Halbesleben, 2006), one's affective network (Totterdell, Wall, Holman, Diamond, & Epitropaki, 2004), and particularly one's mentors (Allen, Eby, Poteet, Lentz, & Lima, 2004). In addition, the aging employee in a boundaryless career setting may be cut off from his or her protégés, or more generally, those employees who the employee was supervising, instructing, or taking care of. Theory by Rau and Adams (2005) and empirical findings by Dendinger, Adams, and Jacobson (2005) indicated that generativity was a strong predictor of job satisfaction. *Generativity* describes an individual's need to pass on skills and knowledge to following generations (Mor Barak, 1995). If the mentor or the protégés are separated in the course of a boundaryless career, this affordance may be lost, as well.

Episodic Careers and Job Attitudes

Ekerdt correctly points out that successfully self-managing a protean career may be suitable to produce a stimulating work arrangement that fits the individual's needs. These circumstances may certainly be satisfying for the individual. However, maintaining a protean career may be a daunting and challenging task that not all individuals may be ready to perform, even though protean career management has been shown to have benefits. Career research has indicated that some individuals can successfully adapt to a rapidly changing economy (New Zealand) and transform their careers (Arthur, Inkson, & Pringle, 1999). A recent study of executives showed that those pursuing a boundaryless career and changing employers experienced higher increases in compensation and reached higher increases in organizational status (Cheramie, Sturman, & Walsh, 2007).

However, not all individuals may be able to successfully engage in a protean career. Raabe, Frese, and Beehr (2007) demonstrated that goal commitment, the quality of career plans, and the knowledge of one's strengths and weaknesses were predictive of the career self-management behavior. Not all participants were equally successful in this self-management behavior (e.g., seeking alternative solutions for a career plan, how actively do you work on overcoming barriers), indicating that career management may be a task that is not just a behavior that can be chosen to be performed or not to be performed, but a task that requires skill and commitment. Similarly, O'Mahony and Bechky (2006) found that contract workers in the IT industry had to have considerable skills, ranging from acquiring new skills and getting referrals to using mild forms of deception, to appear capable of doing the required job. In addition, Briscoe, Hall, and Frautschy-DeMuth (2006) showed that protean and boundaryless career orientations are correlated with personality traits such as openness to experience, learning goal orientation, and proactive personality. Hall (2004) conceptualized protean career orientation as a combination of adaptability and self-awareness, both of which are not based on volition, but rather on predisposition. In other words, some of the factors that allow an individual to have a malleable career are not malleable themselves.

Few studies have assessed whether older workers are differentially affected by the episodic career and if they are less or more capable to engage in protean or boundaryless careers. A rare empirical study (Currie, Tempest, & Starkey, 2006) suggested that, in particular, older workers may be more resistant to boundary and protean careers. In an interview study of employees of TV production companies and a pharmacological company, Currie and colleagues found that older employees who were established middle-level managers were invested in organizational careers and felt threatened by the introduction of an episodic career model. Van Buren (2003) advanced the similar notion that older workers are more physically bounded through their expanding families and therefore less interested in boundaryless careers. Again, we emphasize that the current literature does not provide clear guidance whether and how episodic, protean, and boundaryless careers differentially affect older employees. For example, in contrast to van Buren's (2003) assumption, it is conceivable that older employees, whose parents are likely to be deceased and whose children are likely to have left the house, are very mobile and able to engage in boundaryless careers. Episodic careers also have implications for older workers as they face retirement. We turn now to consider some aspects about retirement within the context of this type of career.

RETIREMENT: PLANNING, DECISION MAKING, AND EMPLOYMENT BEHAVIOR

A central need of employees as they approach retirement is to financially prepare for the time after retirement. Whereas the financial preparation may be an issue for all employees, recent survey data indicate that individuals may not consistently monitor whether retirement preparation is sufficient, so it is likely that a lack of financial resources may only be detected toward the end of one's career (Helman, Greenwald, Van-Derhei, & Copeland, 2007).

To the extent that an episodic career involves part-time work, the financial preparation for retirement may be obstructed by the fact that only rarely are part-time employees eligible for defined benefit (9% of all workers) or defined contribution retirement plans (25% of all workers) (U.S. Department of Labor & U.S. Bureau of Labor Statistics, 2006).

Similarly, among part-time employees, health care is infrequently provided by the employer (22% for part-time employees vs. 85% for full-time employees). Therefore, if episodic careers would be equated with some or much part-time employment, as suggested by Ekerdt, these employees may have more difficulty acquiring sufficient resources for retirement. Increasingly, aging employees choose bridge employment over full retirement (Adams & Rau, 2004; Rau & Adams, 2005; Weckerle & Shultz, 1999), which often constitutes some form of part-time employment. However, it is unclear whether this form of employment is suitable to provide sufficient retirement benefits, due to its transient and part-time nature.

The potentially limited access to retirement benefits in episodic careers becomes even clearer for retirement health care benefits, particularly if the episodic career resembles a boundaryless career (Arthur & Rousseau, 1996). Researchers using the term *boundaryless career* stress the fact that individuals need to be physically mobile and that the career does not take place in the same organizational setting (Briscoe & Hall, 2006; Eby, 2001). Thus, if the episodic career (Ekerdt, this volume) can be equated with a boundaryless career, retirement health care may be in jeopardy. Therefore it may be essential to understand the health care situation of older employees.

Recent survey data from AARP (Burton & Binette, 2007) suggest that access to health insurance and the qualification for retirement benefits are critical factors that drive the decision to continue working or seek new work. Concretely, the AARP survey indicated that 65% of respondents regarded access to health insurance as extremely or very important and that 56% of respondents regarded qualification for retirement benefits as very or extremely important.

However, survey data from the Employment Benefit Research Institute (Fronstin, 2006) indicate that due to changes in accounting rules in the early 1990s, employers drastically decreased their participation in retirement health care benefits. Whereas in 1997, 22% of private sector employers provided health insurance for retirees, in 2003, only 13% provided these benefits. These numbers may be even more problematic as many employers have capped their contributions, so that retirees may have to cover some of the insurance costs themselves (McArdle, Atchison, Yamamoto, Kitchman Strollo, & Neuman, 2006). Although Medicare is available in the United States to all individuals older than 65, it only covers 51% of expenses associated with health care services (Helman et al., 2007). Thus health insurance provided by employers is often important to close the gap between available and necessary health insurance. Given that health care costs can be substantial and are also frequently underestimated by those planning for retirement (Helman et al., 2007), the limited access to health care is equally likely to lead to a prolonged stay in the workforce or to a return.

In addition to the limited availability of retirement health care plans, health care benefits for retirement are often tied to employment durations. In 2004, 60% of employees had to have at least 5 years of service in the organization to qualify for retiree heath benefits. For 35% of all retirees, a person was required to be older than 55 years and employed for at least 10 years (Fronstin, 2006). These eligibility criteria may limit the feasibility of voluntary job mobility and pose structural boundaries to the otherwise boundaryless career (Arthur & Rousseau, 1996). If all retirement health care benefits are lost when service is interrupted or prematurely ended, employees are likely to prefer to remain with their current employers, regardless of job satisfaction and developmental prospects. Similar consideration may be relevant for retirement benefits in general. How likely are retirement benefits vested, and how easily can retirement plans (especially defined benefit plans) be lost when an individual exits the organization?

Immobile benefits in an episodic career setting may lead to employees being trapped in an organization, despite the fact that they would prefer to move on, either to retirement or into other organizations. Being trapped may reinforce a self-fulfilling prophecy described by Greller and Stroh (2004): Older workers may be discouraged to learn and develop, which leads older workers not to invest in development. The subsequent lack of skills reinforces younger workers' stereotypes that older workers are lacking skills. If employees are forced to stay in an organization to protect their health care eligibility but are not having a traditional, organizational career (in the sense that they are trained, developed, and promoted), it is plausible that older employees will be perceived by others in the organization as being less skilled, less up-to-date, and obsolete. Therefore, if organizations want numerically and functionally flexible workforces, as Ekerdt describes, their retirement organizational policies must provide structural prerequisites that provide a feasible alternative to the traditional, organizational career.

So far, we have described an admittedly bleak picture of the older worker in episodic careers: Workers may be trapped in unrewarding organizations, perceiving little developmental support, or alternatively, we describe them as uprooted and separated from mentors and social support. However, as we have indicated, research has not delivered an indication that episodic, protean, or boundaryless careers are any less suitable for older employees. In fact, Greller and Richtermeyer (2006) indicated that age is not a primary determinant of how much support for development an employee receives, but rather, the individual's career-related beliefs and intentions are important.

We advance the notion that for some individuals, the episodic career may indeed offer substantial benefits and opportunities. If health care and retirement benefits are locked in, and if sufficient retirement funds are available, older employees may behave freely and use the spot market of employment as an opportunity to try various jobs, without career pressure, but with the opportunity to capitalize on expertise. To summarize, episodic careers can be rewarding for older employees who can be generative through the mentoring of less experienced coworkers or subordinates and who can experience the intrinsic motivation that can be derived from relatively varied and novel work experiences. However, employees without these opportunities may find such careers to be stressful, especially if financial and health concerns exist.

Charness raises an issue that has negative implications for the ability of older workers to implement successfully an episodic career. He notes that there exists a technology gap based on age; that is, older individuals less frequently use the communication and information technologies that are common to many work settings (e.g., e-mail and the Internet). Such technologies also can facilitate an episodic career by increasing access to both information sources and social networks, which are relevant to skill development and job availability. Some recent data suggest that the current technology gap is lessening, and we look briefly at this topic.

TECHNOLOGY AND OLDER WORKERS

Recent data (Pew Internet and American Life Project, 2007) from a national sample support earlier findings that computer usage decreases substantially in older cohorts. Close to 90% of those surveyed under the age of 43 reported that they had used a computer at least occasionally in the recent past, whereas only 27% of those age 72 and older had. But more relevant to our focus on older workers, about 80% of those aged 43–61 reported computer use, as did 57% of the individuals aged 62–71. If we look more specifically at computer usage at work (excluding the youngest age range, where many respondents may be students, and the older two ranges, where many or all respondents may be out of the workforce), we see that frequent e-mail or Internet use was reported by 59% of the 31- to 42-year-olds, 57% of the 43- to 52-year-olds, and 44% of the 53- to 61-year-olds. An interesting finding from this data set is the interactive effect of education and age range on computer usage at work. While education level has a strong relation to computer use at work across the entire sample, with frequent e-mail or Internet use for about 30% of those with a high school degree or less, 39% of those with some college, 62% of those with at least a college degree, there is relatively little drop-off in usage at work for older workers with college degrees. While about 75% of those with college degrees aged 25–44 report frequent computer use at work, so do 70% of those aged 45–54 and 53% of those aged 55–64. Add to these data the finding that about 30% of the population now in their 40s and 50s have college degrees, compared to about 25% of those in their 60s (U.S. Census Bureau, 2007), and the extent of the technology gap with older workers, especially in the next decade, appears to be less serious than previously thought.

Recent research concerned with technology adoption also has promise for increasing our understanding of factors that may enable the development of effective interventions to assist older individuals with technology implementation. Czaja et al. (2006) found that level of computer self-efficacy (belief that one can successfully use computers) and computer anxiety predicted computer use. These authors also discussed types of training programs that may help to alleviate the negative impact of low efficacy and high anxiety, including programs with supportive learning environments, few time deadlines, and the provision of positive feedback about learning. Morris, Venkatesh, and Ackerman (2005) found that the adoption of a new software package in a work setting was primarily driven by perceptions of its value for enhancing work performance for older men, while older women were influenced strongly by their perceptions of whether their coworkers were adopting the software. Finally, Melenhorst, Rogers, and Bouwhuis (2006) found that the decision by older persons to adopt e-mail as a communication tool was related primarily to perceived benefits of its use and that perceived costs of its usage had little impact on the adoption decision. These findings suggest that organizations can develop effective strategies to encourage technology adoption and implementation among older workers as one way to decrease the technology divide based on age cohort.

As we thought about the chapters written by Charness and Ekerdt and about various work-related changes being discussed in the fields of industrial–organizational psychology and management, several issues not directly linked to the Charness and Ekerdt chapters emerged that we think can help direct research, theory, and practice in the coming decade, as organizations and employees continue to deal with changing and aging workforces. We close our comments with brief discussions of several of these issues.

ADDITIONAL WORKPLACE AND WORKFORCE CHANGES THAT MAY AFFECT OLDER WORKERS

Organizations face ever-increasing global competition, and many have shifted toward enhanced innovation as their primary strategy for developing and maintaining competitive advantages in their marketplaces. Innovation has been identified as more likely to be a sustainable strategic advantage for an organization in comparison to efficiency (or cost control) and quality as competitors can more easily produce an existing product for a lower cost or at higher levels of quality than bring a new product to market (Lawler, 2007). Unfortunately, what is an innovation today is a old market within a short time, so organizations and their employees must continually innovate. Innovative organizations must embrace change and make it an important value central to the culture of the organization, that is, a value whose attainment is committed to by its workforce. This will place added pressure on employees to adapt, learn, and change. These are not behavioral styles associated with stereotypes about older workers. Such stereotypes may consciously and unconsciously lead to ageist bias in organizations. With many occupations and organizations possibly facing shortages in skilled workers, as the older baby boomers begin to retire in large numbers, organizations cannot afford to reduce their potential labor pool by not considering tomorrow's older workers.

Innovation does also increase the importance of the *knowledge worker* (Lepak & Snell, 2002) for achieving organizational goals. This should benefit many older workers as research has consistently shown that job knowledge is accumulative and, further, that domain knowledge is critical for creativity and innovation (Amabile, 1983). Earlier remarks about the need to consider the time course of knowledge obsolescence in various knowledge domains are again relevant to the question of the value of previously learned knowledge for current application.

Changes in organizational structure, especially downsizing and reducing layers of hierarchy, also have variable consequences for the nature of work. A critical question following such structural changes relates to the amount of intrinsic motivation in the new jobs: Put simply, challenging, varied, and relatively whole tasks over which the employee has considerable control are more interesting and intrinsically motivating than tasks that are prescribed, routine, repetitive, and fragmented (Hackman & Oldham, 1980). With fewer people to do the work, organizations that have experienced a reduction in workforce size may follow a strategy of creating new jobs that require more decision making by the employee and offer more challenge and variety, as well. These enriched jobs are more motivating and perhaps especially attractive to older workers, whose greater experience and knowledge lead them to desire more responsibility and control over their work activities. However, organizations can also follow a strategy of just increasing the amount of work to be done by each individual, without adding responsibility and control. Increased workload often leads to stress and dissatisfaction, reducing work motivation. Since older individuals frequently have reduced capacities related to response speed, an increased workload may negatively affect them to a greater extent than younger workers.

The final organizational change that we will consider is the increased use of work teams for both day-to-day task accomplishment and for special assignments via task forces, cross-functional teams, and so on, which typically are fixed-term groups created to deal with a problem or opportunity. A concern related to older workers is that research has shown that age diversity within work groups can lead to increased conflict (Farr & Ringseis, 2002). But, as also noted by Farr and Ringseis, older workers have also been found to be higher in organization citizenship behaviors, such as helping coworkers, that should enhance team performance. At this point, we simply do not have sufficient research evidence to know whether increased use of work teams will increase or decrease the value of older workers to organizations, but this is a topic for which research is needed.

REFERENCES

Adams, G., & Rau, B. (2004). Job seeking among retirees seeking bridge employment. *Personnel Psychology, 57*, 719–744.

Allen, T. D., Eby, L. T., Poteet, M. L., Lentz, E., & Lima, L. (2004). Career benefits associated with mentoring for proteges: A meta-analysis. *Journal of Applied Psychology, 89*, 127–136.

Allen, T. D., & Finkelstein, L. M. (2003). Beyond mentoring: Alternative sources and functions of developmental support. *Career Development Quarterly, 51*, 346–355.

Amabile, T. M. (1983). The social psychology of creativity: A componential conceptualization. *Journal of Personality and Social Psychology, 45*, 357–376.

Ang, S., & Slaughter, S. A. (2000). The missing context of information technology personnel: A review and future direction for research. In R. W. Zmud (Ed.), *Framing the domain of IT management* (pp. 305–327). Cincinnati, OH: Pinnaflex Educational Resources.

Arthur, M. B., Inkson, K., & Pringle, J. K. (1999). *The new careers: Individual action and economic change.* Thousand Oaks, CA: Sage.

Arthur, M. B., Khapova, S. N., & Wilderom, C. P. M. (2005). Career success in a boundaryless career world. *Journal of Organizational Behavior, 26*, 177–202.

Arthur, M. B., & Rousseau, D. M. (1996). *The boundaryless career.* New York: Oxford University Press.

Briscoe, J. P., & Hall, D. T. (2006). The interplay of boundaryless and protean careers: Combinations and implications. *Journal of Vocational Behavior, 69*, 4–18.

Briscoe, J. P., Hall, D. T., & Frautschy-DeMuth, R. L. (2006). Protean and boundaryless careers: An empirical exploration. *Journal of Vocational Behavior, 69*, 30–47.

Burton, C., & Binette, J. (2007). *What older workers want: A survey of AARP members in New Mexico.* Retrieved November 6, 2007, from http://www.aarp.org. research/work/employment/nm_worker_06.html

Callahan, J. S., Kiker, D. S., & Cross, T. (2003). Does method matter? A meta-analysis of the effects of training method on older learner training performance. *Journal of Management, 29*, 663–680.

Cheramie, R. A., Sturman, M. C., & Walsh, K. (2007). Executive career management: Switching organizations and the boundaryless career. *Journal of Vocational Behavior, 71*, 359–374.

Currie, G., Tempest, S., & Starkey, K. (2006). New careers for old? Organizational and individual responses to changing boundaries. *International Journal of Human Resource Management, 17*, 755–774.

Czaja, S. J., Charness, N., Fisk, A. D., Hertzog, C., Nair, S. N., Rogers, W. A., et al. (2006). Factors predicting the use of technology: Findings from the Center for Research and Education on Aging and Technology Enhancement (CREATE). *Psychology and Aging, 21*, 333–352.

Dendinger, V. M., Adams, G. A., & Jacobson, J. D. (2005). Reasons for working and their relationship to retirement attitudes, job satisfaction and occupational self-efficacy of bridge employees. *International Journal of Aging and Human Development, 61*, 21–35.

Dubin, S. S. (1990). Maintaining competence through updating. In S. L. Willis & S. S. Dubin (Eds.), *Maintaining professional competence: Approaches to career enhancement, vitality, and success throughout a work life* (pp. 9–43). San Francisco: Jossey-Bass.

Eby, L. T. (2001). The boundaryless career experiences of mobile spouses in dual-earner marriages. *Group and Organization Management, 26,* 343–368.

Farr, J. L., & Ringseis, E. L. (2002). The older worker in organizational context: Beyond the individual. *International Review of Industrial and Organizational Psychology, 17,* 31–76.

Friedman, E. A., & Havighurst, R. J. (1954). *The meaning of work and retirement.* Chicago: University of Chicago Press.

Fronstin, P. (2006). *Savings needed to fund health insurance and health care expenses in retirement* (Issue Brief No. 295). Washington, DC: Employee Benefit Research Institute.

Greller, M. M., & Richtermeyer, S. B. (2006). Changes in social support for professional development and retirement preparation as a function of age. *Human Relations, 59,* 1213–1234.

Greller, M. M., & Stroh, L. K. (2004). Making the most of "late-career" for employers and workers themselves: Becoming elders not relics. *Organizational Dynamics, 33,* 202–214.

Hackman, J. R., & Oldham, G. R. (1980). *Work redesign.* Reading, MA: Addison-Wesley.

Halbesleben, J. R. B. (2006). Sources of social support and burnout: A meta-analytic test of the conservation of resources model. *Journal of Applied Psychology, 91,* 1134–1145.

Hall, D. T. (2004). The protean career: A quarter-century journey. *Journal of Vocational Behavior, 65,* 1–13.

Hall, D. T., Briscoe, J. P., & Kram, K. E. (1997), Identity, values, and learning in the protean career. In C. L. Cooper & S. E. Jackson (Eds.), *Creating tomorrow's organizations* (pp. 321–335). London: John Wiley.

Hall, D. T., & Mirvis, P. H. (1995). The new career contract: Developing the whole person at midlife and beyond. *Journal of Vocational Behavior, 47,* 269–289.

Helman, R., Greenwald, M., VanDerhei, J., & Copeland, C. (2007). *The retirement system in transition: The 2007 Retirement Confidence Survey* (Issue Brief No. 304). Washington, DC: Employee Benefits Research Institute.

Howard, A. (1995). *The changing nature of work.* San Francisco: Jossey-Bass.

Karp, D. A. (1986). Academics beyond midlife: Some observations on changing consciousness in the fifty to sixty decade. *International Journal of Aging and Human Development, 22,* 81–103.

Kram, K. E. (1983). Phases of the mentor relationship. *Academy of Management Journal, 26,* 608–625.

Kram, K. E., & Isabella, L. A. (1985). Mentoring alternatives: The role of peer relationships in career development. *Academy of Management Journal, 28,* 110–132.

Lawler, E. E., III. (2007, October). *Built for innovation: Organizational excellence in a changing world.* Paper presented at Society for Industrial and Organizational Psychology conference "Enabling Innovation in Organizations: The Leading Edge," Kansas City, KS.

Lee, K., Carswell, J. J., & Allen, N. J. (2000). A meta-analytic review of occupational commitment: Relations with person- and work-related variables. *Journal of Applied Psychology, 85,* 799–811.

Lepak, D. P., & Snell, S. A. (2002). Managing the HR architecture for knowledge-based competition. In S. E. Jackson, M. A. Hitt, & A. S. DeNisi (Eds.), *Designing strategy for effective human resource management* (pp. 127–154). San Francisco: Jossey-Bass.

Maurer, T. J., Wrenn, K. A., & Weiss, E. M. (2003). Toward understanding and managing stereotypical beliefs about older workers' ability and desire for learning and development. In J. J. Martocchio & G. R. Ferris (Eds.), *Research in personnel and human resources management* (Vol. 22, pp. 253–285). New York: Elsevier.

McArdle, F., Atchison, A., Yamamoto, D., Kitchman Strollo, M., & Neuman, T. (2006). *Retiree health benefits examined: Findings from the Kaiser/Hewitt 2006 Survey on Retiree Health Benefits* (Publication No. 7587). Menlo Park, CA: Kaiser Family Foundation.

Melenhorst, A.-S., Rogers, W. A., & Bouwhuis, D. G. (2006). Older adults' motivated choice for technological innovation: Evidence for benefit-driven selectivity. *Psychology and Aging, 21,* 190–195.

Mor Barak, M. E. (1995). The meaning of work for older adults seeking employment: The generativity factor. *International Journal of Aging and Human Development, 41,* 325–344.

Morris, M. G., Venkatesh, V., & Ackerman, P. L. (2005). Gender and age differences in employee decisions about new technology: An extension to the theory of planned behavior. *IEEE Transactions on Engineering Management, 52,* 69–84.

O'Mahony, S., & Bechky, B. A. (2006). Stretchwork: Managing the career progression paradox in external labor markets. *Academy of Management Journal, 49,* 918–941.

Pew Internet and American Life Project. (2007). *February–March tracking survey.* Retrieved November 1, 2007, from http://www.pewinternet.org/dataset_display.asp?r=64

Raabe, B., Frese, M., & Beehr, T. A. (2007). Action regulation theory and career self-management. *Journal of Vocational Behavior, 70,* 297–311.

Rau, B. L., & Adams, G. A. (2005). Attracting retirees to apply: Desired organizational characteristics of bridge employment. *Journal of Organizational Behavior, 26,* 649–660.

Richter, A. W., West, M. A., Van Dick, R., & Dawson, J. F. (2006). Boundary spanners' identification, intergroup contact, and effective intergroup relations. *Academy of Management Journal, 49,* 1252–1269.

Schaie, K. W., & Schooler, C. (1998). *Impact of work on older adults.* New York: Springer Publishing.

Simpson, P. A., Greller, M. M., & Stroh, L. K. (2002). Variations in human capital investment activity by age. *Journal of Vocational Behavior, 61,* 109–138.

Steers, R. M., & Porter, L. (1979). Work and motivation: An evaluative summary. In R. M. Steers & L. Porter (Eds.), *Motivation and work behavior* (pp. 635–644). New York: McGraw-Hill.

Sverko, B., & Vizek-Vidovic, V. (1995). Studies of the meaning of work: Approaches, models, and some of the findings. In D. E. Super & B. Sverko (Eds.), *Life roles, values, and career: International findings of the Work Importance Study* (pp. 3–21). San Francisco: Jossey-Bass.

Totterdell, P., Wall, T., Holman, D., Diamond, H., & Epitropaki, O. (2004). Affect networks: A structural analysis of the relationship between work ties and job-related affect. *Journal of Applied Psychology, 89,* 854–867.

Tsai, H.-Y., Compeau, D., & Haggerty, N. (2007). Of races to run and battles to be won: Technical skill updating, stress, and coping of IT professionals. *Human Resource Management, 46*, 395–409.

U.S. Census Bureau. (2007, March 15). *Current Population Survey, 2006 Annual Social and Economic Supplement*. Retrieved November 1, 2007, from http://www.census.gov/apsd/techdoc/cps/cpsmar06.pdf

U.S. Department of Labor & U.S. Bureau of Labor Statistics. (2006, March). National compensation survey: Employee benefits in private industry in the United States. Summary 06-05. Retrieved November 9, 2007, from http://www.bls.gov/ncs/ebs/sp/ebsm0004.pdf

Van Buren, H. J. (2003). Boundaryless careers and employability obligations. *Business Ethics Quarterly, 13*, 131–149.

Weckerle, J. R., & Shultz, K. S. (1999). Influences on the bridge employment decision among older USA workers. *Journal of Occupational and Organizational Psychology, 72*, 317–329.

Sociocultural Change and Historical Context

11

Aging, History, and the Course of Life: Social Structures and Cultural Meanings

THOMAS COLE, W. ANDREW ACHENBAUM, AND NATHAN CARLIN

A STRANGER IN A STRANGE LAND

As we were rereading the 20 volumes that constitute the series Social Structures and Aging, we felt like strangers in a strange land. We started with Volume 1, *Social Structure and Aging: Psychological Processes* (Schaie & Schooler, 1989), noting Matilda White Riley's (1989) comment that "this book is the first in a series that will be adapted from conferences on biological as well as social and psychological aging" (p. xiii). She also mentioned that the "conference grew out of several planning meetings of the Social Science Research Council," and those meetings, in turn, grew out of "10 years of work done by the Council's Committee on Life-Course Perspectives" (p. xiii). The advantage of this approach, as Riley pointed out, is that these volumes were "engaged in a scientific effort that has been and continues to be cumulative" (p. xiv).

Researchers on aging would take seriously any agenda set by Riley (cf. Achenbaum & Albert, 1995). She had been a masterful executive director of the American Sociological Association from 1949 to 1960, while affiliated with Rutgers University (1950–1973). In the mid-1960s, Riley accepted an invitation from Orville Brim, head of the Russell Sage Foundation, to undertake a summary of research findings in gerontology generated in its formative stages. (It is worth noting that Brim did not ask a gerontologist to do this task; he wanted someone he trusted, someone he knew was a tough-nosed methodologist and rigorous theorist. He knew Riley would be able to translate disparate ideas and data into an interdisciplinary agenda for framing future investigations.) It took Riley 7 years to complete the task, with the assistance of her husband, Jack, and five associates. Riley discarded most of the work published to date. She issued her report in three pathbreaking volumes under the Russell Sage imprint: *An Inventory of Research Findings* (Vol. 1, with Anne Foner, Mary Moore, Beth Hess, & Barbara Ross, 1968); *Aging and the Professions* (Vol. 2, with John W. Riley Jr., & Marilyn Johnson, 1969); and *Sociology of Age Stratification* (Vol. 3, with Marilyn Johnson & Anne Foner, 1972).

This trilogy presaged themes that set the agenda for Social Structures and Aging. The process of aging, Riley contended, was not primarily biological in nature. Nor were declines in physiological and cognitive functioning inevitable. Rather, senescence was a biological and psychosocial process open to intervention and change.

By the time Schaie was launching his series, Riley had challenged prevailing notions of the mechanisms of aging. She was well placed to do so, given her reputation, her work on the Social Science Research Council, and, since 1979, her position as associate director of the National Institute on Aging. To put it bluntly, Riley was in the innermost band of the inner circle of gatekeepers who could ensure quality control as gerontology emerged as a science.

Reading Riley enabled us to understand the estrangement we felt. These volumes were committed to a perspective and paradigm that we do not share. It is not that we disagree with the perspective and paradigm of the series, or that we are uncomfortable with this language; it is simply that we ask different questions, we think differently, and we write differently.

As we were working our way through the volumes, we noticed a standard structure of how most of the articles were written—namely, they identify a problem, survey the existing literature, propose a method (usually one psychosocial in nature) and apply it, give the results, and finally, call for more study. Then there would often be an acknowledgment for the grant that had funded the research. And while this approach yields new insights and new knowledge, it seems to leave the most important questions—that is, questions concerning *meaning*—unanswered. But such is the nature of scientific research, theoretical and empirical.

It occurred to us that our retrospective essay in this series probably would not quite fit any better than earlier attempts to insinuate historical perspectives into a scientifically grounded, theoretically driven psycho-social model. Take the two essays that two of the authors of this chapter contributed to the sixth volume of the Social Structures and Aging series, *Societal Impact on Aging: Historical Perspectives* (Schaie & Achenbaum, 1993).

Cole (1993) opted to write a biography, one of the most popular modes of historical discourse among the reading public and, increasingly, once again appealing to professional historians. "The Prophecy of *Senescence*: G. Stanley Hall and the Reconstruction of Old Age in Twentieth-Century America" delivered what its title promised: it put the ideas and languages of one of gerontology's progenitors into historical context. The repeated references to biomedical experiments in the 1920s as well as to the writings of clergy underscored Cole's characterization of Hall as a wise investigator who believed that "scientists and helping professions would become the new 'initiators' into the last stage of life" (p. 174). Cole then moved forward, teasing out Hall's legacy in basic science and social services. In so doing, the essay took a critical turn: "in spite of himself, Hall did not allow the scientific search for explanation and control to suppress his human search for meaning" (p. 177). Note that it was precisely the potentially good and bad meanings of late life that Cole wanted his audience to hear. Historians share the lessons of the past so that those in the present make different mistakes than their intellectual forebears. Hence, in his last paragraph, Cole limned a postmodern pathway, one that eschewed the mistakes that Hall made. Cole cited Martin Kohli, whose sociological work drew on the work of historians and philosophers but was aimed at social scientists who do aging-based research over the life course.

Maciel and Staudinger (1993) clearly got the message: "Cole leaves us with a dilemma: the very forces in 'professional science' to which G. Stanley Hall appealed to turn their attention toward 'the last stage of life' are proving to undercut their own purpose" (p. 182). The pair then proceeded to discuss how life span psychologists would deal with the subject matter: "Aging is more than decline [to which they devote two sections of their commentary]." Their affirmation that "different individuals age differently" leads to observations of "strategies and mechanisms of dealing with the gains and losses of aging" before concluding with a fascinating discussion of (empirical studies of) wisdom and wise personages. "The prophecy of old age has not been fully explored from a scientific vantage point," concluded Maciel and Staudinger. "It might be too early to conclude that the picture painted by science is unconvincing" (p. 192). It seems that Cole succeeded in joining the issues, but not in bridging the two cultures. Achenbaum's (1993) essay in the same volume, "(When) Did the Papacy Become a Gerontocracy?," was a more deliberate effort (by a non–Roman Catholic who knew little about church history but had spent much of his career pondering the connections between aging structures and graying individuals) to write history like psychologists and sociologists write science. He began, as do most contributions to this series, with a literature review—in this instance, comparative approaches to institutional changes that are sensitive to continuities and shifts in the demography. Taking advantage of a long temporal baseline and a wealth of historical data, he constructed biographical sketches and marked changes in the structure and power base of the papacy. His chapter included two figures plotting time lines. He ended with references to the work of other historical gerontologists and to students of wisdom.

In his comments on Achenbaum's (1993) chapter, van Tassel (1993), the dean of historical gerontologists, noticed that the subject was an unusual one for a U.S. historian to write about, but quickly added that Achenbaum (1993) knew much about gerontocracies. However, van Tassel (1993) had reservations about Achenbaum's (1993) construct and methods. Van Tassel (1993) wrote, "I am leery of numbers, for they answer few questions, although they do have the effect of raising questions" (p. 233). (It is worth noting that this comment comes from a scholar who advocated quantitative approaches to historiography but hews to the hallmark of traditional history—the posing of provocative questions.) And Van Tassel was unconvinced that bio-sketches of popes *really* yielded fruitful data on the papacy as an institution. It was a trenchant yet fair critique, which might be read as a warning about what happens when specialists stray too boldly (foolishly?) from their data, from paradigms they know, and from questions that fit the task.

Ransom (1993), an economic historian, searched for a hook. He found it in Achenbaum's (1993) references to Douglas North's pathbreaking work on comparative analyses of institutions. So, replicating Achenbaum's general strategy, Ransom (1993) traced (a) the ascension of queens and kings to the British throne since 800 and (b) the history of the U.S. presidency based on the age of incumbents on inauguration. In so doing, he found Achenbaum's (1993) analysis more robust than did van Tassel (1993), and he added some more variables to consider. But a larger issue remains: Was the original essay simply too orthogonal to the purposes of the series to contribute significantly to the advancement of science? If so, investigators face a tough paradox: Disciplinary-specific research at best reaffirms what has been done and adds to our knowledge base incrementally; radical work can provoke paradigm shifts (Kuhn, 1962), but it is more likely to miss the mark than pose new questions or shake accepted theoretical and methodological verities.

Since Achenbaum (1993) and Cole (1993) used historical methods, we could not escape the feeling that historical perspectives were not included sufficiently in these analyses—despite occasional claims for doing so. Now we do have voices saying that they are taking history into account, and they are even using some of the key words (e.g., *context*), but there is no real sense of what Geertz (1973) called *thick description*.[1] We could not help but wonder if the template of research was set in 1980—or perhaps even in 1970—with the National Institute on Aging's (NIA) blessing. Is this why, in other words, there is a certain kind of discourse in these volumes that seems, by and large, to exclude historical analysis? In point of fact, the volume that dealt with history in this series overemphasized socioeconomic perspectives—that is to say, even the volume devoted to history was committed to doing a certain kind of history, one that was driven by quantitative analyses. Now, there is no point in taking this opportunity to lament what might have been (though the flyer for this conference stated that the "speakers will review both the accomplishments and omissions of the series, as a fitting capstone for twenty years of effort and to provide guidelines for future research and theoretical explanations"). So we would like to take this opportunity, however briefly, to explore new questions for future research.

Since we consider ourselves academic humanists, the questions that we routinely deal with are perennial in nature, and one such question that we have been especially interested in is, *What Does It Mean to Grow Old?* (see Cole & Gadow, 1986). Most of the scholarship in these volumes, in contrast, is scientific and empirical in nature. In a way, it is odd to be commenting on the history of this conference for two reasons: First, we all hope, of course, that the science has evolved since we first

---

[1] In Volume 1, for example, Atchley (1989) refers to *migration history* as a factor in cognition, and Featherman (1989) invokes historical sources to note the changing context of socialization and calls this *thumbnail interpretive history*. But perhaps our point is best illustrated by a comment by Lawton (1989): "The terms *situation, milieu,* and *context* have often been used to represent aspects of environment," however, "these situations are too complex to be treated as entities" (p. 62). There are other references to history in this volume, and indeed in subsequent volumes, that we noted, but these references are enough to point out that this conference has not included historical analysis in such a way that most historians would recognize as sufficient. At best, what we have here, as Featherman noted, is thumbnail history.

began, and second, we cannot say that history has been sufficiently included in these volumes. So what does it mean for humanities scholars to look at these volumes? The title of our chapter is "Aging, History, and the Course of Life." Aging, of course, was the topic for all of these volumes, and so far in this chapter, we have argued that history has not been taken into sufficient account in these analyses, and now we want to turn to the course of life portion of our title to raise some questions for future reflection. As we come to the end of this 20-year course, what might we—primarily, Cole—have to say about the life course?

AFTER THE LIFE CYCLE

In almost 30 years of reading and writing about later life, Cole's favorite book is still a slender volume by the Catholic theologian Nouwen (Nouwen & Gaffney, 1976), titled *Aging: The Fulfillment of Life*. Like many books on aging in the 1970s and 1980s, Nouwen struggled against negative stereotypes and attitudes toward older people, offering images and ideals emphasizing our shared humanity in the universal process of growing older. The book's central motif is a large wagon wheel leaning against a birch tree in the white snow. The photo invites each of us to think of ourselves as a spoke on the great wheel of life, part of the ongoing cycle of generations. It also implies that each of us has our own cycle to traverse, a moving up and a going down, moving forward, yet also somehow returning to the beginning. Nouwen's wagon wheel resembles the Christ-centered liturgical life cycle, which his medieval forbears rendered on stained glass cathedral windows. Nouwen set the issue of a good life squarely in the province of ordinary living. Leaning heavily on Erikson's work, Nouwen wrote that our "greatest vocation" is to "live carefully and gracefully." Aging, then, becomes the gradual fulfillment of the life cycle, "in which receiving matures in giving and living makes dying worthwhile" (p. 14). With elegant simplicity, he described the three-stage life cycle as it cogwheels with previous and future generations:

> The restful accomplishment of the old wheel tells us the story of life. Entering into the world we are what we are given, and for many years thereafter parents and grandparents, brothers and sisters, friends and lovers keep giving to us, some more, some less, some hesitantly, some generously. When we can finally stand on our own feet, speak our own words, and express our own unique self in work and love, we realize how much is given to us. But while reaching the height of our cycle, and saying what a great sense

of confidence, "I really am," we sense that to fulfill our life we are now called to become parents and grandparents, brothers and sisters, teachers, friends, and lovers ourselves, and to give to others so that, when we leave this world, we can be what we have given. (p. 13)

We love the lyrical beauty of this passage and its view that an individual's personal development naturally entails self-transcendence and moral responsibility in later life. As Nouwen put it, "receiving matures in giving" (p. 14). But contemporary Americans seem to emphasize individual development without a clear consensus—even a rich debate—about the meanings of later life and the responsibilities of older people to future generations. With the rise of mass longevity—and ever-lengthening life expectancy—the roles, responsibilities, virtues, vices, and meanings of an extended old age take on new urgency in both private and public life. Strangely, there is virtually nothing written on this subject.

Now, there is a plethora of literature focusing (appropriately) on the ethics of caregiving, on private and public responsibilities to older people, and on the rights of older people. But there is virtually no discussion of the reciprocal responsibilities of older people. In the bioethics literature, older people (or their proxies) are viewed solely as bearers of rights, as individuals entitled to make their own choices regarding health care. But there is precious little work on the content of those choices—or on the larger issues of the accountability, responsibilities, virtues, and vices of older people.

To address these issues, we will first provide a brief interpretation of Nouwen and Erikson, focusing on the normative dimension of their views on aging and the life cycle. Next, we will offer a historical argument that we are living after the life cycle, both normatively and structurally. We will then tentatively sketch the moral challenges of later life—both for healthy, active older people and for those who are frail, sick, and dependent. And finally, we will consider some moral and spiritual aspects of dependency.

NOUWEN AND ERIKSON ON THE LIFE CYCLE

Let me begin with a brief analysis of Nouwen's perspective and that of his more famous counterpart, Erik Erikson. Philosophically, Nouwen's view rests on an ancient doctrine shared by Greeks, Romans, and Christians alike—that the human life span constitutes a single natural order and that each stage possesses its own characteristics and moral norms. "Life's race course is fixed," wrote Cicero in *De Senectute*, "nature has only a single path and that path is run but once, and to each stage of existence has been allotted its appropriate quality" (Cole, 1991, p. xxxii). With the rise of Christianity, this normative life cycle was set within a divinely ordained natural order—and the Stoic ideal of rational self-mastery was replaced by a journey toward salvation.

While Nouwen writes as a Catholic priest, his view of the life cycle is couched mostly in secular psychological terms, which echo Erik Erikson's famous psychoanalytic formulation of the eight *Ages of Man*, each with its own psychosocial conflict and its corresponding virtue. First formulated at mid-century, Erikson's version of the life cycle virtually dominated American academic thought and public imagination for over 25 years. Erikson's theory is actually a restatement of the Stoic ideal, supplemented by evolutionary and psychoanalytic theories. Like the Stoics, Erikson argued that the cycle of human life contained its own stages, each with its own moral virtues and norms. Erickson saw virtues not as lofty ideals formulated by theologians and moralists, but rather as essential qualities rooted in human evolution. As Erickson (1964) put it, "man's psychosocial survival is safeguarded only by vital virtues which develop in the interplay of successive and overlapping generations, living together in organized settings" (p. 114).

According to Erikson, the central psychosocial conflict in old age is integrity versus despair. (After his death, his wife, Joan, added a stage of emptying; Erikson, 1997.) Wisdom is the corresponding virtue arising from successful resolution of that conflict. Integrity for Erikson (1963) is "an experience which conveys some world order and spiritual sense. No matter how dearly paid for, it is the acceptance of one's one and only life cycle as something that had to be and that, by necessity permitted no substitutions" (p. 269). Wisdom is described as "detached concern with life itself, in the face of death itself. It responds to the need of the on-coming generation for an integrated heritage and yet remains aware of the relativity of all knowledge" (Erikson, 1964, p. 133).

Erikson understood that the life cycle itself does not biologically generate the prescribed virtues, values, and behaviors associated each stage; rather, every version of the normative life cycle is created by the combined prior forces of biology, culture, demography, history, social structure, and patterns of family life. While many of Erikson's followers have treated the eight Ages of Man as if it were a universal paradigm of human development, we believe that Erikson's model represents culmination of the ideal life cycle in modern Western culture. This ideal of a long, orderly, and secure life cycle first emerged during the Reformation and became fully realized in the middle third of the 20th century (see Cole, 1991, chap. 1). Ironically, modernization removed the traditional structural underpinnings of the normative life *cycle* and replaced it with the life *course*.

In both modern and postmodern society, old age emerges as a historically unprecedented, marginal and culturally unstable phase of life. Herein lies the poignancy of our situation. We are living after the life cycle (cf. MacIntyre, 1984). In this context, Erikson's extensive life cycle writings take on an almost numinous quality. They offer hope for an ideal of the life cycle we desperately want to believe in (cf. Moody, 1986). But however attractive, Erikson's ideal cannot accommodate the social, cultural, and demographic complexities of our era. To say that we are living after the life cycle means, in part, that we are living after Erikson.[2] We need a richer, pluralistic dialogue about how to live the ever-lengthening years of later life. But first, let us sketch the historical context of our uncertainty about the roles, responsibilities, purposes, and meanings of old age.

Modernization: From the Cycle of Life to the Course of Life

The modern life course began to take shape with the rise of urban, industrial society. Set free from older bonds of status, family, and locality, aspiring individuals increasingly came to view their lives as careers— as sequences of expected positions in school, at work, and in retirement. In the 20th century, this pattern of expectations became both statistically and ideologically normative, constituting what Martin Kohli (1987) aptly called a moral economy of the life course. By the third quarter of the 20th century, Western democracies had institutionalized this moral economy by providing age-homogenous schools for youthful preparation; jobs organized according to skills, experience, and seniority for middle-aged productivity; and employment-based and publicly funded retirement benefits for the aged, who were considered too slow,

---

[2] In her own 90s, Joan Erikson began to address these issues by adding short chapters on "The Ninth Stage" (chapter 5) and "Gerotranscendence" (chapter 6) to a new edition of Erikson's (1997) *The Life Cycle Completed*.

too frail, or too old-fashioned to be productive (see Cole, 1991, p. 240). This stable sequence is sometimes referred to as the three boxes of life: education for youth, work for adulthood, and retirement for old age (cf. Bolles, 1978). Old age was roughly divided into a period of active retirement supported by Social Security, pensions, and private insurance and a period of frailty supported additionally by Medicare, Medicaid, and health insurance.

During this transition to modernity, the cycle of life was effectively severed from the course of life. In premodern society, when generations of people lived on farms, in villages, and in small towns, local traditions of practice, belief, and behavior provided external moral norms, as each generation visibly cycled into the next; the problem of identity as we know it did not arise. In Germany and Austria, for example, the burial plot of the older generation (even today) was often reused when their children died, just as houses, farms, and businesses were passed down. "The idea of the 'life cycle,'" writes Anthony Giddens (1991), "makes very little sense once the connections between the individual life and the interchange of the generations have been broken" (p. 146). In a modern, mobile society, life stages are disembedded from place; the individual "is more and more freed from externalities associated with pre-established ties to" (p. 147) family, individuals, and groups. Under these conditions, the life course becomes a career, a trajectory in which individuals choose their projects and plans; segments of the life course are marked by open experience thresholds, rather than ritualized passages. Life course transitions are often accompanied by crises of identity; individuals are socialized to confront and resolve such crises, and identity becomes an ongoing, reflexive project.

For many older people in an urban, mobile, and rapidly changing society, achieving a stable identity, knowing one's obligations, one's place in the cycle of generations and in a worldview of ultimate meanings, becomes problematic. At a practical level, for example, many skills that parents and grandparents knew are no longer useful in the information age, although emotional balance, love, and wisdom are still in short supply. Grandmothers have little need to tell granddaughters how to bake bread . . . except as a story of the past. There is little utility in having a grandfather show his grandson how to sharpen a tool on a grindstone.

Even as older people in the last half of the 20th century experienced vastly improved medical and economic conditions, they encountered a culture with no clear consensus about the meanings and purposes of later life. For the first time in human history, mass longevity became the norm in developed countries. Contemporaneously, the dominant social identities available to older people had been narrowly confined to the roles of patient, pensioner, and consumer. Consumer culture, the leisure industry, the welfare state, and the medical establishment each had their own interest in shaping the culture of aging.

In the last quarter of the 20th century, this relatively stable institutionalized life course began to unravel. The 1970s witnessed a powerful movement of older people and their advocates to overcome negative stereotypes of older people as frail and dependent. Mandatory retirement was challenged under the banner of age discrimination. The 1980s initiated a rebellion against the bureaucratized life course and against restrictive age norms. Writers and scholars called for an age-irrelevant society that allowed more flexibility for moving in and out of school and the workforce. At the same time, serious doubts about the proportion of the federal budget devoted to old people were voiced in the name of generational equity. Others voiced specific fears of an unsupportable public obligation to sick and dependent older people. Political support for the welfare state began to erode. And finally, the transition to an information economy—spurred by the rise of computers and the decline of industrial manufacturing—accelerated the pace of life and the speed of technological and social change. Amid a globalizing economy, declining corporate commitment to long-term employment, seniority and defined pension benefits undercut expectations for income stability during retirement. Postmodern or late modern society confirmed with a vengeance Marx and Engel's (1978) famous observation about capitalism: "All that is solid melts into air" (p. 476).

The Moral Challenges of Later Life

In his seminal work *After Virtue*, MacIntyre (1984) argued that we no longer possess a commonly shared moral language; in a world of moral strangers, MacIntyre claimed that the only alternatives are Aristotle or Nietzsche—that is, tradition or chaos. By analogy, we think that we are living after the life cycle—after the collapse of widely shared images and socially cohesive structures and experiences of the life cycle. But we do not think we are forced to choose between idealized tradition or exaggerated chaos. First of all, the lack of a scholarly literature or articulated norms does not imply that most older people are leading morally incoherent lives. And second, the very search for identity itself holds important moral promise. Here we are drawing on the work of Taylor (1989,

1992), who argued that despite the moral limitations of liberal individualism, the biblical tradition lives on as a kind of background cultural inheritance. For Taylor, selfhood or identity is inextricably bound up with some historically specific (and often unarticulated) moral framework or notion of the good. The quest to become one's authentic self need not degenerate into self-indulgence, emotivism, or moral relativism. It can (and logically does) entail becoming aware of and articulating the implicit moral framework of one's family, community, or religious tradition, which provide standards of conduct against which the fully developed person must measure himself or herself. In Taylor's (1992) view, human life and identity are fundamentally dialogical, meaning that we should not, in other words, view the search for identity in old age as a narrowly personal quest. Of course, we are all familiar with examples of late-life narcissism. Yet the effort to live an authentic life is itself a moral ideal—an attempt to understand and fulfill the uniqueness of each human life. Older people trying to make sense of their past through various forms of life review, spiritual autobiography, reminiscence, storytelling, or life story writing groups are often doing important moral and spiritual work, with genuine implications for others. And those who are passionately involved in the arts, public service, religious communities, and new forms of self-exploration exemplify models of elderhood.

Authenticity in itself, however, cannot provide standards of conduct and character to guide moral development in later life. Authenticity alone provides no reasons to restrain the person who authentically chooses selfishness or evil. It contains no intrinsic moral norms or prohibitions. The dominant ideal of late life today seems to be what the Austrian sociologist Rosenmayr (1990) called *Die Späte Freiheit*—"the late freedom." Free from social obligations, retirement—for those who possess good health and adequate income—is equated with leisure activities (visiting family or friends, golf, mahjong, bridge, travel, taking up new hobbies, attending classes at Elderhostel or Institutes for Learning in Retirement). The problem here is not that these activities are wrong or bad; rather, they are based on the concept of freedom *from*—that is, the obligations of midlife—with little or no attention paid to what the freedom is *for*—that is, which principles or commitments should govern the choices being made. Today, senior marketing and advertising specialists have a primary influence on activities, programs, and products for seniors looking for ways to spend their free time. While maintaining one's health necessarily occupies more time and energy as one ages, the commodification of the body has elevated health from a *means* to and *end in itself.*

Services, products, and programs for healthy aging are perhaps the most lucrative segment of the senior market. Health is increasingly construed as physical functioning, divorced from any reference to human meaning or purpose. The reduction of health to physical function fits hand-in-glove with the notion of freedom as unfettered free choice. In today's consumer culture, drug companies, peddlers of over-the-counter products, and antiaging hucksters make billions of dollars selling the false hope that aging is an option or a treatable disease. Before the 20th century, health was understood as a means to an end—living a good life according to the standards embedded in religious traditions. Rarely now does one hear the question, What do we want to be healthy *for?* A medicalized consumer society crowds out the cultural space necessary for grappling with the most important questions of all: To whom am I accountable? What makes life worth living? Am I living a life I can look back on with pride and satisfaction? What legacy am I passing on to my family? How can I prepare for my death in ways that minimize disruption and give hope to my children?

In approaching the moral challenges of aging from the individual's point of view, Cole has always appreciated Rabbi Hillel's ancient three questions in *Ethics of the Fathers* (1:14): "If I am not for myself, who will be for me? If I am only for myself, what am I? If not now, when?" Cole takes each of these questions to stand for a phase of the life cycle, harkening back to Nouwen's formulation. As children and adolescents, there is a natural tendency to see the world as one's oyster. In midlife, we realize that to mature, we must attend to the needs of others. And in later life, with time running out, we must learn to how balance our own needs with the needs of future generations. Interestingly, whereas Nouwen speaks only of giving as we age, Hillel speaks of balancing competing needs and interests. If we take Hillel's questions and apply them to later life today, we can begin to specify key questions that demand careful and balanced responses: As citizens, what responsibilities do we have to our community, the larger society, the environment? To the poor and vulnerable? To our communities of faith? How do we balance these against our personal interests? What are our responsibilities to our children, grandchildren? What level of caregiving and economic support do we owe them? How do we balance these against our own needs and interests? What responsibility do we have for older parents who may be in their 80s or 90s? How do we balance these against responsibilities to our children? To our own personal interests and well-being? What responsibilities do we have to future generations to minimize the national debt they will pay?

To help safeguard the environment, to work for sustainable sources of energy? What responsibility do we have for a spouse who is permanently disabled, perhaps by the later stages of dementia? Can we say, this is not the person I married, and I need to live my own life? Do we owe a degree of loyalty that includes daily visits and care? What responsibilities do we have to shoulder, depending on circumstances, the burden of our economic support? What responsibility do we have for our own health? For exercising prudence in using limited health care resources? What responsibility do nursing home residents have to assist each other? What responsibility do we have to pursue a path of continued growth and spiritual development that aims at self-transcendence, compassion, commitment to others, acceptance of physical and mental decline, and preparation for death?

We will not here attempt to answer these questions. But we believe they are urgent and call for personal wrestling, public debate, academic inquiry, and perhaps public policy. A careful study, for example, of advice literature about aging over time would reveal much about the changing values and norms conveyed to a reading public of older people (see especially Cole, 1991, chap. 7; Haber & Gratton, 1994, chap. 6). We need a great deal of social and behavioral study of what older people think about these issues as well as how they act. We need studies of the moral and spiritual lives of older people in various geographic, ethnic, racial, gender, and class situations. We need diverse religious reflections and their translation into practical programs in congregational life. We need philosophical inquiry and public conversation. And we need to listen carefully to the life stories of both ordinary and exemplary old people.

We do not think we can expect universally true, decontextualized norms and values to which all elders should be held accountable. In a pluralist society, we need to hear from various religious, ethnic, racial, and political groups. We need to hear, for example, from AARP, which is typically perceived mainly as a powerful lobbying group for older people. We think we need new models and ideals. One example is Rabbi Zalman Schacter's spiritual eldering program, which sponsors a series of workshops around the country for older people who would like to grow into genuine elders (Shalomi & Miller, 1995). Another is the civic engagement project currently under way in the Gerontological Society, or Freedman's (1996) efforts to generate strengthening voluntary movements of older people offering their care and their skills with underprivileged urban youth.

The paradoxes and contradictions of aging are not solvable problems to be mastered with competence and expertise. They must be worked through by each individual in search of spiritual growth; yet this rarely happens without guidance and community. Our society, therefore, needs to support various multicultural contemplative practices, including prayer, meditation, self-reflection, yoga, Tai Chi, new religious rituals, and so on. And then we run up against the ancient problem of the active versus the contemplative life—another contradiction that needs revisiting. Some of the most difficult and important questions concern the paradox of physical decline and spiritual growth: How can we learn to work hard maintaining our physical health, while at the same time preparing for our own decline and death? How do we learn to hold on and let go at the same time? One of the central obstacles to wrestling with the challenges of old age lies in the intractable American hostility toward and denigration of physical decline, decay, and dependence. Rather than acknowledge these harsh realities, we pretend that we can master them, and we feel like failures when we do not, hence the elevation of physical functioning to the criteria of successful aging and the virulent fear and denial of frailty and dependency. Let us turn next to the moral and spiritual aspects of dependency.

The Moral Contours of Dependency

When Cole's grandmother became demented in 1986, he asked if she would consider going into an excellent Jewish home for the aged. "What do you think I am," she replied, "a no-goodnik?" This woman, who had postponed marriage to care for her own mother, lost her husband and her only son and still managed to scrape together enough money to leave her grandchildren an inheritance. Stripped of an acceptable identity and the ability to be useful, she tried to jump off her 12th-story balcony. Before slipping into deep dementia, she agonized as the money intended for her grandchildren was spent on her round-the-clock health care. It is often a terrible burden to be a burden to others. What Lustbader (1991) called the *alchemy of successful frailty* depends on finding ways to turn "the 'nothing' of empty time into the 'something' of good days" (Cole, 1991, p. 15). The possibilities of successful frailty depend on innumerable factors, not the least of which is reciprocity.

In her book *Counting on Kindness: The Dilemmas of Dependency*, Lustbader (1991) made an unusual and controversial point about mercy.

The Old French word *merci* originally meant compassion and forbearance toward a person in one's power. In Latin, *merces* signified payment or reward, referring to aspects of commerce. *Mercy*, writes Lustbader, is based entirely on exchange:

> Giving help eventually embitters us, unless we are compensated at least by appreciation; accepting help degrades us, unless we are convinced that our helpers are getting something in return. As much as we might prefer to reject this stark accounting, we discover in living through situations of dependence that good will is not enough. [There is] a delicate balance at the heart of mercy . . . reciprocation replenishes both the spirit of the helper and the person who is helped. (p. 18)

We seem to lack language to acknowledge the difficulty of receiving. Hence the dependent person may feel doubly burdened, "disliking the help that cannot be repaid and feeling guilty for the dislike" (p. 36). Increasing frailty shrinks the opportunities to be useful, eliminating external obligations: "No one expects our presence and no one needs our efforts" (p. 30). Finding ways to be useful requires imagination and willpower, for example, among nursing home patients who figure out ways to look after one another. For a resident to feel useful, this sometimes requires special sensitivity on the part of the caregiver.

Despite an extensive literature search in English, we have been able to find only two contemporary articles on the virtues and vices of dependent older people: one by the theologian, culture critic, and ethicist William May (1986); and the other by the feminist, secular philosopher Sally Ruddick (1999). Before we turn to the topic of virtue and age, we want to offer three words of caution: (a) although we will be discussing ideals of virtue in a relatively decontextualized way, any full exploration must take into account differences in culture, gender, race and ethnicity, and social class; (b) contrary to Cicero's exclusive emphasis on character, exercising virtue is not simply a matter of individual will—virtues occur amid social conditions and relationships that foster or inhibit them; and (c) a given person's capacity for exercising virtue (especially the more subtle and demanding virtues) also depends on his or her prior level of emotional and spiritual development. For some people, obeying the thou-shalt-nots of our society may be a more reasonable expectation. Such important caveats lie beyond the scope of this chapter.

In "The Virtues and Vices of Aging," May (1986) contextualized his discussion by reminding us of the power imbalance between older patients and health professionals. He observed that caregivers who unwittingly display their health and youth are "like a bustling cold front that moves in and stiffens the landscape" (p. 42). They cannot see that their vocation depends on patients, which compounds the power imbalance and obscures the moral significance of reciprocal dependency. Writing across the boundaries of psychology, ethics, and theology, May warned against the common confusion of infirmity with moral failure. He emphasized that virtues do not emerge automatically with age; rather, they "grow only through resolution, struggle, perhaps prayer, and perseverance" (p. 50). The upshot of his analysis, for our purposes, is that May aptly criticized academic ethicists who focus chiefly on moral dilemmas and provide critical guidelines to professionals. It has been over 20 years since he observed that ethics "does not offer much help to patients facing the ordeal of fading powers. [The aged] need guidelines for action, to be sure, but more than that they need strength of character in the face of ordeals" (p. 49).

We have been able to find only one significant essay that takes up May's challenge. In her essay "Virtues and Age," Ruddick (1999)—who did not cite May—argued that there are indeed virtues especially salient in the lives of people "situated between a lengthening, unalterable past and short future, where loss is predictable, but its timing and form is not" (p. 45). Ruddick wrote as a secular, feminist philosopher who was quite wary of articulating ideals that become burdensome to those who are meant to be governed by them. She stated, quite convincingly, that the elderly, like people at any age,

> struggle to maintain conceptions of themselves as good people. Many also try both to preserve relationships and to do well by the people to whom they are importantly related. These efforts of virtue are intrinsically rewarding for the elderly themselves, confirming their sense of agency, accountability, and moral standing. (p. 46)

These efforts also benefit "the people they care for and who care for them" (p. 46).

Ruddick's (1999) account of virtue focused particularly on the vulnerable, needy elderly and those who care for them. She drew not only on philosophical reasoning, but also on her experience of caregiving and witnessing in nursing homes. Ruddick acknowledged that being virtuous is sometimes beyond the control of demented elders, but she insisted that mental deterioration, which occurs slowly, allows time for adaptation and rarely makes efforts of virtue impossible. She criticized theories that characterize virtue primarily as a characteristic of individuals, a charge that may be leveled against May (1986). Such theories, Ruddick (1999) argued, show little tolerance for so-called outlaw emotions such a righteous anger, and they are conceptually unable to guide the moral challenges facing receivers and givers of care. Ruddick was also wary of the stereotypical vices that shadow any list of virtues. She therefore spoke of ongoing efforts of virtues (rather than achieved dispositions or traits) that individuals strive to acquire and maintain. Reversing traditional theological arguments, Ruddick argued that "being virtuous is something one *sometimes* does, not something one is" (p. 54). She not only focused on process, rather than achievement, she also believed that virtue is created between and among people and is therefore inherently relational. Ruddick also took pains to avoid creating an unrealistically burdensome account of virtues that requires continuous and unremitting effort, which she criticized as another form of the masculine Protestant work ethic—perhaps another challenge to May (1986). She reformulated her definitions this way:

> So being virtuous is something people *sometimes* do together. . . . There are days when one isn't up to creating virtue alone or with others. Hours, days, even weeks of sadness, sloth, and apathy are an integral part rather than an interruption of ongoing efforts to be virtuous. They do not mark a person as bad; processes of doing virtue are marked by vicissitude, not failure. Over a period of time, a virtuous person may do more rather than less. . . . But no one needs to be counting or judging. (p. 54)

Ruddick (1999), then, presented a secular feminist account that was rooted in experience. She emphasized process over achievement, relationships over individual virtue, behavior over character. She avoided discussion of the vices by waiving off surveillance or the moral judgment of others. May (1986), on the other hand, offered both secular and theological theories of virtue, emphasized individual character, and did not shrink from light-handed and contextually sensitive moral judgment.

We believe that moral development in midlife and later life must include cultivating reverence for the human life cycle, and especially for future generations—a reversal of the reverence upward tradition. We also believe that human beings at all ages have a basic spiritual need for expansion and liberation of the self. This universal human need for transcendence has implications for human development amid frailty and the process of dying. By consciously and actively working toward an embrace of loss and death (when they are unavoidable), we may be able to embody beauty and spiritual development amid decline. In Rilke's (1998) words, "For beauty's nothing but the beginning of Terror we're still just able to beat, and why we adore it so is because it serenely disdains to destroy us" (p. 12).

What can we expect from this kind of analysis of character and action among the frail elderly? What is missing from these accounts? Can we educate caregivers on the importance of acknowledging reciprocity and fostering relationships that allow their patients to be useful? What would relationships look like if moral language and reciprocity of dependent patients was introduced in nursing homes or home care? How can we educate clergy, both in the pulpit and at the bedside, in the moral challenges of aging? Seminaries have only recently begun to provide some gerontological education to their students, focusing entirely on the needs of older people. What should be added to revitalize religious understanding of older people as moral agents? Finally, with the proliferation of lifelong learning through Elderhostel and Institutes for Learning in Retirement, can older people be engaged in seminars and workshops about moral issues in their lives? We are skeptical about this latter idea since older people notoriously avoid classes in aging. But the use of biblical material, films, fiction, and theater might slip behind psychological defenses and open up new moral and spiritual horizons. Think of the old King Saul, or King David, King Lear, Oedipus at Colonnus, or *Driving Miss Daisy*, *Cocoon*, and *The Trip to Bountiful* approached through the lenses of ethics and the human spirit.

CONCLUDING THOUGHTS

Where do these thoughts about life cycle norms, mass longevity, postmodernity, moral obligations, spiritual development, vices, and virtues leave us? Personally, we feel a sense of awe and amazement at the sheer abundance of life made possible by the gift of mass longevity. But what is the price of that gift? Perhaps, as Theodore Roszak (1998) argued in *America the Wise*, the wisdom of a maturing population promises to be our richest resource. Or perhaps, as a voice from the Talmud suggests, a man who is a fool in his youth is also a fool in his old age, while a man who is wise in his youth is also wise in his old age. We believe that the answer to the gift versus burden of mass longevity will depend in no small measure on how well we learn to identify, support, and accomplish the moral and spiritual work of aging in our era. As Plato understood, one of the best ways to learn is by listening to those who have traveled this road ahead of us. Let me close by listening again to one of Cole's favorite elders, Florida Scott Maxwell (1978). Writing in her 80s as a Jungian analyst, she encouraged us to learn

> that life is a tragic mystery. We are pierced and driven by laws we only half understand, we find that the lesson we learn again and again is that of heroic helplessness. Some uncomprehended law holds us at a point of contradiction where we have no choice, where we do not like that which we love, where good and bad are inseparable partners to tell apart, and where we—heart-broken and ecstatic, can only resolve the conflict by blindly taking it into our hearts. This used to be called being in the hands of God. Has anyone any better words to describe it? (pp. 24–25)

REFERENCES

Achenbaum, W. A. (1993). (When) did the papacy become a gerontocracy? In K. W. Schaie & W. A. Achenbaum (Eds.), *Societal impact on aging: Historical perspectives* (pp. 204–231). New York: Springer Publishing.

Achenbaum, W. A., & Albert, D. M. (1995). *Profiles in gerontology.* Westport, CT: Greenwood Press.

Atchley, R. C. (1989). Demographic factors and adult psychological development. In K. W. Schaie & C. Schooler (Eds.), *Social structure and aging: Psychological processes* (pp. 11–34). Hillsdale, NJ: Erlbaum.

Bolles, R. (1978). *The three boxes of life and how to get out of them: An introduction to life-work planning.* Berkeley, CA: Ten Speed Press.

Cole, T. (1991). *The journey of life: A cultural history of aging in America.* New York: Cambridge University Press.

Cole, T. (1993). The prophecy of *Senescence*: G. Stanley Hall and the reconstruction of old age in twentieth-century America. In K. W. Schaie & W. A. Achenbaum (Eds.), *Societal impact on aging: Historical perspectives* (pp. 165–181). New York: Springer Publishing.

Cole, T., & Gadow, S. (1986). *What does it mean to grow old? Reflections from the medical humanities.* Durham, NC: Duke University Press.

Erikson, E. (1963). *Childhood and society* (Rev. ed.). New York: W. W. Norton.

Erikson, E. (1964). *Insight and responsibility.* New York: W. W. Norton.

Erikson, E. H., & Erikson, J. M. (1997). *The life cycle completed.* Philadelphia: W. W. Norton.

Featherman, D. (1989). What's development in adulthood? In K. W. Schaie & C. Schooler (Eds.), *Social structure and aging: Psychological processes* (pp. 41–56). Hillsdale, NJ: Erlbaum.

Freedman, M. (1996). *The kindness of strangers*. New York: Jossey-Bass.

Geertz, C. (1973). Thick description: Toward an interpretive theory of culture. In *The interpretation of cultures* (pp. 3–30). New York: Basic Books.

Giddens, A. (1991). *Modernity and self-identity: Self and society in the late modern age*. Stanford, CA: Stanford University Press.

Haber, C., & Gratton, B. (1994). *Old age and the search for security: An American social history*. Bloomington: Indiana University Press.

Kohli, M. (1987). Retirement and the moral economy: An historical interpretation of the German case. *Journal of Aging Studies, 2*, 125–144.

Kuhn, T. (1962). *The structure of scientific revolutions*. Chicago: University of Chicago Press.

Lawton, M. P. (1989). Behavior-relevant ecological factors. In K. W. Schaie & C. Schooler (Eds.), *Social structure and aging: Psychological processes* (pp. 57–78). Hillsdale, NJ: Erlbaum.

Lustbader, W. (1991). *Counting on kindness: The dilemmas of dependency*. New York: Free Press.

Maciel, A., & Staudinger, U. (1993). Commentary: What became of the prophecy of *Senescence*: G. Stanley Hall and the reconstruction of old age in twentieth-century America. In K. W. Schaie & W. A. Achenbaum (Eds.), *Societal impact on aging: Historical perspectives* (pp. 182–197). New York: Springer Publishing.

MacIntyre, A. (1984). *After virtue: A study in moral theory*. Notre Dame, IN: University of Notre Dame Press.

Marx, K., & Engels, F. (1978). The communist manifesto. In *The Marx-Engels reader* (pp. 469–500). New York: W. W. Norton.

Maxwell, F. (1978). *The measure of my days*. London: Penguin Books.

May, W. (1986). The virtues and vices of aging. In T. R. Cole & S. Gadow (Eds.), *What does it mean to grow old?* (pp. 41–62). Durham, NC: Duke University Press.

Moody, H. (1986). The meaning of life and the meaning of old age. In T. R. Cole & S. Gadow (Eds.), *What does it mean to grow old?* (pp. 11–40). Durham, NC: Duke University Press.

Nouwen, H., & Gaffney, W. (1976). *Aging: The fulfillment of life*. New York: Bantam Doubleday Dell.

Ransom, R. (1993). Commentary on (when) did the papacy become a gerontocracy. In K. W. Schaie & W. A. Achenbaum (Eds.), *Societal impact on aging: Historical perspectives* (pp. 237–243). New York: Springer Publishing.

Riley, M. W. (1989). Foreword: Why this book? In K. W. Schaie & C. Schooler (Eds.), *Social structure and aging: Psychological processes* (pp. xiii–xv). Hillsdale, NJ: Erlbaum.

Rilke, R, M. (1998). *Duino Elegies*. (Originally published in 1923; translated by S. Cohen). Evanston, IL: Northwestern University Press.

Rosenmayr, L. (1990). *Die späte Freiheit*. Paris, France: Atelier.

Roszak, T. (1998). *America the wise: The longevity revolution and the true wealth of nations*. Boston: Houghton Mifflin.

Ruddick, S. (1999). Virtues and age. In M. U. Walter (Ed.), *Mother time* (pp. 45–60). New York: Rowman and Littlefield.

Schaie, K. W., & Achenbaum, W. A. (Eds.). (1993). *Societal impact on aging: Historical perspectives*. New York: Springer Publishing.

Schaie, K. W., & Schooler, C. (Eds.). (1989). *Social structure and aging: Psychological processes*. Hillsdale, NJ: Erlbaum.

Shalomi, Z., & Miller, R. (1995). *From age-ing to sage-ing*. New York: Warner Books.

Taylor, C. (1989). *Sources of the self*. Cambridge, MA: Harvard University Press.

Taylor, C. (1992). *Ethics of authenticity*. Cambridge, MA: Harvard University Press.

Van Tassel, D. (1993). Commentary: Institutional gerontocracies structural or demographic: The case of the papacy. In K. W. Schaie & W. A. Achenbaum (Eds.), *Societal impact on aging: Historical perspectives* (pp. 232–236). New York: Springer Publishing.

Cultural Transformations, History, and the Experiences of Aging

12

CHRISTINE L. FRY

In this, the 20th and penultimate volume in the Penn State Social Structures and Aging series, we should reflect on themes introduced earlier in the series of conferences and the resulting volumes. The annual succession of seminars has produced an incredible wealth of material. The importance of this body of information and ideas is threefold. First, it has a vision that incorporates diversity. Second, it attempts to take the larger picture into its perspective. Third, it is truly multidisciplinary. Three of the past conferences have focused on historical forces on lives, societies, and aging: (a) *Age Structuring in Comparative Perspective* (Kertzer & Schaie, 1989), (b) *Societal Impact on Aging: Historical Perspectives* (Schaie & Achenbaum, 1993), and (c) *Historical Influences on Lives and Aging* (Schaie & Elder, 2005). In this chapter, we will reconsider these themes in an anthropological way. As an anthropologist, I view my role as providing the most comprehensive or big-picture understanding of what has happened in history and how it has impacted the experiences of aging. Our focus is on what happened to humans after the ice receded about 12,000 years ago. We will not just focus on Europe and North America but will include the entire globe.

As we embark on this task, we first will consider theories of change in gerontology, especially modernization. Second, we examine evolutionary theory within anthropology. Third, a brief overview of a universal history of humankind is presented. Fourth, we examine the consequences of long-term evolutionary trends on the experiences of aging within this framework by taking a somewhat different view of life courses and lives lived, as shaped by different modes of production. Finally, we conclude with a discussion of culture and the experiences of aging.

BEYOND MODERNIZATION

When discussing societal transformations and consequences for older people, one is immediately drawn to the ideas of Donald Cowgill and Lowell Holmes (Cowgill, 1986; Cowgill & Holmes, 1972). However, in the three decades since the formulation of those ideas, we have moved way beyond modernization. Aging and modernization theory sets forth a web of explicit hypotheses linking urbanization, education, health technology, and economic factors to a diminished status and marginalization of older adults. The strength of this theory is that it clearly constitutes a logical set of hypotheses that could be tested and evaluated. It was, in fact, one of a handful of such theories in a data-rich and theory-poor gerontology. It stimulated much research. When data failed to support the hypothesis, we searched for alternative processes. We finally realized we were dealing with a phenomenon more complex than modernization.

When we look back, we realize that the Cowgill and Holmes theory is a product of its time. The middle of the 20th century was one of faith in economic development and modernization to solve world problems, especially poverty. We also now realize that the processes associated with modernization were far too narrow and specific for a very narrow time frame. The narrowness of the time frame also tells us much about modernization theory. Modernization is the moral force of history. To be modern is to be good: life, liberty, and the pursuit of happiness. To be modern is to be a nation state with a political democracy, highly industrial and with a capitalistic free market: the United States. We need a theory which is less value charged and more comprehensive. We need to account for a far larger span of time and for change all around the globe.

Here I am going to make a revolutionary, or perhaps reactionary, suggestion to return to those thinkers of the 19th century who were seeing the transformations that were triggering the tumultuous changes in their times. These are scholars such as Henry Maine, Louis Henry Morgan, Edward Tylor, Emile Durkheim, Alexis de Tocqueville, and Karl Marx. They saw the economic changes brought about by capitalism and industrialization and realized the profound consequences for families. They saw the formation of nation-states. They saw the great transformation into the contemporary world and the hastening of globalization. Before we return to their observations, I want to do some theoretical stage setting. We need to explore an evolutionary paradigm to explain both the cultural processes and historical records.

EVOLUTION AND ANTHROPOLOGICAL THEORY

Anthropological theorizing began as speculation about a universal history of humankind. The hopes were to use ethnographic data to discover the laws of evolution. Tylor (1871) and Morgan (1877) were the champions of this effort. They did discover a law of progress through the stages of savagery to barbarism to civilization. This was a rather sterile and unilineal endeavor since it simply classified people into one of the three categories or subdivisions. It, too, reflected the time period since Europe was spilling out into the rest of the world in the later days of mercantilism. Also, like modernization, it, too, gave a moral force to history, with civilization being much better than savagery or barbarism.

For rather obvious reasons, this framework fell out of favor in anthropology. However, by the mid-20th century, evolution was resurrected and redefined using energetics and ecology. By the end of the century, evolutionary theory had developed in anthropology into a behavioral ecology to investigate the microworld of everyday life and decision making and strategies of behavior. The more macroevolutionary theory attempts to explain the long-term trends operative around the globe that have resulted in cultural complexity (Boyd & Richardson, 2005). It is this latter theory of general evolution (Sahlins & Service, 1960) that we will use to develop a universal history of humankind.

How does evolution and culture work? Evolutionary theory uses Darwinian natural selection (Richardson & Boyd, 2005). Of all known evolutionary processes, natural selection is by far the most nonrandom. Explanatory power is a result of strong and direct linkages between an environment, subsistence strategies, economy, population, and political organization. Unlike our 19th-century pioneers, natural selection does not assume a progressive transformation. Instead, change is a product of humans accommodating to an ecological context, which itself may be in transition, or figuring out new solutions to continuing problems. Natural selection favors certain cultural forms, until another cultural arrangement is invented. Our cultural evolutionary record is one of continuing diversification of cultural forms. Similar to the biological world, more complex cultural units compete with and often replace simpler ones, and may even themselves fall back to simpler forms. Thus we do see an evolutionary pattern of smaller scaled cultures enveloped by larger scaled cultures.

A UNIVERSAL HISTORY OF HUMANS

Our story begins with the diaspora from Africa some 1,000,000 years ago. Humans soon occupied the warm parts of Europe and Asia, subsisting by foraging. By as early as 60,000 years ago, Australia was occupied, and humans made their appearance in the Americas by 25,000 years ago. The Pacific Islands were colonized as recently as 3,000 years ago. Foraging had proved to be so successful that by the end of the last ice age, humans were occupying and exploiting the frigid environments of northern Europe and Asia. When the climate moderated at 12,000 years ago, the ice receded, and those humans faced another crisis of environmental change. In the readaptations, humans would invent a new lifestyle. Foraging, especially in favorable environments, would be replaced by farming villages.

By 9,000 years ago, in the Near East and in Asia, humans experimented with a system of production that involved the domestication of plants and animals. In the Americas, this took place about 4,000 years later. The Agricultural Revolution is both a technological and a social departure from foraging. Technologically, by controlling the life cycles of plants and animals, humans invented a subsistence that was resilient. It could be increased by expanding fields, herds, and the required labor. Sociologically, human labor became not only valuable, but it had to be organized systematically on a seasonal basis. This revolution set the seed for the rapid transformations and diversification of human societies all over the world.

Within a few thousand years, we begin to see a demographic expansion, accompanied by an increase in wealth and settlement size. Small villages nucleate into larger towns and eventually become cities. Domestic architecture sees the addition of monumental temples, administrative palaces, and glorious tombs. These societies use stratification and hierarchy to increase wealth and security. Political and economic institutions form the public arenas of these societies. Domestic units and their productive activities are linked to the administrative core through a redistributive economy and taxation and rents. In the Near East, the city-states of Mesopotamia appear by 5,000 years ago, along with Egypt in northern Africa. In Asia, the states form in India between 5,500 and 4,500 years ago, and the Shang Dynasty sets the course of Chinese civilization around 4,000 years ago. When the Spanish begin their colonization of the Americas in the 16th century, they discover the Aztecs in central Mexico and the Incas in the Andean Highlands and on the west coast of South America. Likewise, when the Portuguese begin the exploration of the African coast, they discover the kingdoms of Benin and Kongo. On each continent, we find societies that are increasingly complex. Egalitarian societies are replaced by small chiefdoms, which become larger and evolve and diversify into city-states, kingdoms, empires, feudal states, nation-states, and the like. Some remain small and disappear. Others grow quite large, such as Rome or the Inca Empire, and then fall apart. Others have considerable durability such as China.

Our cultural evolutionary sequences are well established. Since the 19th century, we have added only in detail and completeness. Why would natural selection favor the strong parallelisms we see in the evolutionary sequences all over the globe? Foraging is humanity's most enduring and most flexible adaptation. However, foraging has a flaw. If the environment in which one is foraging fails, entire populations may be eliminated through starvation. As a forager, there is not much one can do other than move to another environment and hope the collecting is better. Reliance on domesticates, on the other hand, involves direct manipulation of production through work, technology, or expanding cultivation. This resilience places the productive economy less into the hands of the vicissitudes of nature and more into the hands of the cultural capabilities of humans. However, economies based on domesticates are not without their dilemmas. Underproduction is the most profound and most difficult to resolve. In resolving the issues of a secure productive base, natural selection has favored the formation of a hierarchy, subsistence intensification, and political integration.

Hierarchy is a direct result of production based on domesticates. Work increases and becomes valuable. Some men become superordinate, as they control the work and life courses of others. The most common way of solving the issues of underproduction is to overproduce. With a resilient productive strategy involving increased work inputs and technology, subsistence expands and intensifies. More food is produced in less space, and population grows as more workers are needed.

Surpluses become the wealth of a polity as first big men, and then chiefs, and then a wide variety of rulers become the managers of risk and the organizers of a redistributive economy.

We now turn our attention to the consequences of hierarchy, intensification, and political integration on the life strategies of individuals living within different evolutionary circumstances. We will do this by examining what we know about different political economies and by exploring the actual lives of a person or family living in that context, largely drawn from the anthropological literature.

EVOLUTION AND THE CONSEQUENCES FOR LIFE STRATEGIES

With life expectancies of 40 years or less, one might conclude that old age is not a relevant topic until the 20th century. Quite to the contrary, many people did live into their 60s. The vast majority of the mortality occurred in the first decade of life. As far back as Neanderthal times, some 90,000 years ago, we have evidence of individuals surviving with disabilities into their sixth decade of life, although these individuals are rare. Since a significant number of individuals survived into older years, we will examine the consequences of different political and economic conditions for old age and the strategies people used to survive under diverse circumstances.

To accomplish this task, we will examine specific ethnographic contexts and the lives of people who lived under very different circumstances. Instead of looking at life courses defined in culturally different ways, we ask, What is it that individuals do as they pass from childhood to old age? What strategies can they use to maximize opportunities and to minimize risks that their cultural circumstances present? In this section of the chapter, we simplify the existing diversity by exploring life strategies in three contexts, organized by different modes of production:

1. Societies in which kin units organize production (this includes foraging bands, which are the smallest and simplest of human societies), and also, societies in which kin units base their production on the cultivation of plants and herding of animals
2. Societies in which kin units are organized into a system of tribute (these societies have a hierarchy, and the tribute flowing to the top echelon of tribute takers constitutes a surplus created by intensification)

3. Societies where production is organized through capitalism, where workers no longer control their production, but must work for wages in highly structured and technological workplaces owned by entrepreneurs

Although these contexts can be construed as evolutionary types, ranging from foraging societies, which dominated the earth prior to the melting of the ice some 12,000 years ago, to the invention of capitalism only a little over 200 years ago, they do not constitute a true evolutionary sequence. We must use the ethnographic present since that is when anthropologists or other observers collected information about cultures and lives. Most of the data come from the 20th century and hence are parallel in time, but not in space and context. These contexts are not selected to represent different life ways around the globe. Instead, the specific cultures and lives are *illustrative* of the issues we know that people must negotiate across their lives in different political and economic contexts created by the modes of production. Although specific cultures create opportunities and constraints for individuals to figure out as they traverse their life courses, it is possible to make generalizations of an evolutionary nature. First, lives become far more complicated as the world is less dominated by kin. Second, with institutional differentiation, individuals are faced with more choice and decision making in constructing their life strategies. Third, as societies become more politically integrated, a communal or political arena constitutes the major stage to which lives are oriented, as differentiated from the domestic world. Fourth, as wealth and politics dominate life, individuals must work harder, and usually, their labor becomes controlled by others.

Historically, the modes of production do have a temporal sequence. Kin-dominated production was the only mode of production until 5,000 years ago, when societies based on tribute began their expansion. Likewise, capitalism is very recent, but until the 20th century, it interacted with kin-ordered production and continues to interact with tribute-ordered production.

Kin-Dominated Production

Kin-dominated production is by far the most ancient and durable of human productive modes. It began as humans became human and has endured in some places of the world into the 21st century. Simply, groups of related individuals work together, exchange, marry, reproduce, and consume the products of their labor. Kin production is very adaptable to most circumstances and environments. Two subsistence strategies dominate cultures that predicate their economy exclusively on kin units: (a) foraging bands and (b) small-scale cultivators and herders. Each of these subsistence systems shapes the way kin units must operate.

Foraging Bands

Foraging lasted well into the 20th century, with examples such as the !Kung of the Kalahari, Inuit groups of Canada, the Hadsa of eastern Africa, and other groups in marginal habitats in Australia, Asia, South America, and Africa. The !Kung, who we will focus on, live in scattered bands across the Kalahari Desert. Since 1968, they have been the object of anthropological study because they are one of the few societies that continues to subsist by the collecting of vegetable foods and the hunting of animals. Foraging is the least labor-intensive of all subsistence strategies, involving the gathering of nondomesticated plants and the hunting of wild animals. Work estimates range around 20 hours a week in even the most difficult seasons. Individuals simply take what they need from the environment (immediate return), consume it, and go get more as needed, sharing with an extended kin network.

Lives in foraging societies are structured, but only informally, around the world of kin. Because of the repetitive and intermittent nature of the food quest, life is punctuated only by seasonal variation. There is only a minimal division of labor based on skills and ability. Ceremonial life consists primarily of healing ceremonies known as *trance dancing*. Nisa, a !Kung woman (Shostack, 1981), describes her life as follows: "We lived, and we lived" (p. 235). Nisa was born in 1921, and, as recently as 2005 (Konner, 2007), is still doing well, in northern Botswana. Although respectful of individuals older than her, Nisa's life is not organized into stages. As a child, Nisa spent much of her time in play groups that mimicked the adult world. As she matured, she helped her mother with expeditions to the bush with other women to gather food and eagerly awaited the return of her father and his brothers with the rewards of the hunt. As an adult, she is assisted by her daughter collecting bush foods for consumption and sharing. Reciprocal giving and taking sounds idyllic but presents its own challenges in the accounting of long-term reciprocity and linkages to others who are related by degrees of kinship. In fact, a prevalent theme in Nisa's account of her life is being *stinged*. She frequently reminds others that she feels she is not getting her fair share of food or other material goods.

The quest for food requires groups to move frequently as the areas used get depleted. Populations are usually very small, ranging between 30 and 50 individuals per band. Flexibility tends to favor bilateral descent and social mechanisms to extend social networks as far as possible. Nisa's arranged marriage illustrates the strategy of her parents to select a hard-working partner for Nisa and to obtain another contributor to the collective food supply, especially a hunter. Nisa was 12 when she first married and was a most reluctant bride. This marriage brought her husband, who was some 10 years older than Nisa, into her parents' encampment in bride service, where he hunted for her parents. This would be the first in a series of trial marriages that would be unstable since Nisa was not yet sexually mature and did not want a husband. After her first menstruation at the age of 16, she settled into a stable relationship with another man and moved into the world of adults. She and her husband would live with her parents for several months and then move to visit and live with his people. Nisa had her first child around the age of 18, a girl, whose father was a lover. Illness took her daughter just as she was learning to walk. In her 20s, Nisa had two more children, a girl and a boy, along with a couple of miscarriages. Then, her husband died quite suddenly. Following his death, Nisa had a number of lovers, and finally, she settled into a long-term relationship with yet another man. Together, they grew old, fighting, arguing, making up, and living among kin and friends.

Although remarkably productive with little labor input, foraging has downsides, which are mostly felt by the very old. First, the premium placed on mobility is a hardship for individuals who are incapacitated. Second, exchange through sharing or reciprocity places older people in an unfavorable position since they no longer can collect enough to reciprocate. The main way to control other people is through one's generosity. Otherwise, one can only complain about being stinged to embarrass others to share or to silence the complaint by sharing. The very old rely on the generosity of surviving children. Unfortunately for Nisa, by the time she was 37, she experienced the deaths of her two surviving children. Her daughter died in a fight with her husband when he pushed her and broke her neck, and her son died at the age of 15 from a lingering respiratory illness. Seasonality combined with mobility can make for a difficult life, sometimes ending in abandonment. On the positive side, older people are recognized as having accumulated knowledge through a lifetime of experience. Nisa would frequently comment that as a young person, she knew nothing. It was her older relatives who knew and taught her.

Tribal Societies

Village societies of up to 300 people who live together in related kin units without a centralized leadership are what anthropologists call *tribal cultures*. Unlike foragers, who collect from an environment, the subsistence is based on controlling life cycles of plants and/or animals. This strategy involves far more work, especially on a seasonal basis, around planting and harvesting (delayed return). It also involves far more cooperation and interdependency regarding work. Similar to foragers, it is still difficult to control others. Don Talaysva (1942), the Sun Chief of the Hopi in the pueblo of Orabi, wrote his autobiography, illustrating his life strategies in a horticultural tribal society. In northern Arizona, just to the east and slightly south of the Grand Canyon, we find the Hopi Mesas. Here are nine Hopi villages located in defensible locations around three mesas. The Hopi are desert horticulturalists (corn, beans, and squash), who farm near washes and also herd sheep as well as hunt smaller game. Each village consists of a number of permanent apartment-style residences owned by matrilineal clans. The fields are also owned by clans but are worked by the men who marry into the clan. The annual cycle of the Hopi is known for its rich ceremonial life of Kivas and Katchinas, mostly directed to the bringing of rain.

Don's life is a little more structured than that of a forager because of the ceremonial cycle and the matrilineal clans. There are clear transitions at points of initiation into the Katchina cult, the tribe, and marriage. A Hopi man is expected to work hard for his mother's and then his wife's clan and to work for the good of his village. Don Talaysva was born in March 1890 in Orabi, on the Hopi Third mesa. He reports a childhood filled with mischief and trouble. His parents could not discipline him. His mother's brother would be summoned, and he would be smoked (his head held under a blanket with smoldering juniper). The important things he learned in childhood were the importance of food, especially corn, and sexuality. His childhood was filled with helping his parents by protecting fields by chasing birds and other predators with his bow and arrow. He also removed blown-in sand that choked the corn, beans, and squash. When he was older, he often remained away from the village, herding sheep or horses for his father. Don was initiated into the Katchina cult around the age of 9, which was when his maternal uncle thought him ready. He made a significant step toward adulthood by the discovery that the mysterious Katchinas were only men he knew dressed in costume. This was a secret Don had to keep from younger Hopi. After initiation, Don learned to sing Katchina songs and dance as a Clown Katchina for both Orabi and Mohenkopi. Around the age of 20, Don was initiated into the Hopi tribe and became eligible to take the next step to full Hopi manhood and marry.

When Don married, his life changed considerably. After a year of ceremonial preparation by the two clans, Don and Irene were married and set up housekeeping in her clan's house near her mother. At this point, Don knew he was trapped into a world of serious labor because he now had to farm in what is a marginal environment. He also had to give everything to Irene, who would use it to run the household. After a few years, Irene became pregnant. Don's first child, a daughter, was sickly and soon died. This was to happen to three more children, who died within a few months of birth. The loss of the four infants led to accusations of witchcraft and assumptions that Don was not good with children. Irene's sister Jean was having trouble with her husband and feared the quarreling was making her child ill. Norman was given to Irene and Don, and he was nursed back to health. They raised him successfully to adulthood. As a successful parent, Don's life now was dominated by the village community. Don became even more active in the ceremonial life of Third Mesa, and because he was the recognized father of Norman, he became a Ceremonial Father to a number of Hopi boys, as they were initiated into the societies and into manhood. In a few years, the chief of the Sun Clan (a maternal uncle) realized he was too old and ill to continue as chief. He taught Don the proper ways of doing the essential rituals, and Don became the Chief of the Sun Clan and a respected Hopi leader.

Life Strategies in a Kin Mode of Production

In a kin mode of production, kin are paramount. Even if the social landscape is populated with kin, it is not a one-dimensional world. First, there is an opposition between kin and nonkin. Second, there are different kinds of kin. There are more important and less important kin. In a foraging society, such as Nisa's, kinship is bilateral, designed to give an ego the greatest number of kin connections. Controlling other people and their work is not easy. Nisa's primary economic strategy is that of an immediate return. She collects food and other things from the environment and consumes to meet her needs. To keep goods in circulation, she uses reciprocity to give goods when she has them in the hope the equivalent will be returned when she does not have them. For instance, in the Arctic, older Inuit males will overhunt the easier-to-kill caribou in late summer to give the skins to related families, with the hope of receiving seal meat, requiring more physical effort in extremely harsh conditions, from younger men during the winter (Guemple, 1980). Another strategy is the use of a leveling mechanism, such as an accusation of stinging, to embarrass another into giving. One also can complain to remind others of his or her needs and what the world would be like without reciprocity (Rosenberg, 1997). Parents can also arrange the marriages of their children to increase the pool of allied families and to get the labor of a son-in-law in bride service. If one pushes too hard, however, kin either fight back or move away and take up residence with another relative. This, indeed, not only reduces conflict, but it is a major life strategy to move people to parts of the habitat where foraging is more productive. In old age, with diminished capacity to forage, one can only rely on the generosity of relatives, most likely children, if they have survived. Indeed, we see high rates of mortality for children and even infanticide to prevent early weaning and certain death. With more distant relatives, the experience of aging may be rough simply because one cannot direct and control their labor.

For tribal groups such as Don's Hopi, the primary economic strategy is that of a delayed return. One plants in one season with the anticipation of a return several months in the future and storage into an even more distant future. Interdependency is more controlled simply because of work effort increases on a seasonal basis in cultivating crops and managing domesticated animals. Kin with the familiar generation and gender are still the basis for interdependency. However, kin are extended into lineages. For the Hopi, the matrilineal clans own the fields and houses. The elder males, uncles (mother's brothers), manage clan affairs and direct the work effort. Likewise, this can be difficult since people will just leave when conflict arises and go to relatives in another village. Old age is not the best time of life in either society, but because one is a member of a kin unit, one is seldom denied access to food and material goods.

One should note that the level of violence is quite high in bands and tribal societies. The reason is that everyone is his or her own leader, and justice is do it yourself with the help of kin affairs. Nisa's daughter died as a result of a fight. The Hopi, who have been described as Apollonian by Benedict (1934), have high levels of violence. The most dramatic was the destruction of the pueblo of Awatovi and the massacre of all the adult males in this village around 1700 because of feuds with other Hopi villages. Violence often results in premature deaths, which clearly prevent the experience of old age.

Production Ordered by Hierarchy and Tribute

Our second mode of production involves tribute and a hierarchy between tribute givers and tribute receivers. Tribute production uses the kin mode of production to increase the amount of wealth in a society. The tribute mode of production is much more recent, appearing about 5,000 years ago and diversifying throughout most of the world, with the exceptions of Australia and much of North America and the lowlands of South America. Through tribute, kin units are stimulated to produce a surplus, which is given to a big man, chief, or ruler. Thus kin units produce for their own consumption and for tribute and for commodities. The ruler uses this surplus in feasting, redistribution ceremonies, trade, infrastructure improvement, or warfare. With the increase in wealth comes greater security and the ability to invest in technology to reduce the risks associated with production (i.e., irrigation, storage, or rain magic). Tribute-based societies encompass a wide variety of social forms, ranging from those that use the surplus in feasting to archaic and feudal states.

Despite the diversity in specific societies, a common thread in life strategies is shaped by hierarchy and political centralization. Kin units are no longer autonomous. The social world is more complicated. Kin units have to intensify either by working harder or by using technology to produce a surplus. Lives in tribute societies are also more structured since more of life is oriented to a public culture of wealth and prestige. For instance, societies in the Pacific Northwest Coast of Canada are devoted to prestige and redistribution of wealth. Although technically, the subsistence is based on foraging, the peoples of the Northwest Coast are known for their economies of abundance, with feasting, extensive material culture, and social stratification. Florence Edenshaw Davidson was born in 1896 into Raven Moiety in the Haida village of Masset on the Queen Charlotte Islands off the coast of British Columbia. She was the 9th of 11 children of Charles and Isabella Edenshaw. Charles Edenshaw was a hereditary chief of the populous and powerful Eagle Moiety. He was also a well-known artist, who made numerous innovations in Northwest Coast art. Florence reports in her biography *During My Time*, by Blackman (1982), that her adult life was filled with hard work and the creation of wealth. Florence's childhood ended with her first puberty seclusion and, shortly thereafter, her arranged marriage to Robert Davidson of the Eagle Moiety. Robert Davidson was a commercial fisherman and a skilled carpenter. Robert was also 20 years older than Florence. Not only did she work hard in raising nine surviving children, but Florence earned extra money for the family and for the *potlatches* her husband organized by baking bread and pastries for the commercial fisherman, and for a while, she ran a small restaurant out of her home. She also labored in the canneries during the summers. She was an active and elite member of her Haida community through her activities in the Anglican Church and the Women's Auxiliary. Her husband built a large house, in which numerous celebrations were held. A successful potlatch not only organized the public life of her community but elevated the prestige of her husband and kin and guaranteed that there would be future feasting and redistribution. Florence gave a good many very large church socials, in which large quantities of food and other valuable items were given away. In 1991, Florence celebrated her 95th birthday with a potlatch, with 400 people in attendance and baskets of food to be taken home by the guests.

The quest for wealth and prestige can tax a family to the breaking point, as is illustrated by the House of Lim, observed by M. Wolf (1968). The House of Lim was the wealthiest family in a small farming village in northern Taiwan. This family had realized the Chinese ideal with a three-generation joint family of 14 people living as a domestic unit, under one roof, with one kitchen. Han-Ci Lim had died in the 1950s an old man. He began his life like his father, a tenant farmer who was destined to a life of poverty. However, because of his hard work, he managed to purchase small parcels of land and, with the profits, slowly increase his holdings. By the time he died, Han-Ci owned the house, 5 acres of farmland, a small cement bag factory, and a dozen pigs. All of his life, Han-Ci Lim worked very hard and saved his money, and left his family operating several enterprises.

Lives in the context of Taiwanese peasantry are also more structured in dealing with a largely nondomestic world. The family had to negotiate complicated marriages and even adopting women to become wives to sons as they matured. Adulthood is filled with responsibilities for family and hard work to support dependent family members. Han-Ci Lim had six children, of whom two died in infancy. One daughter was adopted out and one daughter married out. Two sons remained to form the joint household. The eldest son was strong willed, and in his late teens, he launched a very successful career in an underground organization, the *lo mua*, and became a very powerful and wealthy man locally and regionally. In his late 20s, he returned to his father's house and married, as expected, even taking a second wife. During a business deal, he was assaulted, severely injured, and within a couple of years, died. Thus his half of the family fell on hard times.

The youngest son had the onerous task of managing the family business and actually had improved its wealth beyond the hopes of Han-Ci Lim. However, he was facing an economy that was not favorable to family-run enterprises. He had to borrow to meet the payroll at the cement bag factory and had difficulties paying it back. He had married a wife who had expectations of greater wealth, and he engaged in a lifestyle of a man of importance, with mistresses, entertaining, drinking, and gambling. One of the reasons for the wealth and prestige of the Lims is they did keep the inheritance together. With hard work, they could afford taxes, rents, and the repayment of debt. However, the stresses became too great, and they split the wealth. The Lims live in the same house, but doors are nailed shut, and a new kitchen has been added, and they are no longer the most respected family in the village.

The public sphere of the culture becomes more prominent in rituals and in the display of wealth. The story of Shaka Zulu illustrates the domination of the intrigue of the kingdom. The Zulu are actually a lineage that allied themselves with other lineages to form a kingdom in South Africa in response to the slave trade. The subsistence of the Zulu was based on herding and horticulture. Shaka was born around 1785, one of many children in a chief's polygamous household (Thompson, 1969). He reports an unhappy childhood and adolescence in one of the regimental age sets. On the death of his father, Shaka defeated his brother and assumed leadership around 1812. By 1816, he seized power over the then insignificant Zulu clan by killing his brother. Shaka then began to make alliances with a number of other clans, and victory on the battlefield cemented his reputation. He continued to innovate with the military organization of the kingdom by organizing the age sets into formal regiments. In addition, he made modifications in weaponry with the short stabbing spear, and he refined the famous buffalo horns formation, by which he could encircle the enemy. Most significantly, he centralized the first fruits ceremonies (tribute) into the kingship. To keep the tribute flowing, there has to be linkages between the producing unit and the chief or king. There may be a series of ranked lineages and lesser chiefs working politically to amass the tribute. Most likely, there is coercion. Shaka took over the magic of the kingdom by becoming responsible for the rain magic, thus reinforcing his power through the supernatural. By 1820, he had consolidated power and was king of all the territory of Natal and South Africa. At the height of the Shakan

Empire, it encompassed over a quarter of a million people. Sometime in September 1828, Shaka was assassinated by his half brothers, one of whom assumed leadership. Later, in the 19th century, the Zulu would be one of the few African peoples who managed to defeat the British Army.

Life Strategies in a Tribute Mode of Production

In these societies, the chief delegates power to those beneath him to control the lives of their villagers and kin to deliver tribute. In this division of labor, there is far more control over the work and lives of others. In spite of the visibility of the elites and nobility, production still takes place within domestic units. There is incredible diversity in the way these units work internally and the linkages to the public arena of display. On the Northwest Coast, the nobility celebrate their rank by mobilizing kin to underwrite the feasting that accompanies the potlatch. Kin units may be ranked both internally and relative to each other, with goods flowing through the highest ranked male and upward to the chief, who technically owns everything. Another alternative is some kind of feudal arrangement involving rents or sharecropping. Regardless of variation, kin control production and manage it for themselves and for tribute. We should note that tribute is not necessarily a negative feature. Tribute increases wealth, which in turn is redistributed in various forms to provide infrastructure improvements and greater security.

The experience of aging in these societies is a little different than in foraging bands and tribal societies. Life strategies involve manipulating the hierarchical order and, often, negotiating higher rank. Because of the increase in wealth and the reduction of risk, life is more secure. Violence is managed by the hierarchy, and revenge is no longer a legitimate concern of individuals and kin. These kin units also have to deal with issues that are irrelevant to lineages and clans in a kin mode of production that worked the land. The House of Lim, for instance was a house of work and control. They had to work to pay taxes and to repay debt. Ownership of land and resources is a major issue primarily to retain the labor of younger kin and the productivity of property. In Europe, older individuals remained in the productive unit, possibly protected by a retirement contract or residing in more modest accommodations supported by the children, who manage production, for example, the West Room in Ireland (Arensberg, 1968).

Industrial Capitalism

We can view the capitalist mode of production as a radical departure from the past. On the other hand, it is the next step in the long evolutionary trend of intensification. What is different about capitalism is that the means of production has been removed from kinship. Capitalists rationalize and forever intensify production by organizing technology, raw materials, energy, labor, and transportation to the market. Labor is recruited from kin units through wages to give those kin units money through which to meet their needs. Capitalism is unlike tribute-based societies in that over time, it replaces the kin mode and the tribute mode of production. The economy becomes organized along different lines and shapes the lives of workers in very different ways. Work moves out of domestic units into factories and firms, where it is much easier to supervise. Families function as reproductive and consumption units. Lives become oriented to the labor market and are structured into the familiar three stages of preparation, working, and retirement (Best, 1980). Life strategies are further conditioned by the segmentation of the labor force. We will examine some of the life strategies in capitalism through the lives of two men from Momence, Illinois, studied as a part of Project AGE (Keith et al., 1994). Momence is a town of a little over 3,000, located about 50 miles south of Chicago. Both men indicate that work is very important, but in different ways. They also see schools shaping their life experiences. Their lives are very definitely staged from childhood/adolescence to adulthood to older adult.

George is very proud of his success in the corporate world. George was born in 1917 in Pennsylvania. He was the only child of older parents. His dad invested all he had in a hotel, which burnt shortly after completion, and he died soon after that. Just before Pearl Harbor, George got an accounting job in the aviation industry, exempting him from service in World War II. He also married Sarah around this time. He claims she was one of two important people in his life, primarily because she encouraged him to return to school and complete 3 years to get ahead in the business world. Together, they had a son and a daughter. After a couple of job changes, he took a senior position in a book-distributing company (in New Jersey), where he eventually became president. The former president of this company was the second most important person in his life, taking him under his wing and promoting him in the company. He was relocated to Momence, Illinois, where he bought one of the biggest houses in town, and has remained there ever since. This was 1964, and he was president of the entire company. Through the 1960s, the company kept expanding, with plants in Nevada and Georgia as well as New Jersey and Illinois. In 1971, the W. R. Grace Company bought out the book distribution company. Within a year, there was conflict, and George was fired. Fortunately for George, he had an employment contract and sued and won $100,000 per year for 15 years. He was lured out of his retirement several times to be a personnel director at a regional corporation and, finally, the vice president of a local bank. He served for over 12 years as vice president of the Momence Gladiolus Festival Association.

Eldon also talks about work, but his theme is the ability to endure hard labor and provide for his family. Eldon was born in St. Anne, Illinois, in 1905. He was the first son in a family of five. His father was a laborer, who moved to where work was available, including southern Illinois, where he made props for coal mines. Eldon attended rural schools until the age of 15, when he began a life of hard work around 1920: "They took me out of school and put me to work. This is when my youth ended and the best stage of my life" (Fry, n.d.). He began with the construction of the Dixie Highway (Illinois Rt. 1) by throwing bags over the side of a coal car and then spreading the contents to make the shoulders of the first hard road in the area. He had other jobs as a farm laborer, constructing township roads, and as a greenskeeper at a local golf course. Until 1930, he lived at home and gave his wages to his parents (the family fund) to care for his younger siblings. The work was hard, and a number of accidents began to take their toll, including broken limbs and lost teeth.

In January 1930, Eldon married Eileen. Life was difficult. They rented a three-room house south of Momence for $4.50 a month but were so poor they had to borrow furniture. He picked nearly 100 bushels of cucumbers a day for a dollar, while Eileen picked 3,000 carnations, also for a dollar. The work in the high temperatures and damp mornings in the fields made him sick, and he could no longer work until he regained his health. Eldon and Eileen moved to Momence in a real crisis by going on relief and begging for food and clothing for their three small children in the depths of the Depression. After 2 years, he could hold a job and landed steady work until the end of the war. Eldon is very proud of the fact they were able to purchase their home in 1943 and pay off the $1,600 mortgage within a year. Then he became a self-employed carpenter and, finally, worked in a local spring factory. At the age of 62, he was injured in two industrial accidents within a month. The company claimed his injuries were old, but with the help of his physician, they were forced to make a small settlement. "I thought nothing could stop me. It wasn't the work that stopped me, it was the accidents. It was just too heavy work for the conditions" (Fry, n.d.). In summing up the important things in his life, Eldon stated,

> The most important things about my life is that I have raised three kids. They are the most important things in my life. I have eight grandchildren and two great-grandchildren. They are the most important things of my life. Without a family, if you die tomorrow, you would have nothing to leave behind. I also own my own home. (Fry, n.d.)

Life Strategies in a Capitalist Mode of Production

Both of these men did not work within a domestic unit, nor did their families own the workplace. Their main economic strategy was one of immediate return in the form of wages. With cash, they both could forage in the marketplace to purchase consumer goods to meet their needs. Like people in a tribute mode of production, they had to pay taxes and repay debt, especially mortgages on their homes. Because of the immediate return of wages and salaries, they are expected to anticipate times when they are not working such as being laid off, being too ill to work, or when they retire. Only by deferring income in the form of savings, capital investment, insurance, or pensions can they expect to have income without a job. The effects of the segmentation of the labor market are quite clear. George had the opportunity to enter upper level management in a small corporation and eventually to oversee the expansion to a national corporate entity and was protected by an employment contract. Eldon was in a different segment of the labor force, where he had difficulty accumulating capital and changed jobs frequently. Families are important to both men, especially for Eldon. Obviously, families are smaller, and all the children survive. It is clearly the world of work that was a major axis in both men's lives, especially George's.

The genius of capitalism is the ability to grow wealth through an ever-expanding cycle of investment and production of commodities. To expand wealth, capitalism alters the relationships between people in production and their control over workers. This change is made possible through the invention of labor as a commodity, which can be sold for wages. Workplaces shift to nondomestic settings, such as factories, where discipline is easier to administrate. Life becomes regulated by the clock since wage work is performed on a schedule. The capitalist mode of production involves the most effective way of controlling the life course and the work of others. A worker may spend upward of one-third of his or her waking life doing something for someone else. Populations first in England, then in Western Europe and the United States became divided into working classes and into the owners and managers of capital. Working classes became further segmented by historic race and ethnic classifications. The lowest of these classes were denied the best jobs or the information that would allow them to perform them. Labor became highly mobile, as witnessed by the diasporas from Europe to North America in the 19th and 20th centuries and from India and China after the abolition of slavery. Slavery was in part abolished and replaced by so-called free labor because wages were a more effective means of control than whips.

As capitalism expanded, other changes were fast in coming. States nurturing capitalism instituted changes creating contemporary nation-states. Nation-states set out to create national identities and cultures by promoting a uniform language and knowledge through universal education. Previously remarkably heterogeneous populations in a short time were homogenized into French, Italians, Germans, or Americans. Laws were created, favoring capitalists, concerning taxation, regulation, contracts, and labor. States developed the institutional infrastructure for capitalism, including transportation, standardized weights and measures, currency, and financial institutions. The nation-state began to function to politically stabilize the nation and to organize the economy. Nation-states became the main building blocks of the world economy.

As nation-states began the rationalization of their economies and trade, they created a new citizenship for their workers and consumers. A significant part of citizenship involves age and life strategies that are enacted by age. Life strategies entail preparation to get well positioned in the labor market. Once positioned, one provides for family and saves and accumulates capital for the end of life.

Capitalism creates a new problem for growing old. Once a person loses a job, quits, or is no longer able to work, there is no longer income. For industrial workers, there is no return to the family farm or the domestic mode of production. The period of life that became known as *retirement* needs to be financed. Old age rapidly became associated with the almshouse and poverty (Haber, 1993). Throughout the 19th and early 20th centuries, families used the traditional family fund strategy to economize, with multigenerational households and pooling the income of working adults. This worked to the advantage of older people but was inherently unfair to younger family members. Earlier, we saw Eldon work for over a decade to provide for his siblings, only to enter marriage with only his income, which was not enough to buy furniture. Family funds triggered intergenerational conflict, which only intensified with the Depression of the 1920s and 1930s. Social Security or the Old Age Assistance part of the program stabilized the incomes of older people, thus effectively ending the strategy of the family fund (Gratton, 1993).

Our evolutionary story has been one of a quest for power and wealth. It has been one of changing demographics, intensification, and new modes of production to achieve greater economic expansion. Modes of production also involve a division of labor and the interdependency that involves the control of other people's lives. Kin production was harnessed by systems of tribute, which received surplus from kin producers. Capitalism was a departure from kin and tribute production. Our story has involved shifts in economic strategies. The immediate return of foraging was replaced by the delayed return of horticulture. Regardless of subsistence strategy, the fruits of one's labor were for consumption within a kin unit. Tribute systems required kin units to produce beyond their needs to pay taxes and debts. Capitalism reverted to an immediate return through wages, but required an additional strategy to defer a part of that income for future use. In this section of the chapter, I argue that the most important thing we can know about the experiences of aging is the mode of production and the political economy in which life experience and life strategies unfold. The mode of production structures relationships between groups of people as they transform nature into culturally useful things: food, technology, goods, services, luxuries, and so on. A division of labor and exchange is created that defines lines of interdependency and responsibility. Humans use these relationships to accommodate to an ever-changing environment and historical circumstances.

In many respects, the returned emphasis on political and economic relationships runs countercurrent to the directions of the social sciences composing gerontology. Sometime in the early to middle 20th century, these disciplines took a turn to minimize the importance of the political and economic context in which social life takes place. The net effect of this disassociation is that we have lost holism from our efforts to build theory about aging. Our inattention to the larger context and the interconnectedness of that context has limited our interest in, and even our ability to ask, certain kinds of questions. Gerontology, on the other hand, has considerable promise, with an established scholarship on resources, pensions, and savings. Critical theory, with its focus on inequities rooted in race, class, and gender (Estes, Biggs, & Phillipson, 2003), is opening a vista into the way political economies shape old age. The loss of holism has rendered a very detailed, but fragmentary, understanding of the workings of the social world (Bass, 2006; Hagestad & Dannefer, 2001). Ironically, we live in a globalized world that is highly integrated through financial and legal arrangements (Nader, 2007).

WORLDS LOST, WORLDS GAINED

When we place things in an evolutionary order, we invite making value judgments about the quality of life in various cultures so ordered by these modes of production. In relative terms, each culture has its strengths and weaknesses. Each culture presents different kinds of risks for people of all ages. Each culture has ways of providing for the needs of its members and enabling a secure life. Foraging provides a steady intake of diverse foods, but there are obvious risks associated with the inability to accumulate wealth. Tribal groups relying on domesticates can accumulate food but must work harder and face the risks of crop failure. Both foragers and tribal people face potential famine and must deal with conflicts, which can rapidly become a feud. Tribute modes of production pretty much resolve issues associated with production failure simply because the tribute is surplus and can be used, if needed, and invested in infrastructure to increase production. However, as populations grew and nucleated, other problems of sanitation and disease were created. Capitalism seems to have resolved production issues with the intensified creation of commodities, including food. However, capitalism is known for expansive periods of growth and contractive periods of depression. Also, capitalism uses social stratification in the creation of wealth. Consequently, the gaps between the wealthy and the poor have markedly increased.

The worlds we left behind with the dawn of the 20th century were societies where life was precarious. Infant mortality was high, with around 50% of children dying before the age of 10. Less than 5% of adults survived beyond their 60th birthdays. Plagues could not be dealt with in an effective way. Famines were all too common until late in the 19th century. It is only with improved sanitation and more secure water supplies and the industrialization of medicine that we see improvements in longevity. These negative features are best left in the past.

What kinds of societies has capitalism created, as this mode of production spread from England in the late 18th century to the rest of the world? This part of our story goes back to the 1400s, when Europe began its mercantile expansion. European traders encountered peoples in Africa, Asia, the Americas, and the Pacific who were involved in established polities and trading networks (Wolf, 1982). By the 19th century, Europe had created a global mercantile trading economy. By the end of the 19th century, this economy was being transformed into a capitalist market in the large-scale production of commodities such as wheat, cotton, cod, tea, coffee, sugar, bananas, meat, and metals.

Globalization has been happening for a long time, but the intensity of a globalized economy is fairly recent. The world order is usually defined following a major war. After the Second World War, the financial and political basis for the global world was established. In the absence of a world government, the Bretton Woods Conference established the global economic agenda by creating the International Monetary Fund, the World Bank, and the GATT agreement. The intent was to design the international financial and trade institutions to stabilize capitalism on a global scale. The United Nations was the political portion of this international world. Globalization has proceeded and was increased when, in 1971, President Nixon removed the backing of U.S. gold from the U.S. dollar, which effectively removed the linkage to gold for all currencies of the world. The money supply increased, and globalization further intensified. In the past three decades, corporations have become increasingly controlled by their CEOs and have focused only on short-term profits. This has been called *CEO capitalism* (Bogle, 2005). By way of contrast, in *stakeholder capitalism*, corporate directors take into account factors other than maximizing stockholder value in reaching their decisions.

How has globalization shaped the experience of aging? Should we in gerontology be concerned about it? Globalization has and definitely will shape the experience of aging. All the people we met in the life histories outlined previously had their lives shaped by globalization. The !Kung of the Kalahari are not isolated but have been involved in trading networks for hundreds of years. An entire band was featured in the movie *The Gods Must Be Crazy*. Nisa's old age was much improved when Marjorie Shostak gave her the royalties from her best-selling book about her life to buy cattle. Don experienced boarding schools for Indian children to remove them from parents to educate them and provide skills for the dominant Anglo society. Florence welcomed Queen Elizabeth and Prince Philip to the Queen Charlotte Islands, representing the Canadian government and local people. Shaka Zulu prepared his kingdom to confront and defeat the British. The House of Lim faced a globalizing economy that was not friendly to small, family-run enterprises. Both George and Eldon felt the direct effects of globalization. George's position changed when his corporation was bought out by a larger conglomerate. The carnations that Eileen picked for a dollar a day are now imported from Holland, arriving daily in Chicago on a cargo jet.

Global capital, as all capital, uses all the factors in production, but most of all, it involves labor. The global assembly line has been created to cut the costs of labor. Globalization increases the competition between laborers all over the world. Workers in Tennessee must compete with workers in Mexico. Workers in California must compete with workers in the Philippines or in Singapore. There are some who foresee David Ricardo's famous Iron Law of Labor as a real potential. If the experience of old age is sharply conditioned by the presence of an income and economic security, it, too, is an issue of labor. If wages are depressed, how is it possible to adequately save for retirement? Through the 1980s, we have seen a shift in the labor force toward more short-term contract jobs, as compared to the now rare lifetime employment with one firm. We have also seen the shift from production to service economies in the heartland of capitalism. Defined benefit pensions have all but disappeared, with defined contribution benefits taking their place. Wages have stagnated. Savings in the United States is now as low as it was in 1932.

Because the economy is now global, we should examine what is happening around the globe (Phillipson, 2006). What happens in one part has direct effects elsewhere. Although gerontology has always had a strong international component, by and large, it has been Eurocentric. Modernization theory pretty much assumed the rest of the world would become like Europe, but it did not turn out that way. The attempts to increase profits since the 1970s have resulted in so-called offshore production zones in Asia and Latin America. Here assembly of commodities takes place in areas where the commodities are not subject to tariff and shipped all over the world. Even though there are jobs in these zones, wages are extremely low, and workers, mostly women and children, labor long hours in sweatshops. We even see children as young as 12 indentured to work with no way of paying to gain their release (Dannefer, 2003). The conditions we see around the globe are worse than in Europe in the 19th century. One wonders if one should even be thinking about deferred income to support old age when nearly half of the world's workers earn only $2.00 a day. With the changes in pensions and the labor force in the service economies of Europe and North America, we may well return to conditions similar to those of the 19th century. It is clear, with the trends of only three decades in duration, that the 21st century is going to be a much less secure place in which to grow old.

Economies are remarkable institutions, organizing humans to transform nature into usable cultural goods. Capitalism is still very new when compared with the domestic mode of production, which has over 1,000,000 years of history, and tribute modes of production, which have thousands of years of history. Capitalism harnessed fossil fuels, redefined labor, and created large corporations, which rival and shape the nation-states in which they operate. Capitalism has demonstrated its adaptability by spreading production and markets across the globe and has demonstrated its ability to work with other modes of production. We still have much to see happen with capitalism in the centuries ahead. This economy is not without its problems. First, there is the cyclical boom and busts, which can be devastating. There are major questions about sustainability and world population growth. Because of the increased polarization in the labor market, segmentation, poverty, disease, and hunger remain, in spite of the greatest amount of wealth ever created. Finally, many peoples of the world have resisted capitalism. From the revolutions of 1848 in Europe, to the Mau Mau Rebellion in East Africa, to the Malaysian resistance, to the Green Revolution, to the rebellion in Chiapas, to the resurgence in Islamic and Protestant fundamentalism and liberation theology in Latin America, and even to the terrorism that destroyed the World Trade Center, we see that the global economy is not as unified as we might think.

CULTURE AND THE EXPERIENCES OF AGING

The experience of aging is a personal experience. It is the culmination of life experience and all the opportunities and strategies that one has played out during life. The importance of the life review is that one seeks the pattern of what has gone before. The blueprint for lives is culturally scripted. Across the life span, one learns through interaction with others of differing ages, one figures out what makes life good and what makes it bad. Humans have the remarkable ability to develop into unique personalities that endure and change into late life. The blueprints for lives are only rough guidelines. Like most things cultural, lives are self-organized. In spite of potential wide-ranging variation, the answers to what makes life good are not random. We should listen to what people have been telling us for nearly a half century about their well-being. The answers center on only a few issues: health; material security; social life, including family; and personal character concerns. Of these, the health and material factors are most likely to see agreement across cultures. The social and character factors are likely to see more variation since they are played out in variable local contexts. However, all are shaped by the political economy and one's position in that context.

By taking a look at life stories, we can see how these issues play out in people's lives. Nisa, as a forager in the family mode of production, is concerned with material security and getting her fair share. Don learned early about the importance of food and sex. As he matured, he married and began to work his wife's clan's fields. He also was initiated into the Hopi tribe, becoming involved in ceremonial life, and eventually became the Sun Chief and a leader of Orabi. Florence worked hard for the welfare of her large family and assisted in accumulating the necessary goods for potlatching. She was active in her community and took responsibility for others who were not highly ranked. Shaka Zulu welcomed the opportunity to innovate and to compete with his half brothers for leadership of the Zulu kingdom, leading a very successful army. The Lim family, as a tribute giver, struggled to hold the family and its resources together, instead of splitting. Theirs is a house full of responsibility, work, and complaint. Eldon, who was in the lower segments of the labor force, saw his achievement in his family being raised and their house paid for. His major life tasks had been completed. George was very pleased with his corporate success and continuing involvement in the corporate world and in formal community organizations. Do any of these qualities have anything to do with age? These are issues associated with living. Kaufman (1986) reported that contrary to what gerontologists expect, older people, when talking about their lives, do not see old age as a unique stage of their lives. They just continue living, playing out their strategies with whatever challenges or opportunities arise.

What does our evolutionary story tell us about the experiences of aging and their possible meanings? It is clear that the political and economic contexts set limits and define opportunities. It is also clear that as the exclusively kin mode of production is replaced by tribute and capitalism, the social arenas in which people play out their lives become more diverse. With institutionalized hierarchy, individuals can negotiate an expansive world free of leveling mechanisms, such as complaints of stinging, to keep them in their place. With more wealth production, risks are somewhat reduced, and starvation is less of a threat. There are some positive things to be said, as the political economy is transformed from kinship to tribute to capitalism, that directly relate to increased life spans and security.

There are also some negative things. The leisurely life of foragers is left behind, as labor becomes valuable and the demand for it increases. Institutionalized hierarchy results in not only status differences, but in differentials of wealth and lifestyle. Hierarchy itself is unstable because concentrations of wealth and excessive demands from the tribute takers produce conflict and rebellion both internally and externally. In the 5,000 or so years since the advent of tribute economies, we have seen them come and most of them go, including the powerful Roman Empire. Even youthful capitalism is unstable. Since its inception, we have seen seven major depressions. Expanding or contracting social systems alter life strategies and life chances, especially for those transitioning into adulthood. For instance, we have seen a whole generation of Chinese disadvantaged when they were sent to work with the peasants during the Cultural Revolution (Ikels, 1989). Within capitalism, it is an expanding or unstable labor market that shapes lives. Major depressions (Elder, 1974), altering political and economic systems (Titma & Tuma, 2005), and major wars (Laub & Sampson, 2005) have lasting effects on individuals positioning themselves in the labor market during the event and its aftermath. Likewise, the structuring of inequality within nation-states has long-term effects on individuals of different classes following periods of change (Featherman, Selbee, & Mayer, 1989).

Let us return to the question of old age. Let us also return to the thinkers with whom we began this chapter: Morgan (1877), Maine (1861), Durkheim (1893/1933), Marx (1967), and de Tocqueville (1835/1994). What is it they were seeing shortly after the creation of capitalism? In contrasts such as status–contract, *societas–civitas*, and mechanical–organic solidarity, they saw the tremendous expansion and transformation of the economy. They also saw how these changes challenged families to accommodate to their new role. Old age in economies dominated by kin and tribute was not a problem. Age was not without its problems, but kin units resolved those problems positively or negatively. The change in the family is one of the most profound transformations defining old age in the capitalist mode of production. Our 19th-century thinkers saw the loosening of family bonds and filial piety, releasing adults as individuals free of parental control to the labor market. Filial dependency remained only for the immature young. It is the labor market of capitalism that has created old age and the institution of retirement. It is defined as a problem because of increased disability and decreased income.

Leisure and reaching the state where one can just be (no longer under the control of the wage) is not the state of affairs for everyone. Nor will it be in the immediate future. In the United States, less than half of those families approaching retirement expect to see little alteration in their lifestyles once they retire at 65. Many individuals will never see retirement, especially with the growing trend toward defined contribution pensions and voluntary savings. Capitalism has changed and will continue to change. That is expected since the capitalist mode is fueled by competition, as the invisible hand works its magic for innovation and profit. We fixed capitalism after the Second World War to stabilize it to prevent the major swings in the boom and bust cycle. We should be able to also fix capitalism to stabilize the life course wages and consumption abilities for the workers who spend upward of one-third of their waking working lives producing goods and services. Since the 1980s, the short-term profit focus of CEO capitalism has resulted in individualizing risk for workers in old age all over the globe. A form of shareholder capitalism, where the human factors in production are considered in late life, is certainly possible. It is possible, as evidenced by the nation-states of Western Europe, who protect their citizens and keep economic inequality about 40% lower than in the United States (Blim, 2005). Humans have experimented with all sorts of strategies within the opportunities and limitations of the political economy and mode of production in which they are located. Capitalism, with the financial and insurance institutions, has provided a number of solutions. Since the 1980s, however, CEO capitalism has been deregulated to the detriment of the environment, labor, and economic rights.

Unfortunately, a negative consequence of hierarchy is that some have, and others have not. The labor market is segmented and globalized. Just as it takes money to make money, it takes money to save and defer income. Poverty not only continues to plague humankind, but it continues to affect larger and larger numbers of families, especially because of global capital's search for cheaper labor. Impoverishment and immiseration is a problem for people of all ages, children, adults, and older adults. It is also a problem for the nations of the globalized world and the globalized economy to resolve.

REFERENCES

Arensberg, C. (1968). *The Irish countryman.* New York: Macmillan.

Bass, S. (2006). Gerontological theory: The search for the Holy Grail. *Gerontologist, 46,* 139–144.

Benedict, R. (1934). *Patterns of culture.* New York: Houghton Mifflin.

Best, F. (1980). *Flexible life scheduling.* New York: Praeger.

Blackman, M. B. (1982). *During my time: Florence Edenshaw Davidson, a Haida woman.* Seattle: University of Washington Press.

Blim, M. (2005). *Equality and economy: The global challenge.* New York: Altamira Press.

Bogle, J. C. (2005). *The battle for the soul of capitalism.* New Haven, CT: Yale University Press.

Boyd, R., & Richardson, P. J. (2005). *The origin and evolution of cultures.* New York: Oxford University Press.

Cowgill, D. O. (1986). *Aging around the world.* Belmont, CA: Wadsworth.

Cowgill, D. O., & Holmes, L. D. (Eds.). (1972). *Aging and modernization.* New York: Appleton, Century, Crofts.

Dannefer, D. (2003). Whose life is it, anyway? Diversity and "linked lives" in global perspective. In R. A. Settersten (Ed.), *Invitation to the life course: Toward new understandings of later life* (pp. 259–268). Amityville, NY: Baywood.

De Tocqueville, A. (1994). *Democracy in America.* New York: Alfred A. Knopf. (Original work published 1835)

Durkheim, E. (1933). *The division of labor in society.* New York: Free Press. (Original work published 1893)

Elder, G. H. (1974). *Children of the great depression: Social change in life experience.* Chicago: University of Chicago Press.

Estes, C., Biggs, S., & Phillipson, C. (2003). *Social theory, social policy, and ageing: A critical introduction.* Berkshire, England: Open University Press.

Featherman, D., Selbee, L. K., & Mayer, K. U. (1989). Social class and the structuring of the life course in Norway and West Germany. In D. I. Kertzer & K. W. Schaie (Eds.), *Age structuring in comparative perspective* (pp. 55–94). Hillsdale, NJ: Erlbaum.

Fry, C. L. (n.d.). Unpublished field notes. Momence, IL: Project AGE.

Gratton, B. (1993). The creation of retirement: Families, individuals and the social security movement. In K. W. Schaie & W. A. Achenbaum (Eds.), *Societal impact on aging: Historical perspectives* (pp. 45–73). New York: Springer Publishing.

Guemple, L. D. (1980). Growing old in Inuit society. In V. W. Marshall (Ed.), *Aging in Canada: Social perspectives* (pp. 95–102). Don Mills, Ontario: Fitzhenry and Whiteside.

Haber, C. (1993). Over the hill to the poorhouse: Rhetoric and reality in the institutional history of the aged. In K. W. Schaie & W. A. Achenbaum (Eds.), *Societal impact on aging: Historical perspectives* (pp. 90–113). New York: Springer Publishing.

Hagestad, G. O., & Dannefer, D. (2001). Concepts and theories of aging: Beyond microfication in social science approaches. In R. H. Binstock & L. K. George (Eds.), *Handbook of aging and the social sciences* (5th ed., pp. 3–21). San Diego, CA: Academic Press.

Ikels, C. (1989). Becoming a human being in theory and practice: Chinese views of human development. In D. I. Kertzer & K. W. Schaie (Eds.), *Age structuring in comparative perspective* (pp. 109–134). Hillsdale, NJ: Erlbaum.

Kaufman, S. R. (1986). *The ageless self: Sources of meaning in late life.* Madison: University of Wisconsin Press.

Keith, J., Fry, C. L., Glascock, A. P., Ikels, C., Dickerson-Putman, J., Harpending, H. C., et al. (1994). *The aging experience: Diversity and commonality across cultures.* Thousand Oaks, CA: Sage.

Kertzer, D. I., & Schaie, K. W. (Eds.). (1989). *Age structuring in comparative perspective.* Hillsdale, NJ: Erlbaum.

Konner, M. (2007). Dim beginnings. *New York Review of Books, 54,* 26–29.

Laub, J. H., & Sampson, R. J. (2005). Coming of age in wartime: How World War II and the Korean war changed lives. In K. W. Schaie & G. Elder (Eds.), *Historical influences on lives and aging* (pp. 208–229). New York: Springer Publishing.

Maine, H. S. (1861). *Ancient law.* London: Murry.

Marx, K. (1967). *Capital.* New York: International Publishers. (First published in German 1894)

Morgan, L. H. (1877). *Ancient society.* New York: World Publishing.

Nader, L. (2007). Law: The missing link in policy studies. *Anthropology News, 48,* 35–36.

Phillipson, C. (2006). The dynamic nature of societal aging in a global perspective. In D. Sheets, D. B. Bradley, & J. Hendricks (Eds.), *Enduring questions in gerontology* (pp. 131–158). New York: Springer Publishing.

Richardson, P. J., & Boyd, R. (2005). *Not by genes alone: How culture transformed human evolution.* Chicago: University of Chicago Press.

Rosenberg, H. G. (1997). Complaint discourse: Aging and caregiving among the Ju/hoansi of Botswana. In J. Sokolovsky (Ed.), *The cultural context of aging: Worldwide perspectives* (pp. 33–55). Westport CT: Bergin and Garvey Press.

Sahlins, M. D., & Service, E. R. (Eds.). (1960). *Evolution and culture.* Ann Arbor: University of Michigan Press.

Schaie, K. W., & Achenbaum, W. A. (Eds.). (1993). *Societal impact on aging: Historical perspectives.* New York: Springer Publishing.

Schaie, K. W., & Elder, G. (Eds.). (2005). *Historical influences on lives and aging.* New York: Springer Publishing.

Shostak, M. (1981). *Nisa: The life and words of a !Kung woman.* Cambridge, MA: Harvard University Press.

Talaysva, D. C. (1942). *Sun chief: The autobiography of a Hopi Indian.* New Haven, CT: Yale University Press.

Thompson, L. (1969). Cooperation and conflict: The Zulu kingdom and Natal. In M. Wilson & L. Thompson (Eds.), *The Oxford history of South Africa: Vol 1. South Africa to 1870* (pp. 334–390). London: Oxford University Press.

Titma, M., & Tuma, N. B. (2005). Human agency in the transition from communism: Perspectives on the life course and aging. In K. W. Schaie & G. Elder (Eds.), *Historical influences on lives and aging* (pp. 108–143). New York: Springer Publishing.

Tylor, E. B. (1871). *Primitive culture: Researches into the development of mythology, language, art and custom.* London: Murry.

Wolf, E. R. (1982). *Europe and the people without history.* Berkeley: University of California Press.

Wolf, M. (1968). *The house of Lim: A study of a Chinese farm family.* Englewood Cliffs, NJ: Prentice Hall.

The Aging Experience, Social Change, and Television

13

RUKMALIE JAYAKODY

The chapters by Cole, Achenbaum, and Carlin (this volume) and Fry (this volume) emphasize changes in the meaning of old age. Cole and colleagues highlight the increasing uncertainty of old age, particularly given dramatic changes in mortality. As they point out, for the first time in human history, "we are living after the life cycle—after the collapse of widely shared images and socially cohesive structures and experiences of the life cycle" (p. 252). Fry, by discussing the effects of a global economy, also focuses on the changes in the aging experience across cultures. Social changes from a variety of sources, including those discussed by Cole et al. and Fry, have important implications for the meaning of aging. Another pervasive source of change influencing people worldwide since the 1950s is television. However, debates on television's effects are almost uniformly centered on the young, and television's effects are rarely examined in the context of the aging experience. This chapter examines family changes worldwide and discusses why research on television's influence should extend to all phases of the life span, not just children and adolescents.

Acknowledgments: The research described in this chapter was made possible through generous funding from Penn State's Population Research Institute and the Social Science Research Institute.

This discussion utilizes a life course perspective, which examines different influences on experiences across the life span, including historical, cultural, economic, and demographic (Elder, 1998). The life course perspective places special emphasis on the social meaning of age, and two of its themes are particularly relevant to the chapters by Cole et al. and Fry. The first theme highlights the important role of history, pointing out that the life course of individuals is embedded in and shaped by the historical times and places individuals experience over their lifetimes. The impacts of social change are emphasized in this theme, noting that people develop and age in different ways, according to the nature of social change. In the context of television, this first theme specifies that television's effects will likely vary, depending on the age of exposure. Individuals whose introduction to television occurs at age 60 will be impacted differently from those exposed as children. A second life course theme, the concept of *linked lives*, examines how lives are lived independently, noting that social and historical influences are experienced through a network of shared relationships (Elder, 1998). Therefore, besides television's direct impact, the aging experience will also be influenced by other generations' responses. This chapter will highlight family changes across the globe, utilizing these two life course themes to better understand the implications of these changes for the experience of aging today. Research from Vietnam will be used to illustrate how the experience of aging has been affected by television and will offer some hypotheses for further cross-cultural research on television's influence on the aging experience.

INTERNATIONAL FAMILY CHANGE

Family life has changed tremendously over the past century, and especially in the past several decades. These changes have been extensive not only in their geographic scope, covering most of the world's populations, but also in the breadth of family dimensions affected. For example, in many parts of the world, age at marriage has risen dramatically, children's involvement in mate selection has increased, parental authority has declined, premarital sex has increased, contraceptive use has become widespread, and there have been extensive changes in fertility and mortality. Although less thoroughly documented, attitudes and beliefs regarding family life have also changed tremendously. These transformations are so ubiquitous that they are often discussed in global terms, with globalization being increasingly used to describe worldwide changes beyond economics and trade (Jayakody, Thornton, & Axinn, 2008).

Theories of family change include both structural and ideational perspectives. Structural theories emphasize alterations in the cost–benefit calculus, highlighting shifts from agricultural to industrial to a service economy, the movement of populations from rural to urban areas, increases in income, changes in technology, expansions in education, and declines in disease and mortality. The fundamental argument of these theories is that changes in the social and economic circumstances and constraints—for example, industrialization and the expansion of education—have ramifications throughout society. These changes modify the ways in which individuals relate to family members, with implications for husband–wife relationships, parents' influence over children, relationships among siblings, and the family's role in elder care. On the other hand, others argue that cost–benefit changes alone are insufficient to produce the observed changes in family behavior and that other forces must also be in play (Caldwell, 1982; Cleland & Wilson, 1987; Freedman, 1979).

In addition to structural changes, ideational dimensions have also been identified as an important force in understanding family change and are thought to be central in shaping demographic behavior (Axinn, Ghimire, & Barber, 2008; Coale & Watkins, 1986; Lesthaeghe & Wilson, 1986; Thornton, 2001; Watkins, 1991). *Ideation* refers to a new way of thinking, and ideational change requires that individuals are in contact with ideas and information they had not previously encountered. Suggested mechanisms for the spread of new ideas include educational institutions (Caldwell, 1982; Thornton & Lin, 1994); gossip networks (Watkins & Danzi, 1995); increased migration, travel, and tourism (Bongaarts & Watkins, 1996); and the mass media (Bongaarts & Watkins, 1996).

Television, which is specifically designed to transmit new ideas and information, may be a particularly powerful source of ideational change. Television has been described as one of the most powerful idea disseminators, socializing agents, and public opinion molders in the contemporary world (Kottak, 1990), and television's power to change attitudes and behavior has long been assumed (Butcher, 2003; Kottak, 1991; Westoff & Bankole, 1999). Furthermore, the introduction and spread of new ideas through television often transcends traditional barriers of language and literacy. New models of family structure and social arrangements are introduced through television, and these new models are often labeled as modern and defined as good (Hornick & McAnany, 2001). These new ideas, techniques, and values may result in family change.

Television may impact change through both structural and ideational mechanisms, and rather than being competing alternatives, structural and ideational explanations are interrelated and reinforcing (Jayakody et al., 2008). Ideational frameworks that specify approaches for experiencing and living with reality must take into account the economic and social system that bounds that reality. Similarly, ideational frameworks may modify those economic and social systems. Social and economic systems are also vital in facilitating or limiting the spread of beliefs, values, and motivations across geographical and social boundaries. For example, education obviously involves the spread of new ideas (ideation), but access to education can also alter the microeconomic calculus to marriage and childbearing (structural). Similarly, television's impact may operate through the introduction and spread of new ideas or by changing consumption and savings behavior as individuals and families assign priority to a television purchase. My purpose is not to choose between structural and ideational explanations of television's impact; rather, I believe that both are important and fit together in mutually reinforcing ways. Be it through structure, ideation, or more likely a combination of both, television may influence family change by altering social and family relationships, changing aspirations, and introducing new ideas and models of behavior.

TELEVISION AND INTERNATIONAL FAMILY CHANGE

Rapid mass communication development and expansion are prominent mechanisms in both structural and ideational explanations of international family change. In the United States, the first television sets went on sale in 1938 and achieved rapid growth after World War II. By 1950, half the U.S. population was reached by television signals. Television's introduction was accompanied by almost immediate debates on its effects. Congressional hearings on the effects of television violence on children began as early as 1952 (Hoerrner, 1999). This focus on television's effects on children continues today, and there is virtually no discussion on television and the aging experience.

Currently over 99% of U.S. households have television, with the average household containing 2.4 (U.S. Census Bureau, 2006). Table 13.1 provides information on the prevalence of televisions for countries around the world from which recent Demographic and Health Survey data are available. Table 13.1 illustrates that country-to-country and urban–rural differences persist. For example, in the sub-Saharan country of Tanzania, less than 3% of households own a television, while in Gabon and South Africa, over 50% own a television. Despite these regional differences, the pervasiveness of television worldwide is illustrated in the latter three columns of Table 13.1. These columns present data on whether respondents have access to a television in their sampling cluster, showing that in many world regions, especially in urban areas, over 90% of the population has access to a television. Census data from the Integrated Public Use Microdata Series–International demonstrate how rapidly television has expanded. For example, while only 1% of Mexican households owned a television in 1960, by 2000, 86% of households did. In the Philippines, television ownership grew from 35% in 1990 to 54% by 2000 (Minnesota Population Center, 2006). This rapid growth in television means that satellites now beam images into remote hamlets that until recently remained isolated.

The transforming power of international television is widely acknowledged. *Media imperialism* (Schiller, 1998), *media internationalization* (Chan, 2000), and *media globalization* (Robertson, 1992) are all terms used to describe the process involved with the spread of international television. Although there is substantial debate on cultural globalization, both proponents and opponents agree on the powerful role of the media, and international television in particular (McAnany, 2002). For example, Smith (1990) argued strongly against the creation of a global culture but acknowledged the powerful role of the media. Alternatively, Robertson (1992) argued that increasing global interconnectedness will lead to the emergence of a single global consciousness, largely due to increased media access and spread. Similarly, Giddens (2000) highlighted how a series of globalizing forces have reshaped lives and emphasized the media as an agent of change affecting everyone. Television provides some of the most broadly shared messages and images in history (Gerbner, Gross, Morgan, Signorielli, & Shanahan, 2002). Compared to other media forms, such as newspapers, magazines, and radio, television is particularly influential because its image-based format transcends barriers of language and literacy and is therefore accessible to both elites and nonelites. Translation of programs into the local language is often not needed for wide viewership as plots and story lines can often be followed without language proficiency. Television's access to nonelites is also illustrated by the large divergence in many countries between television ownership and access (see Table 13.1). Television ownership is not necessary to television viewing.

Table 13.1

PRESENCE OF TELEVISIONS IN DEMOGRAPHIC AND HEALTH SURVEY HOUSEHOLDS AND SAMPLING CLUSTERS

	TVS IN HOUSEHOLD			TVS IN CLUSTER		
	TOTAL	URBAN	RURAL	TOTAL	URBAN	RURAL
South and Southeast Asia						
Bangladesh (2004)	23.5	48.8	16.2	93.1	98.7	91.4
India (1998)	35.4	71.2	21.0	99.6	100.00	99.5
Indonesia (2002)	66.1	83.4	51.4	98.0	100.00	96.3
Nepal (2000)	13.5	62.6	7.9	53.0	97.4	48.0
Philippines (2003)	65.3	81.9	45.3	96.1	99.4	92.1
Vietnam (2002)	71.9	92.5	67.3	99.3	100.00	99.2
Sub-Saharan Africa						
Benin (2001)	17.3	35.5	5.8	64.9	86.6	51.2
Burkina Faso (2003)	11.9	49.7	2.7	38.8	99.2	24.0
Cameroon (2004)	25.7	44.2	5.0	68.9	93.8	41.1
Chad (2004)	3.0	15.5	0.1	12.7	59.6	1.6

Comoros (1996)	9.9	23.2	4.8	56.2	88.7	43.6
Cote d'Ivoire (1998)	30.1	54.5	13.7	81.1	98.5	69.3
Ethiopia (1999)	2.1	13.3	0.0	10.1	63.9	0.0
Gabon (2000)	56.0	67.2	14.7	91.4	99.6	61.1
Ghana (2003)	27.2	47.8	10.1	68.5	95.3	46.3
Guinea (1999)	9.7	32.4	1.0	29.3	85.6	7.6
Kenya (2003)	22.1	47.7	13.8	70.3	94.2	62.5
Madagascar (1997)	7.1	23.2	1.5	24.7	66.3	10.3
Malawi (2000)	2.5	14.2	0.5	18.1	79.0	7.8
Mali (2001)	17.9	47.0	6.1	62.7	95.1	49.5
Mozambique (2003)	10.3	30.6	0.8	30.0	79.4	6.7
Namibia (2000)	30.2	60.8	9.6	71.1	96.6	54.0
Niger (1998)	5.4	27.9	0.5	24.4	90.8	10.0

(continued)

291

Table 13.1

PRESENCE OF TELEVISIONS IN DEMOGRAPHIC AND HEALTH SURVEY HOUSEHOLDS AND SAMPLING CLUSTERS (CONTINUED)

	TVS IN HOUSEHOLD			TVS IN CLUSTER		
	TOTAL	URBAN	RURAL	TOTAL	URBAN	RURAL
Nigeria (2003)	32.6	62.5	16.7	72.1	96.0	59.5
Rwanda (2000)	2.6	17.0	0.3	15.7	85.3	4.5
Senegal (1997)	21.4	45.1	5.2	62.2	99.7	36.8
South Africa (1998)	60.7	75.3	38.3	96.0	98.1	92.8
Tanzania (1999)	2.7	9.9	0.2	16.1	54.6	2.2
Togo (1998)	16.2	37.9	4.4	71.9	97.5	58.0
Uganda (2000)	6.7	29.4	2.4	31.2	92.4	19.8
Zambia (2001)	21.2	51.0	4.2	50.8	94.9	25.7
Zimbabwe (1999)	27.3	57.4	8.9	79.7	100.0	67.3
Latin America and Caribbean						
Bolivia (1998)	68.5	90.7	21.3	84.9	100.0	52.8
Brazil (1996)	70.8	78.2	39.1	96.4	99.9	81.7

Columbia (2005)	87.6	93.0	69.9	99.2	100.0	96.5
Dominican Republic (2002)	84.0	87.5	76.8	99.4	100.0	98.3
Guatemala (1998)	58.5	80.3	40.2	88.1	100.0	78.1
Haiti (2000)	25.7	58.2	3.2	51.2	94.3	21.4
Nicaragua (2001)	61.1	82.5	29.1	88.5	99.7	71.8
Peru (2000)	72.3	90.6	36.0	92.5	99.9	77.8
Other						
Egypt (2003)	90.6	93.2	88.3	100.0	100.0	100.0
Jordan (1997)	94.8	95.8	89.7	100.0	100.0	100.0
Morocco (2003)	67.3	86.4	37.1	93.9	98.9	85.9
Turkey (1998)	93.9	96.2	88.7	100.0	100.0	100.0

In effecting change, television can influence attitudes and behaviors through two primary mechanisms: content and availability. The impact of television content is most frequently acknowledged. Television content may promote change by informing, enabling, motivating, and guiding individuals. Television appears a particularly effective mechanism for new idea transmission. New ideas that may influence family behavior include information about contraception, smaller family size preferences (Caldwell, 1982), ideas about secularization and individualism (Bumpass, 1990; Lesthaeghe & Surkyn, 1988; Lesthaeghe & Wilson, 1986), consumption as an appropriate orientation (Easterlin, 1987; Freedman, 1979), more egalitarian gender relationships (Hornick & McAnany, 2001; Kottak, 1991), power structures defined less by heredity and more by achievement (Johnson, 2000), and youth autonomy. For example, television programs may show a young couple meeting and falling in love, encountering obstacles such as parental objections, and persevering to form a love match.[1] Program emphasis on youth autonomy and a love match, rather than parentally arranged marriages, may influence young television viewers to follow the same path (Hornick & McAnany, 2001). Similarly, television portrayals of smaller families could introduce ideas that small families are normal and acceptable (Coale & Watkins, 1986; Mason, 1997), altering fertility preferences and behavior.

The mere availability of television can also bring about change by altering the opportunity costs of various activities or by altering social relationships. There is a time competition aspect to television, so that time spent watching television means time not spent on other activities. For example, in *Bowling Alone,* Putnam (2000) argued that the spread of television caused declines in American's social involvement. Community involvement declined not because of what people saw on television, but because they were home watching television, instead of participating in community social activities. Particularly important in family change theoretical frameworks is the extent to which this reorganization of activities alters the activity context from familial to nonfamilial. Expanding from the modes of production framework (discussed in Fry, this volume), the modes of social organization framework examines the extent to which activities (including, but not limited to, production) occur within or outside the family context. Most activities of daily living have been historically organized within the family

---

[1] This is the basic formula of South Korean and Chinese romantic films, widely watched in Vietnam.

(Ogburn & Nimkoff, 1955; Thornton & Fricke, 1987), but television watching may be a leisure activity that increasingly occurs outside the family context, changing interactions with both family and nonfamily. Research has primarily emphasized the growth in nonfamily activities such as educational institutions and wage labor, finding that increases in nonfamily experiences result in greater youth independence, delayed marriage, increased contraceptive use, and reduced fertility (Axinn & Yabiku, 2001; Thornton & Lin, 1994). Reorganizing leisure activities through television's availability may produce similar changes, as activity contexts become increasingly nonfamilial. Therefore the experience of aging and what it means to be elderly may be influenced by television, either/both through television content or alterations in social relationships due to television availability.

The life course framework emphasizes the importance of timing and that the impact of an event is contingent on when it occurs in a person's life (Elder, 1998). In keeping with this life course view, I hypothesize that whether television has effects and what it affects will vary by life course position. Exposure to television early in an individual's life span may influence his or her fertility behavior or his or her attitudes toward intergenerational relationships, with important implications for the individual's aging experience. Additionally, the linked lives life course theme suggests that even if the elderly are not directly affected by television, they may still experience change through television's effects on other generations. Television's emphasis on autonomy and individualism may alter adult children's attitudes toward providing and caring for their elderly parents. The pervasive nature of television and powerful hypotheses on its effects suggest that more attention is needed on how the experience of aging is altered by television. To generate hypotheses on how television affects the elderly, and lay the foundation for future work, I report findings from fieldwork conducted in rural Vietnam during 2005.

VIETNAM, TELEVISION, AND THE ELDERLY

Vietnam's population of 82,000,000 is largely composed of the Kinh ethnic majority group, who make up 86% of the population. Fifty-three different ethnic minority groups compose the remaining 14%. The Kinh primarily inhabit the fertile delta regions—the Red River Delta in the north and the Mekong Delta in the south—and the coastal plains, and with very few exceptions, Kinh settlements are electrified. In contrast, Vietnam's minority groups mainly reside in mountainous areas in the north and central part of the country that largely lack electricity, and therefore television. In preparation for a larger project on television and family change, preliminary fieldwork, in collaboration with the Vietnam Museum of Ethnology, was conducted over several weeks in fall 2005 in Vietnam's Nghe An province. Nghe An is located in the north central region of Vietnam, bordering Laos (see Figure 13.1). About 17% of its population is composed of 51 different ethnic minority groups. We focused on the Khmu, one of the poorest ethnic minority groups in Vietnam. Although Vietnam as a whole has experienced dramatic changes in fertility and mortality (life expectancy is 73.4 and the total fertility rate is 1.8), mortality and fertility remain high among

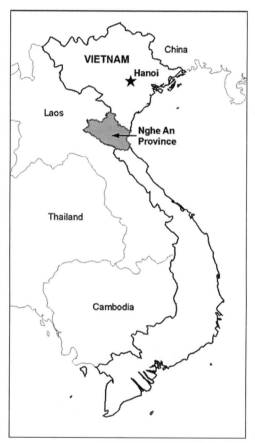

Figure 13.1 Map of Nghe An province, Vietnam. From VIDAGIS, Geographic information system for Viet Nam. (2006), Hanoi, Viet Nam. ESRI World Countries, County Boundaries (2002). ESRI Data. Redlands, CA: Environment Systems Research.

the Khmu. In the four villages we studied, individuals aged 55 and over composed between 4% and 6% of the population. The elderly are well respected in Khmu society, and the ethic of filial piety has been tradition-ally strong. Television's arrival, however, may alter some of these long-held intergenerational patterns.

Our data collections involved a series of focus group interviews and intensive, semistructured interviews in Khmu villages that lacked elec-tricity, and in Khmu villages that had recently (within the past year) been electrified. Because few Khmu speak Vietnamese, interviews were con-ducted in Khmu (no television programs are available in Khmu; most are in Vietnamese). With electrification, some households obtained televisions. Although television ownership was limited to only about 9% to 12% of households, television viewing was widespread. Individuals without televisions routinely went to a neighbor's house to watch. It was not uncommon to find over 60 people crowded into a small house, with some viewers standing on ladders outside windows. Interviews in elec-trified villages focused on how electricity and television had changed family and community life. These qualitative data highlight how the ex-periences of the elderly have been affected by television.

Khmu elderly were very clear that television had brought many changes to their lives and to their village. Many elderly expressed con-cern on how influential television was becoming for the younger genera-tions. In this society, which has no written language, the elderly have had important roles as storytellers, orally handing down stories and informa-tion to younger generations. However, television has replaced the elderly as the storytelling medium, and films, particularly those from China and South Korea, draw far greater interest and attention. Power hierarchies have also been affected, as the elderly are no longer the primary source of information. As one elderly man explained, the agricultural programs on television, which guide farmers on increasing crop yield through the effective use of pesticides and newer farming techniques, are far more instructive than his farming experiences.

Another example of how television's arrival impacted traditional hi-erarchies was illustrated by the fate of one village's shaman. Although our fieldwork in nonelectrified villages highlighted the importance of the shaman, and while we had frequent interactions with them, we were surprised by having spent several days in a recently electrified village where we had yet to meet the shaman. After inquiring where he was, and why he was not present, we were informed that individuals in this village had agreed that the shaman's services were no longer needed.

Television's frequent showings of Tylenol commercials had convinced villagers that Tylenol and other similar modern medicines, which promised quick relief, were more cost-effective and faster than the shaman's traditional cures, which required several days and the killing of chickens. We subsequently interviewed the former shaman, who expressed agreement with the villagers' decision, acknowledging that he was no competition for Tylenol. This 71-year-old man, who just a few months ago had a powerful position in the village, expressed confusion and anxiety over what to do with his remaining days.

Several Khmu elderly felt that television's arrival will result in increasing work and responsibility for them. They described how some adults were discussing leaving the village to find wage employment in cities. Television's portrayals of a better lifestyle and opportunities through wage labor were presenting attractive alternatives to a life of rice farming. Some adults planned to leave child rearing and farming responsibilities to their elderly parents while they went away to find work. A 64-year-old woman described how her son and daughter-in-law had left the village and were working on a road crew. Although she thought she had reached a point in her life when she could relax and enjoy her family, she was now the primary caretaker for her five grandchildren, ranging in age from 1.5 to 9 years.

One of the major areas of alarm expressed by Khmu elderly was the influence television was having on the young. New ideas and ways of behavior were being introduced through program content. For example, one 9-year-old boy we spoke with described how his family was one of the poorest in the village. His father was currently in jail for stealing a neighbor's water buffalo, leaving his mother alone to provide for himself and his four younger siblings. When we asked him what he wanted to do in the future, he was quick to tell us that he was going to be a businessman and drive a nice car. This ambition was expressed by a young boy who had never been to school and who lived in a village where no one owned a bicycle, much less a motorbike or a car. An additional example of change among the younger generation comes from a focus group interview with adolescent girls. While most of the discussion focused on the entertainment aspects of television, one girl insisted that television was very educational. When asked to describe the educational aspects of television, this 16-year-old responded, "Television is very educational. It teaches us how to kiss and do things with boys." These examples illustrate how the elderly have been affected by television and how the experience of aging is being transformed.

CONCLUSION

Although television receives substantial attention for its effects on children and adolescents, rarely do discussions of the aging experience include television. Yet television has grown rapidly worldwide, with substantial implications for all members in a society, including the elderly. In particular, television worldwide is largely Western in content. Even when national programming is available, it still reflects viewpoints and images from the national capital or large urban centers and Western production norms (Hornick & McAnany, 2001). Imported models of family structure are prevalent on television, and television may offer radically different ways of imagining social relationships. The image of romantic love widely disseminated by television has profoundly modified representations of love in societies characterized by an arranged marriage system (Locoh & Mouvagha-Sow, 2008). Individual autonomy, egalitarianism, and independence of thought are also frequently presented on television. These constructs may lead to changing conceptions on youth autonomy and alter intergenerational and gender relationships. The Western/modern/cosmopolitan images and messages in television programs clearly illustrate and define what it is to be modern, and define modern as good (Hornick, 2001). Television portrayals of human nature, family relationships, social roles, power relations, and societal norms shape the public consciousness (Gerbner, Gross, Morgan, & Signorielli, 1994), and television representations gain influence because people's social construction of reality depends heavily on what they see. Other often discussed forces of social change, such as urbanization, industrialization, or modernization, emphasize structural changes. These structural changes are clearly important, but the influence of television in these Khmu villages illustrates the extent of change in the absence of large-scale structural alterations, further illustrating the necessity of incorporating ideational perspectives into social change discussions. Television can have a major impact on the elderly and the experience of aging, and future research should include examining television's effects on the elderly.

REFERENCES

Axinn, W. G., Ghimire, D., & Barber, J. (2008). The influence of ideational dimensions of social change on family formation in Nepal. In R. Jayakody, A. Thornton, & W. G. Axinn (Eds.), *International family change: Ideational perspectives* (pp. 251–280). Mahwah, NJ: Erlbaum.

Axinn, W. G., & Yabiku, S. T. (2001). Social change, the social organization of families, and fertility limitation. *American Journal of Sociology, 106*, 1219–1261.

Bongaarts, J., & Watkins, S. C. (1996). Social interactions and contemporary fertility change. *Population and Development Review, 20*, 639–682.

Bumpass, L. (1990). What's happening to the family? Interactions between demographic and institutional change. *Demography, 27*, 483–498.

Butcher, M. (2003). *Transnational television, cultural identity, and change: When STAR came to India.* New Delhi: Sage.

Caldwell, J. (1982). *Theory of fertility decline.* London: Academic Press.

Chan, J. M. (2000). When capitalist and socialist television clash: The impact of Hong Kong TV on Guangzhou residents. In C.-C. Lee (Ed.), *Power, money, and media: Communication patterns and bureaucratic control in cultural China* (pp. 245–270). Evanston: Northwestern University Press.

Cleland, J., & Wilson, C. (1987). Demand theories of the fertility transition: An iconoclastic view. *Population Studies, 41*, 5–30.

Coale, A. J., & Watkins, S. C. (Eds.). (1986). *The decline of fertility in Europe.* Princeton, NJ: Princeton University Press.

Easterlin, R. (1987). *Birth and fortune.* Chicago: University of Chicago Press.

Elder, G. H. (1998). The life course and human development. In R. Lerner (Ed.), *Theoretical models of human development* (Vol. 1, pp. 939–991). New York: John Wiley.

Freedman, R. (1979). Theories of fertility decline: A reappraisal. *Social Forces, 58*, 1–17.

Gerbner, G., Gross, L., Morgan, M., & Signorielli, N. (1994). Growing up with television: The cultivation perspective. In J. Bryant & D. Zillerman (Eds.), *Media effects: Advances in theory and research* (pp. 17–41). Hillsdale, NJ: Erlbaum.

Gerbner, G., Gross, L., Morgan, M., Signorielli, N., & Shanahan, J. (2002). Growing up with television: Cultivation process. In J. Bryant & D. Zimmerman (Eds.), *Media effects: Advances in theory and research* (pp. 43–68). Mahwah, NJ: Erlbaum.

Giddens, A. (2000). *Runaway world: How globalization is reshaping our lives.* New York: Routledge.

Hoerrner, K. L. (1999). *The forgotten battles: Congressional hearings on television violence in the 1950s.* Baton Rouge, LA: Manship School of Mass Communication.

Hornick, R. C. (Ed.). (2001). *Public health communication: Evidence of behavior change.* Mahwah, NJ: Erlbaum.

Hornick, R. C., & McAnany, E. (2001). Mass media and fertility change. In J. B. Casterline (Ed.), *Diffusion process and fertility transition* (pp. 208–239). Washington, DC: National Academy Press.

Jayakody, R., Thornton, A., & Axinn, W. G. (2008). Perspectives on international family change. In R. Jayakody, A. Thornton, & W. G. Axinn (Eds.), *International family change: Ideational perspectives* (pp. 1–18). Mahwah, NJ: Erlbaum.

Johnson, K. (2000). *Television and social change in rural India.* New Delhi: Sage.

Kottak, C. P. (1990). *Prime-time society: An anthropological analysis of television and culture.* Belmont, CA: Wadsworth.

Kottak, C. P. (1991). Television's impact on values and local life in Brazil. *Journal of Communication, 41*, 70–87.

Lesthaeghe, R., & Surkyn, J. (1988). Cultural dynamics and economic theories of fertility change. *Population and Development Review, 14*, 1–45.

Lesthaeghe, R., & Wilson, C. (1986). Modes of production, secularization and the pace of fertility decline in Western Europe, 1870–1930. In A. Cole & S. C. Watkins (Eds.), *The decline of fertility in Europe* (pp. 261–292). Princeton, NJ: Princeton University Press.

Locoh, T., & Mouvagha-Sow, M. (2008). An uncertain future for African families. In R. Jayakody, A. Thornton, & W. G. Axinn (Eds.), *International family change: Ideational perspectives* (pp. 45–80). Mahwah, NJ: Erlbaum.

Mason, K. O. (1997). Explaining fertility transitions. *Demography, 34,* 443–454.

McAnany, E. (2002). Globalization and the media: The debate continues. *Communication Research Trends, 21,* 3–19.

Minnesota Population Center. (2006). *Integrated Public Use Microdata Series–International: Version 2.0.* Minneapolis: University of Minnesota.

Ogburn, W. F., & Nimkoff, M. F. (1955). *Technology and the changing family.* Boston: Houghton Mifflin.

Putnam, R. D. (2000). *Bowling alone: The collapse and revival of American community.* New York: Simon and Schuster.

Robertson, R. (1992). *Globalization: Social theory and global culture.* London: Sage.

Schiller, H. (1998). Striving for communication dominance: A half century review. In D. Thussu (Ed.), *Electronic empires: Global media and local resistance* (pp. 17–26). London: Arnold.

Smith, A. (1990). Towards a global culture? In M. Featherstone (Ed.), *Global culture: Nationalism, globalization, and modernity* (pp. 171–192). London: Sage.

Thornton, A. (2001). The developmental paradigm, reading history sideways, and family change. *Demography, 38,* 449–465.

Thornton, A., & Fricke, T. (1987). Social change and the family: Comparative perspectives from the West, China, and South Asia. *Sociological Forum, 2,* 746–779.

Thornton, A., & Lin, H.-S. (1994). *Social change and the family in Taiwan.* Chicago: University of Chicago Press.

U.S. Census Bureau. (2006). *Statistical abstracts of the United States.* Washington, DC: Author.

Watkins, S. C. (1991). *From provinces to nations: Demographic integration in Western Europe, 1870–1960.* Princeton, NJ: Princeton University Press.

Watkins, S. C., & Danzi, A. D. (1995). Women's gossip and social change: Childbirth and fertility control among Italian and Jewish women in the U.S. *Gender and Society, 9,* 469–490.

Westoff, C. F., & Bankole, A. (1999). *Mass media and reproductive behavior in Pakistan, India, and Bangladesh.* Calverton, MD: Macro International.

Familial and Societal Context

14

Religion and Intergenerational Transmission Over Time

VERN L. BENGTSON, CASEY E. COPEN,
NORELLA M. PUTNEY, AND MERRIL SILVERSTEIN

How do some families use religion as a solidifying force for connecting individuals between and within generations, while in others, religion is a source of conflict? How do older generations pass down their religious beliefs and practices to younger generations in light of changing social and historical circumstances, and what factors condition their transmission? What are the social and material consequences of continuity in religious orientation and involvement for individuals and their families? These are fundamental questions as we consider the interconnectedness of religious and family structures.

In this chapter, we present some recent analyses concerning continuity and change over generations, focusing specifically on the intergenerational transmission of religion—and the role of grandparents. Using data from the University of Southern California's Longitudinal Study of Generations (LSOG), we look at patterns of religiosity among grandparents, parents, and their young adult children across three decades of dramatic social change. We examine evidence about how much influence parents and grandparents have on their grandchildren's religious

Acknowledgments: The authors would like to acknowledge support for this research from the John Templeton Foundation and the National Institute on Aging (grants 5 R01-AG07977 and 5T32-AG00037).

service attendance, feelings of religiousness, and religious ideology, and how this may have changed over time.

Religiosity can be examined as a personal history or trajectory over the course of life, one that is influenced by family members. But we must also take into account that such influences take place within the context of the changing strength and scope of formal religious authority (Chaves, 1991; Wuthnow, 1988) as well as the demographic shifts in family behaviors and structures that have characterized American society since the 1960s. The dynamics of family influences on an individual's religiosity are multilevel as well as reciprocal. Most religious traditions (particularly those in the Abrahamic legacies of Judaism, Christianity, and Islam) place a high value on family bonds and the imparting of appropriate moral values to children. In addition, religious beliefs and practices represent an important vehicle for defining how families define their relationships to one another and to the larger community over time (Bahr & Chadwick, 1988; Thornton, Axinn, & Hill, 1992).

The LSOG is a 35-year panel investigation involving more than 3,000 individuals from 350 three- and four-generation families. Begun in 1971, family members—grandparents, parents, and their adolescent or young adult children—have been surveyed at regular intervals about their perceptions of family relationships as well as their values, religious beliefs and practices, political and social attitudes, physical and psychological health, work life, and personal goals. This was just after the so-called Decade of Protest—the 1960s—when the generation gap between youth and elders became cause for concern around the world. An important goal of the study was to chart both behavioral and cognitive–affective dimensions of interactions between parents and children, grandparents and grandchildren, across time, and to examine the consequences of close or distant relations between generations. In 1991, we began adding a fourth generation, the great grandchildren of the original grandparents, as they turned age 16. A recent book, *How Families Still Matter: A Longitudinal Study of Youth in Two Generations* (Bengtson, Biblarz, & Roberts, 2002), summarizes some of our findings.

BACKGROUND OF THE STUDY

We know too little about the ways in which religious beliefs and practices are transmitted from generation to generation (Myers, 1996), or how these processes have changed in the context of the massive social and technological changes of recent years. What are the patterns of religious experience in families, and are they still passed on from grandparents, to parents, and to their children? One mark of a religious tradition is its ability to link the past to the present and to foster continuity between past experiences and future events (Hervieu-Leger, 2000). As far back as the biblical and Koranic stories of the Patriarch Abraham, the family has been the primary site for the socialization of beliefs, values, and practices that constitute a religious tradition. Where there is concurrence between generations, religion can serve to solidify emotional ties between family members. These tight social bonds can provide a firm foundation for a family culture that leaves a lasting imprint on younger generations. Indeed, recent research suggests that the influence of religion pervades every aspect of social life, including demographic patterns of marriage and fertility, education and occupational pursuits, and attitudes toward family and gender (Sherkat & Ellison, 1999; Thornton, 1985). The religious belief orientations and rituals enacted within the family have a definable impact on individual choices and trajectories across the life course.

And yet some sociologists have written that the family has lost its moral and religious influence. This perspective has a long history. In advancing his secularization thesis, Berger (1967) suggested that the family as a plausibility structure had become too fragile to serve as the essential underpinning of religious tradition or as the central agent for passing on spiritual capital to the next generation. The decline in the family's religious and moral influence has been attributed to parental divorce (Popenoe, 1993) and to the rampant individualism of postindustrial societies (Bellah, Madsen, Sullivan, Swidler, & Tipton, 1985). Evidence might be seen in the attendant increase in religious *seeking* behavior in American society, which prizes self-exploration and self-fulfillment over religious socialization and social control (Inglehart & Baker, 2000; Roof, 1993; C. Smith, 2005; Wuthnow, 1998). Others have asserted that the devaluing of religion in contemporary families has been a primary force in weakening the relationship between parents and children, which in turn has ushered in a host of social problems (Dobson & Bauer, 1990).

However, recent empirical research affirms the continued importance of families in contemporary society (Bengtson, 2001; Cherlin, 2002) and demonstrates that parental influences on youth's achievement orientations and values have not decreased over time, even in the context of higher divorce rates (Bengtson et al., 2002). Several studies have shown that parents exert a lasting imprint on the religious ideology and commitments of their children (Glass, Bengtson, & Dunham, 1986; Myers, 1996, 2004; Sherkat, 1998). Moreover, the degree of affectual solidarity between parents and children exerts a powerful influence on these socialization processes and is perhaps the best predictor of inter-generational continuity or contrast (Bengtson et al., 2002). From this perspective, the moral agency of American families *has not* declined significantly. Even with the considerable social changes of the latter 20th century, we suggest that today's multigenerational families represent a stock of religious capital sufficient to influence the religious traditions and involvement of successive generations.

Religious Socialization in Families

While religiosity is often considered (and measured) as a characteristic of an individual, it is also a social product forged by early socialization, which primarily takes place in nuclear and extended families. Studies show these early family influences on religiosity are enduring. Sherkat (1998) uses the term *adaptive preference* to describe how people tend to stay in their denomination of origin (childhood), and if people do switch from their childhood religion, they tend to adopt a religion similar to the one with which they are familiar (Sherkat & Wilson, 1995). Following this idea, C. Smith (2005) observed that most adolescents tend to prefer the religion of their parents. Myers (1996) found that religiosity in adulthood is determined largely by parental religiosity, independent of aging and life course effects.

On the other hand, substantial social changes over the past four decades—high rates of divorce, cohabitation, single parenthood, mothers' high labor force participation, the increasing longevity of older adults—have changed the family's structure and functions (Bengtson, 2001; Casper & Bianchi, 2002) such that the socialization of younger generations into a particular religious tradition is more complex and perhaps less likely than for earlier generations. There is also significant variability in how the socialization environment of the home conditions the transmission of religiosity, particularly the marital status and relationship quality of parents. Roof (1999) used the analogy of religion as a multicolored kaleidoscope: How families transmit religious beliefs and practices can take on various configurations, depending on gender, race and ethnicity, marital status, and socioeconomic position. The situation of mixed-faith families, where parents have different religious backgrounds, further complicates the likelihood of religious transmission.

Multigenerational Influences on Religious Socialization

Several studies have shown that the family exerts influence in ways that go beyond the parent–child nuclear family model of value transmission (for a review, see Putney & Bengtson, 2002). Young adults are situated in a complex web of family relationships and receive messages about religious beliefs, values, and expectations from parents, grandparents, and other relatives (Mueller & Elder, 2003). Until recently, grandparents have not been considered in socialization theory and research. They were relegated to the periphery of the nuclear family model, and their influence on youths' outcomes was not explored. However, recent research indicates that in the United States, contemporary grandparents play an increasingly important role in the lives of their grandchildren (Bengtson, 2001), one consequence of the far-reaching demographic changes in the structures of families (Casper & Bianchi, 2002). Because of the increase in life expectancy over the 20th century, grandparents have longer lives than ever before, and grandchildren spend an increased proportion of their lives with living grandparents. This has increased the chances for grandparents to play a significant role in the lives of children (Uhlenberg, 2005). Thus it is not surprising that a majority of grandchildren report being emotionally close to their grandparents as well as sharing similar views and values with grandparents (Silverstein, Giarrusso, & Bengtson, 2003).

Grandparents today have greater opportunities to share stories and experiences with their grandchildren, which will have an impact on how young people enact relationships with their own grandchildren as adults (King & Elder, 1999). Depictions of grandparents as distant or detached family observers run counter to what recent research shows. Many grandparents have a continuing presence in the lives of their grandchildren, providing emotional support and advice as well as being a cultural window into family history, which allows grandchildren to learn more about themselves and their distant kin (Pratt & Fiese, 2004; Silverstein et al., 2003).

Religion is one cultural thread that may bring grandparents and grandchildren closer together—or, on the other hand, cause them to be more apart and distant. Highly religious grandparents report that they have stronger emotional relationships with their grandchildren and are more involved in their lives (King & Elder, 1999). That religion may solidify relationships between grandparents and grandchildren may seem counterintuitive today, as it was a generation ago, because older and younger generations are often seen as having opposing worldviews that are in conflict (Bengtson, 1970, 1975). Recent nationally representative data show, however, that a majority of American teens prefer the religious traditions of their parents, rather than seeking out other religions (C. Smith, 2005). In light of similarities and continuities between parents and children on matters of religious faith, it may also be likely that grandparents and grandchildren are similar in terms of religious beliefs, values, and practices.

Examining Influence Across Several Generations

Over the course of three decades of LSOG data collection, our research team has made periodic assessments of parent–child similarities and differences on a variety of values, opinions, and behaviors (Acock & Bengtson, 1980; Bengtson, 1970, 1975; Bengtson et al., 2002; Glass et al., 1986; Roberts & Bengtson, 1999). Recently, this led to a closer examination of possible transmission effects across multiple generations (Copen, Biblarz, Silverstein, & Bengtson, 2005). We looked at several domains of values, opinions, and behaviors that might indicate cross-generational influences or transmission effects. To our surprise, we found that religion evidenced the strongest transmission effect, stronger than political orientations, socioeconomic status, or indicators of psychological well-being such as depression or self-esteem (see Figure 14.1).

Why? That religion would be the strongest indicator of cross-generational transmission, today, at the beginning of the 21st century, goes against conventional wisdom. Youth throughout history have been the innovators and elders the conservators, particularly in times of rapid social change. We expected this to be true particularly with regard to religious values and practices, with youth branching out in different directions from those of their grandparents. But this was not the case. While grandparent–grandchild similarity was minimal in several dimensions of comparison, it was highest in the area of religious values. Was this simply because the grandchildren were similar to their parents in religious orientation and because of this, appeared to be similar to their grandparents?

Drawing on an expanded model of family socialization, we advance four hypotheses concerning religious continuity in families. We have deliberately formulated these as radical or unconventional statements, countering the conventional wisdom currently heard from politicians and pundits, and unfortunately, from some sociologists, that family influences are declining:

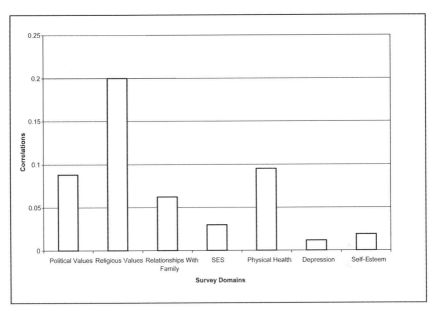

Figure 14.1 Mean correlations between G2 grandmothers (*n* = 194) in 1971 and G4 grandchildren (*n* = 479) in 2000: Longitudinal Study of Generations.

1. Grandparents *do* exert a noticeable effect on the religiosity of their grandchildren as the latter reach young adulthood.
2. Such influence of grandparents on grandchildren *has increased* over time from the 1970s to the 2000s.
3. Grandparents exert influence on grandchildren's religiosity that is *independent* of parental influences, though related to it. Grandparent involvement in children's lives has most often been characterized as a relationship mediated by the quality of the relationship between parent and grandparents (Uhlenberg & Hammil, 1998). However, we suggest that today's grandparents have a role in shaping young adult grandchildren's religious orientations that is independent of the effect of parents.
4. Despite divorce, grandparents' influence *remains significant.* In the context of parental divorce (compared to parents who do not divorce), grandparents' influence on their grandchildren's religiosity will not decline and may even become stronger as a consequence of parents' reduced ability to influence their children's religious beliefs.

METHODS

Sample

Data for analyses are from the LSOG, a study of over 3,000 respondents ages 16–91, from 350 three- and four-generation families (previously described). Individuals eligible for sample inclusion were generated from the families of grandparents randomly selected in 1970 from the membership of a large, 840,000 member health maintenance organization in the Los Angeles area. The sample pool was generally representative of White, economically stable, middle- and working-class families. Self-administered questionnaires were mailed to the grandparents and their spouses (G1s), their adult children (G2s), and their grandchildren who were aged 16 or older (G3s). In 1985, 1,331 of the original sample were surveyed again, and since then, data have been collected at 3-year intervals through 2004. The response rate between 1971 and 1985 was 65% and has averaged 74% between waves since then. Starting with the 1991 wave of data collection, great grandchildren (G4s) have been brought into the study as they turned age 16. The G3s in our sample are members of the baby boom generation, while the G2s are their parents, and the G1s, their grandparents. The G4s in our sample are otherwise known as Generation X. Figure 14.2 summarizes the longitudinal design of the LSOG.

Measures

Dependent Variables

To test our hypotheses, we use three dimensions of religiosity, which have been measured at every time wave: (a) frequency of religious service attendance, (b) self-defined religiousness, and (c) agreement with conservative religious beliefs. Our dependent variables are the *grandchild's* indicators on these three dimensions of religiosity.

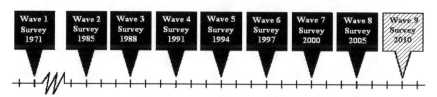

Figure 14.2 Longitudinal Study of Generations survey design: 1971–2010.

Religious service attendance frequency is a single item with six response categories, ranging from 1 (*never*) to 6 (*more than once a week*). Religiousness is a single item, which reads, "Regardless of whether you attend religious services, do you consider yourself to be (1) not at all religious; (2) somewhat religious; (3) moderately religious; or (4) very religious." Agreement with conservative religious beliefs is a four-item scale (based on the religious ideology scale developed by Comrey & Newmeyer, 1965), asking how much the respondent agrees or disagrees with the following statements: (a) "Every child should have religious instruction"; (b) "This country would be better off if religion had a greater influence in daily life"; (c) "God exists in the form as described in the Bible"; and (d) "All people today are descendents of Adam and Eve." There are four response categories, ranging from 1 (*strongly disagree*) to 4 (*strongly agree*). Responses are coded so that a higher score indicates stronger agreement with conservative religious beliefs. Validated in previous research using these data (Glass et al., 1986), this scale has averaged high reliability across all generations and time waves through 2004 (Cronbach's α = .87).

These three dimensions of religiosity, along with religious affiliation (an open-ended question) and religious salience (the importance of religion compared to eight other aspects of life), have been included in LSOG surveys continuously since 1971 and can be used to examine changes in religiosity over time. (See Table 14A for the list of all longitudinal religiosity measures and response categories.) We have analyzed responses to all religiosity items over the entire sample, by generation (G1, G2, G3, and G4), for each data collection time and confirmed that these items are measured with justifiable validity and reliability. In addition, several other religiosity measures have appeared at various data collection times.

Independent Variables

We use the *parent's* and the *grandparent's* frequency of church attendance, self-reported religiousness, and agreement with conservative religious beliefs as the major independent variables. In addition, we control for several grandchild characteristics: (a) grandchild's age, (b) grandchild's gender (1 = female), (c) grandchild's education, ranging from 1 (*grade school*) to 8 (*advanced degree*), (d) grandchild's marital status (1 = married), (e) whether the grandchild has children (1 = yes), (f) whether the grandchild lives with parents (1 = yes) , and (g) whether the grandchild's parents have ever divorced (1 = yes). We also control for frequency of contact with grandmothers and grandfathers. Grandchildren are asked about four types of contact: in person, phone, mail, and e-mail (in 2000) with scores ranging from 1 (*not at all*) to 8 (*daily contact*). A composite mean contact score was calculated.

Religious affiliation, which is included in the summary statistics (Table 14.1), is an open-ended item in the survey that reads, "What is your current religious affiliation? (Please specify the church or denomination. Write "none" if you have no affiliation.).)" Responses are coded based on an index of 80 religious denominations and categories. We collapsed responses into five categories: Protestant, Catholic, Jewish, other (which includes Church of Latter Day Saints), and no religious affiliation.

Analytic Design

For this study, we constructed grandparent–parent–grandchild triads. The subsample consists of G1, G2, and G3 linked family respondents in 1971 (Wave 1) and G2, G3, and G4 linked family respondents in 2000 (Wave 7). This resulted in a multigenerational subsample from the LSOG panel comprising 257 grandparents, 341 parents, and 565 grandchildren. Grandparents and parents are paired with unique grandchildren; that is, if grandchildren have siblings, they are paired with the same parents and grandparents in the sample. While this overrepresentation of some triad members presents the potential for attenuation in the distribution that may not occur otherwise, our previous research with this same data using a similar sampling procedure revealed no significant increase or decrease in predictability (Acock & Bengtson, 1980; Bengtson et al., 2002; Glass et al., 1986).

We utilized a generational sequential design (Bengtson et al., 2002; Roberts & Bengtson, 1999), in which the religiosity of two generations is compared when they are at the same age or life stage, but measured in different historical periods. This allows us to examine change over time and to begin to assess the effects of changing structural conditions.

For grandparents, parents, and grandchildren in 1971 and 2000, we present descriptive information for religious affiliation, frequency of church attendance, religiousness, and agreement with conservative religious beliefs. For each of the dimensions of religiosity, we examined similarities or contrasts between family generations—parents and children, grandparents and grandchildren—and traced changes for each

Table 14.1

SELECTED DEMOGRAPHIC AND RELIGIOSITY CHARACTERISTICS OF GRANDPARENTS, PARENTS, AND GRANDCHILDREN: 1971 AND 2000

	G1		G2		G3	
	GRANDMOTHER (n = 237)	GRANDFATHER (n = 253)	MOTHER (n = 370)	FATHER (n = 309)	GRANDDAUGHTERS (n = 435)	GRANDSONS (n = 369)
			1971			
Mean age (years)	67	70	42	46	19	19
Mean education[a]	3.7	3.4	4.5	5.0	4.1*	4.1*
Religious denomination (%)						
Protestant	66	61	55	55	45	47
Catholic	16	12	19	18	23	16
Jewish	12	12	12	13	11	9
Other	5	8	10	7	9	10
No religious affiliation	1	7	4	7	12	18

(continued)

315

Table 14.1

SELECTED DEMOGRAPHIC AND RELIGIOSITY CHARACTERISTICS OF GRANDPARENTS, PARENTS, AND GRANDCHILDREN: 1971 AND 2000 (CONTINUED)

	G1		G2		G3	
	GRANDMOTHER ($n = 237$)	GRANDFATHER ($n = 253$)	MOTHER ($n = 370$)	FATHER ($n = 309$)	GRANDDAUGHTERS ($n = 435$)	GRANDSONS ($n = 369$)
1971						
Other dimensions of religiosity (means)						
How often do you attend religious services[b]	3.1	3.0	2.8	2.9	2.8	2.4
How religious are you?[c]	3.0	2.8	3.0	2.8	2.7	2.6
Conservative religious beliefs (4 items)[d]	3.5	3.3	3.1	3.0	2.8	2.6
	GRANDMOTHER ($n = 270$)	GRANDFATHER ($n = 177$)	MOTHER ($n = 403$)	FATHER ($n = 298$)	GRANDDAUGHTERS ($n = 341$)	GRANDSONS ($n = 292$)
2000						
Mean age (years)	72	74	48	51	23	22
Mean education	4.1	4.9	5.2	5.6	4.6*	4.1*

Religious denomination (%)					
Protestant	34	32	35	24	30
Catholic	16	13	14	12	8
Jewish	10	11	9	11	7
Other	8	10	9	10	15
No religious affiliation	32	34	33	43	40
Other dimensions of religiosity (means)					
How often do you attend religious services	3.3	3.1	3.1	3.2	2.8
How religious are you?	2.9	2.7	2.8	2.6	2.3
Conservative religious beliefs (4 items)	2.9	2.8	2.9	2.8	2.5

Note: Education may not be finished at time of survey. Data are from the Longitudinal Study of Generations.
[a]From 1 (*grade school*) to 8 (*advanced degree*).
[b]From 1 (*never*) to 6 (*more than once a week*).
[c]From 1 (*not very*) to 4 (*very*).
[d]From 1 (*low*) to 4 (*high*).

generation across three decades of massive social change. Of special interest are the two cohorts of grandchildren, the G3s and G4s, who came of age in two different historical periods. Next, we use OLS regression procedures and partial correlations to examine cross-generational *transmission,* or *influence,* indicated by the degree of correspondence or correlation between parents and their children and between grandparents and grandchildren, controlling for grandchild's age, gender, education, marital and parental statuses, co-residence with parents, and parental divorce. To examine the effects of parental divorce on the intergenerational transmission of religiosity, we also control for grandchild–grandparent contact.

Before turning to our results, we should clarify what we mean by *influence,* or *transmission,* and how we measure this statistically. We are not examining whether grandparents attend religious services more frequently than their grandchildren, or are more religious than their grandchildren, or have stronger conservative religious beliefs than their grandchildren. Rather, we are concerned with how much *influence* grandparents have on their grandchildren's frequency of religious service attendance, or religiousness, or the strength of their conservative religious beliefs. The degree of influence, or transmission, is reflected by the level of grandparent–grandchild correspondence on a given dimension of religiosity, after controlling for other factors. We use partial correlations to represent this correspondence.

RESULTS

Table 14.1 presents descriptive characteristics for grandparents, parents, and grandchildren in 1971 and 2000 on age, education level, and four dimensions of religiosity: (a) religious affiliation (grouped into categories), (b) frequency of religious service attendance, (c) religiousness, and (d) conservative religious beliefs. Focusing on these four dimensions of religiosity, there are several notable changes over time.

First, the religious affiliation categories for grandparents, parents, and grandchildren have shifted dramatically across the 30-year period. For all generations, there was a substantial increase in the proportion who profess no religious affiliation, while there was a marked decline in the proportion who are Protestant (primarily mainline Protestant). The proportion of respondents who reported being Catholic also declined, but not to the same degree. The proportion who reported being Jewish was stable over the period. (While the Jewish percentage is much higher than the national average, T. W. Smith & Kim, 2005, the Los Angeles region is home to a large Jewish community, and the sample reflects this distribution.) In that these changes between 1971 and 2000 affected all generations, regardless of life stage, this suggests a period, or historical, effect. These patterns of change, if not their magnitude, are consistent with national trend data (Hout & Fischer, 2002; T. W. Smith & Kim, 2005; Wuthnow, 1998). For example, the General Social Survey indicates that the proportion of Americans who report no religious affiliation has risen significantly over the past 30 years (T. W. Smith & Kim, 2005).

In 1971, 1% of grandmothers and 7% of grandfathers reported their religious affiliation as none. By 2000, almost one-third of grandmothers and grandfathers indicated none. A similar pattern holds for parents across the 30-year period. This is particularly the case for baby boomer (G3) fathers in 2000, where 43% reported none when asked their religious affiliation. These statistics could be interpreted as reflecting the declining status of organized religion in American society over the past several decades (Chaves, 1991).

Second, in contrast to higher rates of religious disaffiliation in our sample, average religious service attendance rose slightly over the 30-year period for all generations. Notable was the increase in service attendance for grandsons (G3s in 1971 and G4s in 2000). This finding reflects higher service attendance rates over time among those who *do* report a religious affiliation (not shown); that is, the G4s in 2000 who report a religious affiliation attended religious services more often than did their church-affiliated G3 parents, when both generations were adolescents or young adults. These findings are in concert with national church attendance figures (Sherkat & Ellison, 1999). However, as has been found with national data, we caution that there may be considerable overreporting of the frequency of church attendance (Hadaway, Marler, & Chaves, 1998).

Third, self-reported religiousness declined somewhat for all generations between 1971 and 2000, and significantly so for parents and grandchildren. Interestingly, mean religiousness scores for grandsons showed the largest decline over the 30-year period (from 2.6 to 2.3); at the same time, grandsons also showed the largest increase in average religious service attendance. This incongruity lends some credence to the suggestion that Generation X (G4) grandsons in particular may be overestimating how frequently they attend religious services.

Fourth, for both grandmothers and grandfathers, there is a significant decline in their agreement with conservative religious beliefs over the time period ($p < .01$). There is also a decline in parents' and grandchildren's agreement with conservative religious beliefs ($p < .05$ and $p < .07$, respectively). Although there is evidence that the proportion of conservative Protestants in the United States has increased in recent years (Woodberry & Smith, 1998), in our sample, we see a significant overall decline in adherence to conservative religious beliefs over time. While the trends observed thus far for this sample may be less typical than those found for the United States in general (T. W. Smith & Kim, 2005), we are reminded that the cultural patterns occurring in the Southern California area have often served as a bellwether, suggesting emergent trends in religious service participation and denominational dynamics.

We hypothesized that grandparents *do* significantly influence the religiosity of their grandchildren, and furthermore, that grandparents' influence has *increased* between 1971 and 2000. To test these two hypotheses, we use grandparent–parent–grandchild triads (G1, G2, G3 and G2, G3, G4) to estimate a series of OLS regression models, using G1 grandparents in 1971 and G2 grandparents in 2000, to predict the frequency of religious service attendance, self-reported religiousness, and agreement with conservative religious beliefs of G3 grandchildren in 1971 and G4 grandchildren in 2000. For each dimension of religiosity, separate models were estimated for grandparents (combined) and grandchildren (combined) and for each grandparent–grandchild gender configuration. We controlled for parents' religiosity (for each dimension separately) as well as grandchildren's age, education, marital status, parental status, whether living with parents, and parental divorce. Results are shown in Table 14.2. For each religiosity dimension, we examine and contrast the partial correlation coefficients and significance levels, focusing on *patterns* of difference across the 30-year period.

When we consider religious service attendance, results show that in 1971, G1 grandmothers strongly influenced their grandchildren's religious service attendance, and especially that of their granddaughters. Grandparents (combined), and grandfathers, also influenced their granddaughters' religious service attendance. On the other hand, grandparents did not influence their grandsons' religious service attendance. By 2000, however, only grandfathers had any influence on their grandchildren's religious service attendance, and that effect was marginal. What this suggests is that 30 years ago, grandparents, and especially grandmothers,

Table 14.2

COMPARING THE INFLUENCE OF GRANDPARENTS ON GRANDCHILDREN FOR SELECTED RELIGIOSITY DIMENSIONS: 1971 AND 2000, PARTIAL CORRELATIONS

	1971			2000		
	TOTAL G3S (n = 764)	MALE G3S (n = 347)	FEMALE G3S (n = 417)	TOTAL G4S (n = 565)	MALE G4S (n = 275)	FEMALE G4S (n = 290)
Conservative religious beliefs						
G1 Grandparent	0.05	0.12	0.00	0.20**	0.14	0.14
G1 Grandmother	0.05	0.11	-0.02	0.20***	0.15	0.25**
G1 Grandfather	0.07	0.09	0.05	-0.01	0.02	0.00
Religious service attendance						
G1 Grandparent	0.06	0.00	0.16***	0.03	0.08	0.00
G1 Grandmother	0.12**	0.05	0.14**	0.02	0.05	0.00
G1 Grandfather	0.06	0.00	0.13**	0.12*	0.14	0.09
Self-rated religiousness						
G1 Grandparent	0.10*	0.06	0.13*	0.05	0.05	0.05
G1 Grandmother	0.16**	0.18*	0.16**	0.10*	0.02	0.16**
G1 Grandfather	0.04	-0.01	0.09	-0.04	-0.04	-0.05

Note: Controls for parents' religiosity (by dimension) and grandchild's gender (1 = female), age, education (1 = some college or more), marital status (1 = married), has children (yes = 1), living with parents (yes = 1), and parents ever divorce (yes = 1). Data are from the Longitudinal Study of Generations 1971 and 2000.
$*p < .10.$ $**p < .05.$ $***p < .01.$

did influence their grandchildren's, especially granddaughters', religious service attendance. However, by 2000, that influence had largely dissipated.

In terms of the transmission of self-reported religiousness, in 1971, grandparents, and especially grandmothers, had a significant influence on grandchildren's religiousness, and particularly granddaughters' religiousness. In 2000, only grandmothers appear to be influencing their grandchildren's religiousness, again primarily that of their granddaughters. These data show that grandfathers did not influence their grandchildren's religiousness, regardless of historical time.

So far, results suggest a matrilineal tilt when it comes to the intergenerational transmission of religious service attendance and self-reported religiousness from grandparents to grandchildren. We can also say that the influence of grandparents on their grandchildren's religious service attendance and self-reported religiousness has weakened substantially over the past 30 years.

We see a different picture when we examine the intergenerational transmission of conservative religious beliefs. There is no evidence that in 1971, grandparents exerted any influence on their grandchildren's conservative religious beliefs independent of parents' conservative religious beliefs. However, by 2000, grandparents, and especially grandmothers, demonstrated a significant independent influence on their grandchildren's conservative religious beliefs; that is, grandparents who hold stronger conservative religious beliefs are more likely to pass on those beliefs to their grandchildren. The effect of grandmothers on their granddaughters' conservative religious beliefs is especially strong ($b = .25$; $p < .05$). On the other hand, there is no indication of any such influence passing from grandfathers to grandsons in 2000.

Evidence for the first hypothesis, which states that grandparents have a significant influence on the religiosity of their grandchildren, is mixed, depending on the dimension of religiosity being considered, the gender of the grandparent and grandchild, and the social and historical context, as reflected in the time of measurement. In 1971, grandparents did influence their grandchildren's religious service attendance and religiousness, but in 2000, this influence appeared to have waned. Alternatively, grandparents significantly influenced their grandchildren's conservative religious beliefs in 2000, but there is no evidence of such influence 30 years earlier. We found that where there is the intergenerational transmission of religiosity to grandchildren, it is most likely to be that of grandmothers, and the beneficiary is most likely to be a granddaughter.

Hypothesis 2 states that the influence grandparents have on grandchildren's religiosity has *increased,* not decreased, over the past three decades. As before, support for this hypothesis is mixed. We see a significant increase in the passing on of conservative religious beliefs from grandparents to grandchildren between 1971 and 2000. Grandmothers have a particularly salient effect on the conservative religious beliefs of their grandchildren, an influence which increases fourfold from 1971 ($b = .05$, n.s.) to 2000 ($b = .20$; $p < .01$). For this one dimension of religiosity, Hypothesis 2 is supported. We do not observe an increase in the influence of grandparents on grandchildren for the other two dimensions of religiosity; rather, grandparents' influence has declined. This pattern holds regardless of the gender of grandparents or grandchildren.

The third hypothesis proposes that while the transmission of religiosity from grandparents to grandchildren is mediated through the parents, grandparents will exert an influence on their grandchildren's religiosity that is independent of the influence of their parents. This is demonstrated by the analyses shown in Table 14.2. As noted, models regressing grandchild's religiosity on grandparents' religiosity were run separately for the three dimensions of religiosity. In each model, parents' corresponding religiosity indicator is controlled, and is significant (detailed results available from the second author). This means that all significant partial correlations shown in Table 14.2 by definition reflect grandparents' independent influence on their grandchildren's frequency of church attendance, religiousness, or conservative religious beliefs, varying by gender. This suggests that orientations toward religious beliefs and practices that are formed within nuclear and extended families persist into adulthood, with parents and grandparents simultaneously serving as independent and joint agents of religious socialization. On the basis of these analyses, we find qualified support for Hypothesis 3.

We are continuing to test the hypothesis that grandparents influence their grandchildren's religiosity independent of parents' influence using structural equation modeling procedures and different gender configurations. We are also examining lagged effects using this approach (not shown). Preliminary results demonstrate a grandparent transmission effect that is independent of the parents' influence on their children (results available from the second author).

Grandparent Influence and Parental Divorce

In our earlier research, we found that parental divorce does significantly reduce the ability of parents to pass on their achievement orientations and values to their children (Bengtson et al., 2002; Roberts & Bengtson, 1999). Now, when we examine the effect of parental divorce on parents' ability to influence their children's religious service attendance, religiousness, and conservative religious beliefs, we find the same pattern: Divorce diminishes the influence of parents.

However, our previous research did not examine how *grandparent* transmission processes might be affected by parental divorce. While we would expect marital dissolution to compromise parents' ability to influence their children's religious beliefs and practices, we propose that the active involvement of grandparents during this time may have a compensatory function. Therefore our fourth hypothesis predicts that grandparents' ability to influence their grandchildren's religious beliefs and practices will not be negatively affected by parental divorce, and may even increase. This is because grandparents' contact with grandchildren often increases during and after their parents' divorce, at least for the custodial spouse's parents. It is during this time that grandparents may be called on to provide the additional support and comfort needed by their grandchildren as they try to cope with the stresses that accompany their parents' separation and the restructuring of the family environment. This situation may also bring greater opportunity for grandparents to engage in the day-to-day socialization of their grandchildren. Spending more time together and the sharing of experiences can increase the potential for common value orientations.

Using 2000 data, we found that in the context of parental divorce, and controlling for grandparent–grandchild contact, grandparents' ability to influence their grandchildren's religiosity varied by the particular religiosity dimension being considered. Regardless of whether or not parents divorced, grandparents did not significantly influence their grandchildren's religious service attendance (although the direction of the relationship suggests parental divorce weakens grandparents' influence). When we examined grandparents' ability to pass on their conservative religious beliefs to their grandchildren in the context of marital disruption, we found that this transmission effect was stronger when parents did *not* divorce. This pattern changes, however, when we consider the intergenerational transmission of feelings of religiousness. Grandparents' influence on their grandchildren's religiousness is significant and marginally stronger ($p < .10$) when parents *are* divorced, as compared to when parents remain married, even after controlling for frequency of contact between grandparents and grandchildren (shown in Figure 14.3).

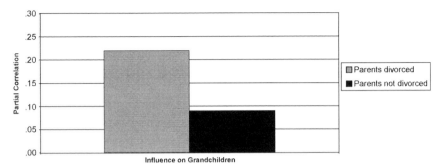

Figure 14.3 Comparing grandparents' influence on their grandchildren's religiousness, by parental divorce: 2000. In 2000: Longitudinal Study of Generations.

Note: Controls for parents' religiousness and grandchild's age, education, marital status, living arrangement, parental status, and contact with grandparents.

In the context of parental divorce, grandparents' ability to influence their grandchildren's feelings of religiousness is somewhat enhanced, suggesting a compensatory effect. For this one dimension of religiosity only, we find partial support for Hypothesis 4.

DISCUSSION AND CONCLUSION

This study takes on an age-old concern—the intergenerational transmission of religion—and addresses it in new ways, applying sociological methods and theory to the issue of religious continuity, and change, in families. Using 30 years of data from 350 multigenerational families participating in the LSOG, we examined the transmission of religious beliefs, values, and practices across four generations. We focused on the cross-generational influences and outcomes of three dimensions of religiosity: frequency of church attendance, self-reported religiousness, and religious belief orientation. Our aim was to learn more about how religion is passed down to younger generations within nuclear and extended family contexts, what role grandparents play in these transmission processes, and how these processes vary across generations and time and by parental divorce.

We tested four hypotheses. First, we proposed that grandparents do influence the religiosity of their grandchildren, and second, that this cross-generational influence has increased over the past three decades. We found partial support for these two hypotheses, depending on the dimension of religiosity being considered, the gender configuration of the cross-generational transmission flow, and historical time. Examination of 1971 data revealed that grandparents played a significant role in influencing their grandchildren's religious church attendance and religiousness. Noteworthy was the transmission effect flowing from grandmothers to granddaughters. Yet by 2000, the grandparents' influence on their grandchildren's religious service attendance and religiousness had largely dissipated. An alternate pattern occurred for the transmission of conservative religious beliefs. Thirty years ago, there was no indication of grandparent–grandchildren transmission of this religiosity dimension, but in the past decade, it is this dimension that we see being transmitted.

We also hypothesized that grandparents will exert an influence on their grandchildren's religious beliefs that is independent of parents' religious beliefs, though also mediated by them. The data support this expectation, particularly between grandmothers and granddaughters, suggesting that grandparents play a direct role in the religious socialization of their grandchildren. Fourth, we hypothesized that in the context of parental divorce, grandparents' influence on their grandchildren's religiosity would not weaken, and may even become stronger.

In proposing that grandparents' transmission processes may actually be stronger in the face of parental divorce, we found this effect for the more subjective dimension of religiousness, rather than for conservative religious beliefs, which is, in essence, a normative dimension of religiosity. In fact, parental divorce tended to reduce grandparents' transmission of conservative religious beliefs to their grandchildren, just as parents' marital stability strengthened transmission. This suggests that we might consider finer distinctions of meaning among dimensions of religiosity. In examining the transmission of religious beliefs across generations, we should pay attention to the nature of those beliefs and to the possibly negative valuation that individuals may give to particular life events (such as parental divorce) or lifestyle choices (such as cohabitation or out-of-wedlock childbearing); that is to say, there may be religious constraints on the ability of parents or grandparents to transmit their religious beliefs and values to their children or grandchildren because of strictures imposed by religious teachings. To the extent that moral interpretations of life events or lifestyle choices run counter to the tenets of one's faith, they may limit the transmission of religious values and beliefs from one generation to another. We suggest that when researchers examine the intergenerational transmission of religious beliefs, it is important to also consider the content of those beliefs, in particular, their proscriptions and rules for social behavior.

We considered the usefulness of traditional models of socialization to explain religious transmission in families. In general, socialization theories have tended to focus almost exclusively on the influence of parents on children, without acknowledging that children are situated within a wider web of family relationships, as represented by the multigenerational family. In this study, we expanded on traditional family socialization theories to explore the magnitude of grandparent–grandchild religious transmission as well as which family contexts facilitate or inhibit intergenerational religious continuity.

In pursuing this research topic, we are reminded that overlying the more immediate focus on the intergenerational transmission of religion across generations are the broader cultural debates over the potential demise or continued resilience and solidarity of the American family. Whether by politicians, social scientists, pastors, or citizens, the contemporary family is under constant moral surveillance (Brooks, 2002). The main concern of critics is whether contemporary changes in the form and function of the family, such as high rates of divorce, cohabitation, single parenthood, alternative partnerships, and the like, have seriously weakened the family's ability to pass down a cogent set of moral values and rules for living to the next generation. They argue that the virtues of religion as a source of social responsibility have been usurped by individualistic pursuits, putting the family at risk for moral decay. It is within this larger framework that the debate between religious idealists and family pragmatists rages on.

We suggest that these findings can serve to revise current stereotypes about the lack of family influence on religion and moral values. Families continue to invest in the moral upbringing of children. For example, today, most teenagers claim the religious affiliation of their parents (C. Smith, 2005), and parents' religious participation continues to have a strong impact on their children's religious participation over time (Sherkat, 1998). In sum, these results affirm the continued resilience and relevancy of families for the passing on of religious traditions and beliefs to younger generations. We also believe that insights from this research concerning religious transmission and socialization can tell us a great deal about the health and functioning of contemporary American families and, by extension, will have considerable import for other institutions such as churches, schools, the legal system, and public policy.

FUTURE DIRECTIONS

Through our examination of the religious transmission processes and out-comes in contemporary families, and particularly the transmission role of grandparents, we contribute to a major aim of the LSOG, which is to ex-amine the causes and consequences of family cohesion and conflict across a wide range of settings and conditions in the context of rapid social change.

We offer several suggestions for future research. Contrary to the predictions of the secularization thesis, the influence of religion appears to be on the rise in American civic life today (Roof, 1999; C. Smith, 2005; Wuthnow, 1998). Thus it is important that we know more about how religious values and practices are socialized in children and how, or whether, family influences have changed over the past decades. We need to understand patterns of religious influence in families across genera-tions and how religion helps or hinders family members to cope with contemporary crises and burdens such as poor health or caregiving for elderly parents or other dependent family members.

We need to examine how the changing family structures so evident today may be related to the new religious forms emerging at the start of the 21st century and whether this portends religious revolution or reformation. We need to translate our research findings on these issues so they can provide insight to parents and congregations attempting to train up a child in the way he or she should go in today's complex and fast-changing society.

Future research on religious identity should put aside the either-or approach and explore how the family intersects with other structures of influence, such as peers, neighborhood, and the media as well as religious and educational institutions, to create different types of religious identi-ties among today's youth.

Large-scale survey instruments have not adequately measured reli-giosity, especially the areas of religious belief and intensity. For the next LSOG survey, we would like to develop and test such measures. We would like to do the definitive work in such measurement.

Research on the intersection between religion and the family is only just beginning, although the close relationship between the two has long existed (Christiano, 2000). Some researchers assert that the family has weakened in the face of social change, claiming that the so-called decay of a moral society is a result of the family's moral ineffectiveness. We propose an alternative view. Our research on multigenerational families and the transmission of religious capital across generations and time indicates that families continue to use religion to define and reinvent their collective purpose. The moral foundation of families is not tenuous, but rather has been reconstituted. Redirecting our research questions to address the new strategies that parents—and grandparents—use to pass down religious beliefs, values, and practices to their children is the next step in understanding how social changes have impacted the moral influence of the family.

REFERENCES

Acock, A., & Bengtson, V. L. (1980). Socialization and attribution processes: Actual vs. perceived similarity among parents and youth. *Journal of Social Research, 68,* 151–171.

Bahr, H. M., & Chadwick, B. A. (1988). Religion and family in Middletown, USA. In D. L. Thomas (Ed.), *The religion and family connection: Social science perspectives* (pp. 51–65). Provo, UT: Religious Studies Center, Brigham Young University.

Bellah, R. N., Madsen, R., Sullivan, W. M., Swidler, A., & Tipton, S. M. (1985). *Habits of the heart: Individualism and commitment in American life.* New York: Harper and Row.

Bengtson, V. L. (1970). The "generation gap": A review and typology of social-psychological perspectives. *Youth and Society, 2,* 7–32.

Bengtson, V. L. (1975). Generation and family effects in value socialization. *American Sociological Review, 40,* 358–371.

Bengtson, V. L. (2001). Beyond the nuclear family: The increasing importance of multi-generational bonds. *Journal of Marriage and Family, 63,* 1–16.

Bengtson, V. L., Biblarz, T. J., & Roberts, R.E.L. (2002). *How families still matter: A longitudinal study of youth in two generations.* New York: Cambridge University Press.

Berger, P. (1967). *The sacred canopy: Elements of a sociological theory of religion.* New York: Anchor Books.

Brooks, C. (2002). Religious influence and the politics of family decline concern: Trends, sources, and U.S. political behavior. *American Sociological Review, 67,* 191–211.

Casper, L. M., & Bianchi, S. M. (2002). *Continuity and change in the American family.* Thousand Oaks, CA: Sage.

Chaves, M. (1991). Family structure and Protestant church attendance: The sociological basis of cohort and age effects. *Journal for the Scientific Study of Religion, 30,* 501–514.

Cherlin, A. (2002). *Public and private families: An introduction* (3rd ed.). Boston: McGraw-Hill.

Christiano, K. J. (2000). Religion and the family in modern American culture. In S. H. Houseknecht & J. G. Pankhurst (Eds.), *Family, religion and social change in diverse societies* (pp. 43–78). New York: Oxford University Press.

Comrey, A. L., & Newmeyer, J. A. (1965). Measurement of radicalism-conservatism. *Journal of Social Psychology, 67,* 367–369.

Copen, C. E., Biblarz, T. J., Silverstein, M., & Bengtson, V. L. (2005, August). *The ties that bind: Intergenerational transmission of religious values within American families.* Paper presented at the American Sociological Association annual meeting, Philadelphia.

Dobson, J. C., & Bauer, G. L. (1990). *Children at risk: The battle for the hearts and minds of our kids.* Dallas, TX: Word.

Glass, J., Bengtson, V. L., & Dunham, C. (1986). Attitude similarity in three-generation families: Socialization, status inheritance or reciprocal influence? *American Sociological Review, 51,* 685–698.

Hadaway, C. K., Marler, P. L., & Chaves, M. (1998). Over-reporting church attendance in America: Evidence that demands the same verdict. *American Sociological Review, 64,* 122–130.

Hervieu-Leger, D. (2000). *Religion as a chain of memory* (S. Lee, Trans.). New Brunswick, NJ: Rutgers University Press.

Hout, M., & Fischer, C. S. (2002). Why more Americans have no religious preference: Politics and generations. *American Sociological Review, 67,* 165–190.

Inglehart, R., & Baker, W. F. (2000). Modernization, cultural change, and the persistence of traditional values. *American Sociological Review, 65,* 19–51.

King, V., & Elder, G. H., Jr. (1999). Are religious grandparents more involved grandparents? *Journal of Gerontology: Social Sciences, Ser. B, 54,* S317–S328.

Mueller, M. M., & Elder, G. H., Jr. (2003). Family contingencies across the generations: Grandparent–grandchild relationships in holistic perspective. *Journal of Marriage and Family, 65,* 404–417.

Myers, S. M. (1996). An interactive model of religiosity inheritance: The importance of family context. *American Sociological Review, 61,* 858–866.

Myers, S. M. (2004). Religion and intergenerational assistance: Distinct differences by adult children's gender and parent's marital status. *Sociological Quarterly, 45,* 67–89.

Popenoe, D. (1993). American family decline, 1960–1990: A review and appraisal. *Journal of Marriage and Family, 55,* 527–555.

Pratt, M. W., & Friese, B. H. (Eds.). (2004). *Family stories and the life course: Across time and generations.* Mahwah, NJ: Erlbaum.

Putney, N. M., & Bengtson, V. L. (2002). Socialization and the family revisited. In R. A. Settersten Jr. & T. J. Owens (Eds.), *New frontiers in socialization: Advances in life course research* (Vol. 7, pp. 165–194). London: Elsevier Science.

Roberts, R.E.L., & Bengtson, V. L. (1999). The social psychology of values: Effects of individual development, social change, and family transmission over the life span. In C. D. Ryff & V. W. Marshall (Eds.), *The self and society in aging processes* (pp. 453–482). New York: Springer Publishing.

Roof, W. C. (1993). *Generation of seekers: The spiritual journeys of the baby boom generation.* San Francisco: Harper San Francisco.

Roof, W. C. (1999). *Spiritual marketplace: Baby boomers and the remaking of American religion.* Princeton, NJ: Princeton University Press.

Sherkat, D. E. (1998). Counterculture or continuity? Competing influences on baby boomers' religious orientations and participation. *Social Forces, 76,* 1087–1114.

Sherkat, D., & Ellison, C. (1999). Recent developments and current controversies in the sociology of religion. *Annual Review of Sociology, 25,* 363–394.

Sherkat, D. E., & Wilson, J. (1995). Preferences, constraints and choices in religious markets: An examination of religious switching and apostasy. *Social Forces, 73,* 993–1026.

Silverstein, M., Giarrusso, R., & Bengtson, V. L. (2003). Grandparents and grandchildren in family systems: A socio-developmental perspective. In V. L. Bengtson & A. Lowenstein (Eds.), *Global aging and its challenges to families* (pp. 75–102). New York: Aldine de Gruyter.

Smith, C. (2005). *Soul searching: The religious and spiritual lives of American teenagers.* New York: Oxford University Press.

Smith, T. W., & Kim, S. (2005). The vanishing Protestant majority. *Journal for the Scientific Study of Religion, 44,* 211–223.

Thornton, A. (1985). Reciprocal influences of family and religion in a changing world. *Journal of Marriage and Family, 47,* 381–394.

Thornton, A., Axinn, W. G., & Hill, D. H. (1992). Reciprocal effects of religiosity, cohabitation, and marriage. *American Journal of Sociology, 98,* 628–651.

Uhlenberg, P. R. (2005). Historical forces shaping grandparent–grandchild relationships: Demography and beyond. In M. Silverstein (Ed.), *Intergeneration relations across time and place* (pp. 77–97). New York: Springer Publishing.

Uhlenberg, P., & Hammil, B. G. (1998). Frequency of grandparent contact with grandchild sets: Six factors that make a difference. *Gerontologist, 38,* 276–285.

Woodberry, R. D., & Smith, C. S. (1998). Fundamentalism et al: Conservative Protestants in America. *Annual Review of Sociology, 24,* 25–56.

Wuthnow, R. (1988). *The restructuring of American religion: Society and faith since World War II.* Princeton, NJ: Princeton University Press.

Wuthnow, R. (1998). *After heaven: Spirituality in America since the 1950s.* Berkeley: University of California Press.

Table 14A

LONGITUDINAL MEASURES OF RELIGIOSITY INCLUDED IN THE LONGITUDINAL STUDY OF GENERATIONS: 1971–2000

ITEM	VALUES	GENERATION	TIME WAVE
1. What is your current religious affiliation?	Nominal	All	1, 2, 3, 5, 6, 7
2. How often do you attend religious services these days?	1 = Never 2 = Once a year or so 3 = Several times a year 4 = About once a month 5 = Once a week or so 6 = More than once a week	All	1, 2, 3, 5, 6, 7
3. This country would be better off if religion had a greater influence in daily life.	1 = Strongly agree 2 = Agree 3 = Disagree 4 = Strongly disagree	All	1, 2, 3, 4, 5, 6, 7
4. Every child should have religious instruction.	1 = Strongly agree 2 = Agree 3 = Disagree 4 = Strongly disagree	All	1, 2, 3, 4, 5, 6, 7
5. God exists in the form as described in the Bible.	1 = Strongly agree 2 = Agree 3 = Disagree 4 = Strongly disagree	All	1, 2, 3, 4, 5, 6, 7

6. All people today are descendants of Adam and Eve.	1 = Strongly agree 2 = Agree 3 = Disagree 4 = Strongly disagree	All	1, 3, 4, 5, 6, 7
7. Rank in order which values you find most important in life: religious participation (working with others in your own church or organization).	1 = Most important 9 = Least important	No G1s at T7	1, 2, 3, 4, 5, 6, 7
8. Regardless of whether you attend religious services, do you consider yourself to be religious?	1 = Not at all religious 2 = Somewhat religious 3 = Moderately religious 4 = Very religious	All	1, 2, 3, 5, 6, 7

333

15

How Have Social Institutional Forces Shaped Family Structure and Well-Being Over the Past 50 Years?

MARK D. HAYWARD

Trends in marriage, divorce, and cohabitation rates have fueled debates about the health of marriage as a fundamental social institution. There is little doubt that marriage has undergone profound changes in the latter part of the 20th century. The debate centers on interpreting these changes. Is marriage in trouble, culturally threatened, and in need of protection by public policy? Are the changes in marriage reflective of long-run changes in other facets of social life that have altered the opportunities for and benefits of marriage? Not surprisingly, given historical proximity to these changes in marriage, social observers lack the benefit of a long-run perspective. Regardless of one's interpretation, however, marriage as an institution has changed, and these changes will undoubtedly have profound implications both for the development of new social policies and the future well-being of families and children. This chapter sheds some light on the possible causes and consequences of the so-called marriage quake in the United States during the latter part of the 20th century.

Acknowledgment: This research was partially supported by an infrastructural grant from the National Institute of Child Health and Human Development (5 R24 HD042849). For additional information about this chapter, please contact Mark Hayward, Population Research Center, 1800 Main, University of Texas at Austin, Austin, TX 78712. E-mail: mhayward@prc.utexas.edu

THE RETREAT FROM MARRIAGE

There is little doubt that the average age of marriage has increased in recent decades. As shown in Figure 15.1, the estimated median age of first marriage has risen rapidly since 1970 for both men and women. Although the median age of marriage in the 1950–1970 period was low relative to what followed, it was also low relative to the median age of first marriage in the earlier part of the 20th century. Nonetheless, the median age of marriage has risen to unprecedented levels over the 100-year period for which we have data and has declined in popularity for over 50 years.

Changes in the median age of first marriage are determined by two demographic processes. The first is the *delay in marriage* among persons who eventually marry. Thus the trend shown in Figure 15.1 reflects changes in the timing of marriage, and there is some evidence that delayed marriage is the primary driving force behind the upward trajectory in the median age of marriage (Goldstein & Kenney, 2001).

The other demographic process that determines the changes in the median age of first marriage is changes in the proportion of persons who never marry—perhaps the starkest indicator of the popularity of marriage. Figure 15.2 shows that although the proportion of men and women never marrying substantially declines with age, there was an increase between 1970 and 1999 in the proportion of persons never marrying. For example, the proportion of men aged 40–44 years never marrying

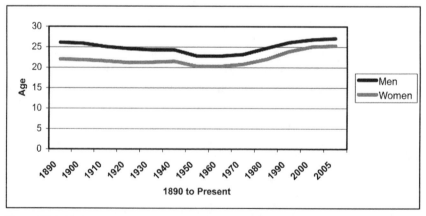

Figure 15.1 Estimated median age of first marriage. Data are from U.S. Bureau of the Census. (2004). Annual social and economic supplement. Current population reports series, 20-553.

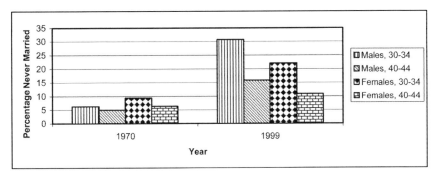

Figure 15.2 Percentage never married by age, sex, and year.

rose from 5% to about 16%. The proportion of same-aged women who had not married by this age rose from about 6% to 11%. A significant segment of the population, though a distinct minority, no longer marries by the end of the prime ages for starting a family (U.S. Bureau of the Census, 2006).

An important study by Goldstein and Kenney (2001) shed some important light on these basic trends in the median age of marriage and the prevalence of never marriage. Using a mathematical forecasting approach and marital history data for a nationally representative sample of adult women, Goldstein and Kenney's forecast models predict that marriage will continue to remain a relatively universal experience among American women: About 90% of women are predicted to eventually marry, regardless of birth cohort. Underneath the aggregate trend, however, are important differences by population subgroup. For example, in Goldstein and Kenney's study, the rates of ever marrying increased for college-educated women from 91.4% for the 1945–1949 birth cohort to 97.3% for the 1960–1964 birth cohort. In contrast, the rates of ever marrying for these cohorts fell for women without a college degree, from 96% to 92%. The increase in ever marrying among college-educated women is being balanced by the decline in ever marrying among women who are not college educated, resulting in what appears to be a stable aggregate trend in ever marrying. A recent study by Schoen and Cheng (2006) supported the educational gap in marriage forecasted by Goldstein and Kenney (2001).

In addition, divorce rates have fallen for college-educated women in recent decades, while divorce rates have been relatively stable or risen among less educated women (McLanahan, 2004). A parallel study on permissive attitudes toward divorce finds similar educational differences:

College-educated women have become less—not more—permissive toward divorce, while the opposite is true among women without a college education (Martin & Parashar, 2006). If we link the trends in ever marrying and divorce by education group, marriage, and its potential benefits, appears to be increasingly tied to education, with the most benefits accruing to college-educated women.

On the whole, then, the statistical evidence suggests that the retreat from marriage as reflected in the aggregate trend is largely a story of delayed marriage. However, underneath the aggregate trend are important subgroup differences that foretell a growing inequality associated with the benefits of marriage. While marriage appears to have become more popular among well-educated Americans, it has become less of a fact of life for poorly educated Americans. It should not be surprising that marriage has become an important topic in contemporary American political debates.

The Causes of the Retreat From Marriage

Changes in Women's and Men's Labor Market Positions

Sociologists and demographers studying marriage trends in the United States have offered a number of alternative explanations for the retreat from marriage. One explanation is based on changes in the labor market positions of women and men in the latter part of the 20th century. Women's labor force participation, and with it, women's economic independence, rose steadily in the latter part of the 20th century. Some researchers have hypothesized that women's economic independence fueled a decline in the marriage rates and an increase in divorce because marriage became less economically desirable (e.g., Goldscheider & Waite, 1986). However, as discussed earlier, the trend data (as well as individual-level studies of marriage behavior; Lichter, McLaughlin, Kephart, & Landry, 1992; Oppenheimer, 1997; Sweeney, 2002) are not consistent with this idea—those women most likely to be economically independent are college-educated women, and they are also the most likely to marry and stay married.

Coupled with women's growing economic independence is the gradual erosion of men's economic position in the latter part of the 20th century—particularly men without a college education and young Black men. Beginning in the 1970s, economic opportunities for men without a college education declined as the manufacturing sector lost jobs due to outsourcing and automation, while low-wage service sector employment expanded. Wages for men without a college education fell in the 1970s and 1980s, and this downward trend was only marginally arrested by the strong economy of the 1990s (Levy, 1998). The downward wage trend potentially had two effects (Cherlin, 2005). First, it undermined men's breadwinner role in the family in the sense that women needed to work. Second, it made men less attractive marriage partners (Lichter et al., 1992).

The Second Demographic Transition

A third and probably complementary explanation is that modernization in the latter part of the 20th century led to a growing cultural emphasis on individualism and self-fulfillment (Lesthaeghe, 1983; Lesthaeghe & Surkyn, 1988) and a shift away from the norm of marriage as a lifelong commitment. Cherlin (2005) characterized this cultural shift as the decline in *companionate marriage as a cultural ideal* to *individualized marriage*. A number of trends are sometimes thought to reflect this fundamental cultural shift in marriage norms: delayed marriage, increased rates of divorce, the rise in cohabitation, increases in nonmarital childbearing, and the growth in women's labor force attachment. A number of scholars have referred to these trends—which occurred over the latter part of the 20th century and may still be occurring—as the *second demographic transition* (Lesthaeghe & Surkyn, 1988; McLanahan, 2004).

The *first demographic transition* started early in the 19th century for most of Western Europe and English-speaking countries elsewhere and continued until the early part of the 20th century. The first demographic transition refers to the dramatic drop in mortality followed by rapid declines in fertility. The societal results of the first transition were widespread and profound over a century, for example, investments in child quality through public education, a demographic bonus favoring economic development and increased life cycle savings during the middle phase, and a shift away from the family toward pension systems to support growing numbers of elderly persons living to advanced ages. McLanahan (2004) posed the question of whether the second demographic transition will have similarly profound consequences for social institutions and policies addressing children's needs, focusing on the trends of growing inequality in parental resources for children.

A recent study by DiPrete and Buchmann (2006) provided compelling evidence of a long-term trend in the latter part of the 20th century of a growing gap in the benefits of a college education among women. For example, college-educated women were increasingly likely to delay childbearing, experience growth in their personal income, have a greater probability of marriage, and achieve a higher standard of living (partly by marrying high-income males). In contrast, women lacking a college education saw falling personal incomes in the latter part of the 20th century, a declining probability of marriage, and a falling standard of living. College-educated women were able to seize opportunities, while less well educated women found themselves falling increasingly behind.

Not surprisingly, the consequence of these trends, combined with growing educational differences in the divorce rate, was growing social class differences in what kind of family environment children grew up in (McLanahan, 2004). Children of poorly educated women were increasingly likely to grow up in single-parent families, experience family instability, and face a declining standard of living, while children born to well-educated women were more likely to live in stable, two-parent families with a rising standard of living. Thus the latter part of the 20th century was a time in which resources available to children were bifurcated along social class lines. Resource advantages and deficits increasingly clustered at the ends of the socioeconomic spectrum. One potential long-term consequence of the bifurcation in family resources is the intergenerational transmission of inequality in terms of children's academic achievement, health and health care, and cognitive and social development, and ultimately, the calcification of social class divisions. The family, for better or worse, is an important but often overlooked force influencing societal stratification.

Older persons are not typically included as part of sociologists' and family demographers' discussion of the retreat from marriage and the growing social divide in family resources and child well-being. This may be an important oversight. For example, a study of decennial census data by Simmons and Dye (2003) reported data showing an upward trend in grandparents responsible for rearing grandchildren. At the present time, there is very little hard empirical evidence for the reasons underlying this trend. Simmons and Dye's study reported a number of anecdotal reasons, which may be related. These reasons include parents' death, mental illness, and substance abuse.

Although the reasons for the trend are not clear, there is evidence about the characteristics of grandparents who are rearing their grandchildren. Only 40% had a job in the last 5 years. Forty percent were over age 60. Twenty percent of the grandparents rearing their grandchildren lived in poverty—a significantly higher rate than parents with related children. Not surprisingly, given the costs associated with rearing children on fixed and low incomes, grandparents were also more likely to fall into poverty than parents with related children. From a policy view, the child-rearing contributions of grandparents are considerable in terms of resources that do not have to be provided by local, state, and federal agencies. Grandparents informally care for about 12 times as many children as the nation's foster care, potentially saving taxpayers $6,500,000,000 per year.

The patterns noted previously are consistent with the other trends associated with the second demographic transition. It appears that children with poorly educated parents are increasingly being reared by someone other than their immediate parents, posing difficulties both for the grandparents and the children. The second demographic transition's effects, therefore, are likely to be felt up and down the age range. The bifurcation of resources available to children may also be contributing to inequality in the resources for older persons to maintain their health and well-being.

Challenges of the Second Demographic Transition for Public Policy

As noted earlier, the first demographic transition provided the impetus for a wide array of societal changes, including the spread of public education, pension systems, increased life cycle savings, and economic development. These societal changes, in turn, contributed to continued improvements in health, reductions in poverty, new technologies, ideological changes such as feminism, and labor market opportunities for women. In this sense, some of the seeds of the second demographic transition can be found in the first demographic transition.

McLanahan (2004) posed a fundamentally important question that defines the challenges of the second demographic transition:

> What policies may encourage mothers and fathers in the lowest [income] quartile to adopt the behaviors of parents in the top quartile? Specifically, how can we get women from disadvantaged backgrounds to delay childbearing, invest in education and training, and form stable partnerships? Similarly, how can we get men from disadvantaged backgrounds to remain committed to their children? (p. 622)

McLanahan (2004) responded to these queries by noting the importance of developing a set of mutually reinforcing social policies:

- Policies aimed at allowing men and women at the low end of the socioeconomic ladder to achieve a standard of living that makes marriage attractive
- Policies that support high-quality child care and education for children that not only make work more attractive for women, but also directly benefit children's health and academic achievement
- Policies enforcing paternal financial responsibilities toward offspring
- Income support policies that encourage marriage, rather than penalize persons for marrying
- Marriage promotion programs that recognize the challenges of the gender trust and sexual infidelity that foster unstable unions

An additional challenge confronting American policy makers is the possible political bifurcation that may have also accompanied the second demographic transition. One issue that is rarely recognized in academic discussions of public policy is the long-term trend in the spatial concentration of families with and without resources. An important exception is Massey's (1996) work on the topic, who argued that a variety of ecological mechanisms in the latter part of the 20th century have reinforced the growing class divide through the spatial segregation of affluence and poverty.

Not only is this pattern reflected in vast community differences in tax revenues and the demand for services, but it is also reflected politically. In a recent article published in *USA Today* (Cauchon, 2006), for example, the marital status of constituents in an election district was reported to be associated with the political party of its representatives. Republicans represented 49 out of 50 of the districts with the highest rates of married people—districts containing large numbers of children. Democrats represented all of the 50 districts containing the highest proportion of single people. Republicans represented 39,200,000 children, while Democrats represented only 32,000,000 children. Republicans represented districts with children with greater family resources compared to children's family resources in districts represented by Democrats. Furthermore, those Republican districts considered to be most vulnerable in the November 2006 elections had considerably fewer married persons than the average Republican district.

The key point is that the development of public policies like those mentioned by McLanahan (2004) will be inimically shaped by a political map of the United States, which is linked to the second demographic transition. Public policy rarely is developed with regard to national referents. In the case of public policies responding to the growing inequality in family resources, policies will be developed and contested in a political arena where the needs of districts with concentrated family resources will be pitted against the needs of districts with concentrated family deficits. While demography is not destiny, the long-term and growing divide in family resources associated with the second demographic transition is nonetheless also linked to the political means of responding to the increasing concentration of resource deficits facing millions of families.

CONCLUSION

The retreat from marriage is an important and long-term demographic trend and a central component of the second demographic transition. However, the trend varies across social classes in a way that contributes to a growing division of resources available to all generations within a family. Social class differences in the trend are also associated with the growing concentration of deficits and advantages in the array of resources at the ends of the socioeconomic spectrum. These patterns have spawned policy debates about family policies and the role of marriage in ameliorating poverty. These policy debates, however, are themselves being contested in a political arena that is reflective of another consequence of the second demographic transition: the spatial and political alignment of family resources.

REFERENCES

Cauchon, D. (2006, September 27). Marriage gap could sway elections. *USA Today*. Retrieved May 2, 2008, from http://www.usatoday.com/news/washington/2006-09-26-marriage-gap_x.htm

Cherlin, A. J. (2005). American marriage in the early twenty-first century. *Future Child, 15*, 33–55.

DiPrete, T. A., & Buchmann, C. (2006). Gender-specific trends in the value of education and the emerging gender gap in college completion. *Demography, 43*, 1–24.

Goldscheider, F. K., & Waite, L. J. (1986). Sex differences in the entry into marriage. *American Journal of Sociology, 92*, 91–109.

Goldstein, J. R., & Kenney, C. T. (2001). Marriage delayed or marriage forgone? New cohort forecasts of first marriage for U.S. women. *American Sociological Review, 66,* 506–519.

Lesthaeghe, R. (1983). A century of demographic and cultural change in western Europe: An exploration of underlying dimensions. *Population and Development Review, 9,* 411–435.

Lesthaeghe, R., & Surkyn, J. (1988). Cultural dynamics and economic theories of fertility change. *Population and Development Review, 14,* 1–45.

Levy, F. (1998). *The new dollars and dreams: American incomes and economic change.* New York: Russell Sage Foundation.

Lichter, D. T., McLaughlin, D. K., Kephart, G., & Landry, D. J. (1992). Race and the retreat from marriage: A shortage of marriageable men? *American Sociological Review, 57,* 781–799.

Martin, S. P., & Parashar, S. (2006). Women's changing attitudes toward divorce, 1974–2002: Evidence for an educational crossover. *Journal of Marriage and Family, 68,* 29–40.

Massey, D. S. (1996). The age of extremes: Concentrated affluence and poverty in the twenty-first century. *Demography, 33,* 395–412.

McLanahan, S. (2004). Diverging destinies: How children are faring under the second demographic transition. *Demography, 41,* 607–627.

Oppenheimer, V. K. (1997). Women's employment and the gain to marriage: The specialization and trading model. *Annual Review of Sociology, 23,* 431–453.

Schoen, R., & Cheng, Y.-H. A. (2006). Partner choice and the differential retreat from marriage. *Journal of Marriage and Family, 68,* 1–10.

Simmons, T., & Dye, J. L. (2003). Grandparents living with grandchildren: 2000. In *Census 2000 Brief.* Washington, DC: U.S. Census Bureau.

Sweeney, M. M. (2002). Two decades of family change: The shifting economic foundations of marriage. *American Sociological Review, 67,* 132–147.

U.S. Bureau of the Census. (2006). *Statistical abstract of the United States 2006.* Washington, DC: Government Printing Office.

Commentary: Marital Trends and Familial Influences—Toward Developing an Understanding of Context

16

CHALANDRA M. BRYANT AND MICHELLE L. BRAGG

The chapters by Bengston, Copen, Putney, and Silverstein (this volume) and Hayward (this volume) focus on two of society's fundamental institutions: family and religion—both of which are private (vs. public) institutions (Anderson, 2001). The chapters underscore important demographic shifts affecting marriage as well as family formation and function.

The work by Bengston et al. is largely concerned with the intergenerational transmission of religiosity. The authors, after identifying the goals of their chapter, discuss the arguments regarding the significance of the family, namely, the central role family plays in the transmission of values, generally, and of religiosity, in particular. The authors discuss three primary models of socialization relative to the transmission of religiosity from parent to child. Additionally, Bengston et al. underscore the fact that the role of grandparents in the transmission of both values and religion has been underinvestigated. However, as life expectancies in America continue to increase, so, too, does the potential role of grandparents in the lives of their children and grandchildren. The data used in their study, the Longitudinal Study of Generations (LSOG), affords the opportunity to examine the transmission of religion across four generations, which is a significant contribution to the existing body of research.

In their study, Bengston et al. examine three dimensions of religiosity (i.e., frequency of church attendance, self-reported religiousness, and religious belief orientation) and outline four assertions: (a) grandparents exert a noticeable effect on the religiosity of their grandchildren as the latter reach young adulthood; (b) such influence has increased over time; (c) grandparents exert influence on grandchildren's religiosity that is independent of parental influences; and (d) despite divorce, grandparents' influence remains significant. Bengston et al. discuss the findings of their research as well as the cross-generational implications of the study. In short, the authors suggest that their findings "affirm the continued resilience and relevancy of families for the passing on of religious traditions and beliefs to younger generations" (p. 327).

Hayward begins his chapter by outlining specific demographic trends that influence marriage, divorce, and cohabitation for men and women in the United States, namely, the *second demographic transition*. He then highlights reasons for the retreat from marriage, which include cultural, economic, and sociological explanations. Finally, Hayward concludes with policy implications and some possible prescriptions for addressing the aforementioned concerns.

Taken together, the two chapters converge on a common point: Demographic shifts since the 1960s to the present have significant ramifications for individuals and families. With respect to marriage, demographic realities generate push and pull factors that influence the stability of the key dyad from which families are built and anchored: the marital unit of husband and wife. From the standpoint of families, the shifts influence the stability (i.e., level and tenure of sustained commitment) as well as the function of families, which are fundamental agents of socialization within society.

The two chapters also highlight normative shifts that can impact individual and collective behavior. Norms emerge from several sources (Fukuyama, 1997): institutions (i.e., the state), spontaneous construction (i.e., those that evolve out of repeated interactions), exogenous construction (i.e., religion), and nature (i.e., kinship). In attempts to provide some historical context as it relates to normative shifts, the work of the noted scholar Francis Fukuyama (1999) is instructive. In *The Great Disruption,* he eloquently outlines the shift in norms from *Gemeinshaft* (or community) in premodern Europe to *Geshellshaft* (or society) in the industrial era up to the postindustrial era, in which norms center more on individualism (i.e., increased personal autonomy); that is to say, norms have been changing (and affecting families) for some time. Presently, the normative shifts, coupled with demographic trends, also influence the definition of *family* in the United States such that the current notion of family is not exclusively so-called traditional (i.e., two-parent, nuclear); rather, so-called nontraditional families (i.e., stepfamilies, multigenerational families) are commonly included in mainstream discussions of family.

Concomitantly, religious shifts have also been occurring in America since the 1960s. As outlined in a recent article by Marler and Hadaway (2002), the decline of Protestant hegemony, the diminished presence of traditional religious institutions, increased intermarriage among Jewish Americans, and the "assimilation of the Catholic ghetto" (p. 289) characterize the changes that have taken place. Moreover, there is a shift toward *spiritual seeking* as well as a shift toward religion being much more personal and self-defined (Anderson, 2001; Kohut, Green, Keeter, & Toth, 2000). Thus the combination of normative and other shifts (i.e., economic), along with religious shifts, presents challenges to both individuals and families, particularly with respect to stability. The individual orientation of norms toward self-actualization as well as with respect to religion certainly influences the ability of families to effectively transmit norms across generations.

The goal of this chapter is to underscore and contextualize the important trends discussed in the aforementioned chapters. With respect to the Hayward chapter, we will specifically highlight the racial and ethnic context of the demographic shifts mentioned. In terms of the chapter by Bengston et al., we will also discuss the individual orientation of religion. In addition, we will highlight the influence of technology on religious practices in particular. More generally, we will comment on the importance of religion and marriage in the United States. While divorce rates in America have risen significantly since the 1950s, persons continue to marry; that is, marriage, in a global or macro sense, is still highly regarded. However, at the individual level, personal happiness plays a greater role in decisions to marry (as well as divorce; Layard, 2005), which is in keeping with the shift to individualism mentioned earlier.

HOW WE ARRIVED AT MARRIAGE AS WE KNOW IT

Let us focus our attention for a moment on marriage. Lately, many discussions have taken place about the institution of marriage changing. Intimate relationships and marriages, as we now know them, did not surface until the early decades of the 19th century (Gadlin, 1977). This indicates that yes, indeed, marriage has changed. However (and this point is very important), the fact that it has changed is not new; marriage as an institution has been changing for hundreds of years. This is clearly evident as we progress from the colonial period through today.

During the colonial period (mid-1600s), privacy was not an aspect of personal life. Households fell under the guidance of the community. For example, if a spouse left his or her home for another partner, that spouse would be punished and forced to return home (Gadlin, 1977). Lack of privacy was even reflected in the physical space; houses were small, with very few rooms. Thus the sexual life of married couples was far from private. Love was not a reason for marrying. On the contrary, love followed marriage. Loving one's spouse was a duty, an obligation. Family was the center of all aspects of life, including church, school, and work. Passions were meant to be controlled, and reason was meant to dominate over passion (Gadlin, 1977).

Unlike the colonial period, the next era, the Jacksonian period (19th century), was not marked by constant surveillance. The home was no longer the center of existence because people's lives became divided between work and home. This division was the result of industrialization, in addition to the development of urban centers. People left their farms and small towns to avoid poverty, but they were ill prepared for life in urban settings, where they were no longer under the strict guidance of their watchful community. These changes contributed to a crisis of personal identity and interpersonal relations. Ironically, the newly acquired personal privacy seemed to threaten their identity. The community, which seemed to have restrained and controlled individuals during the colonial period, also provided social support and warmth. When the firm network ties that bound colonial Americans together began dissolving, that dissolution weakened social support systems, which in turn left couples solely responsible for their own marital relationships. Whereas among colonial Americans, feelings of love followed marriage, during the Jacksonian period, feelings and love now became the reason for relationships. Consequently, when feelings faded, so, too, could the relationship. According to Nissenbaum (as cited in Gadlin, 1977), other changes involved perceptions of sexual behavior:

> Colonial Americans had acknowledged sexual feelings as natural and restricted sexual behavior to marriage where it did not threaten social cohesion. Jacksonian Americans attempted to control the sexual

impulses. . . . In so doing they transformed the nature and meaning of sexuality. Whereas sexual relations had previously been seen as naturally directed at obtaining sexual pleasure, they were now understood as legitimate only as an expression of warmth and intimacy, the ultimate indicator of a deep spiritual bond between people. (pp. 47–48)

Interestingly, during the Progressive era, the larger social order began to regain control, and interpersonal life was once again becoming a public matter. This became evident with the growing popularity of publishing accounts of private matters (e.g., lovelorn column in newspapers).

The responsibility for the success or failure of marriage and family fell on the shoulders of husbands and wives alone. Gadlin (1977) succinctly summarized this change when he stated that couples began to "expect a good deal from one another to sustain the mutual interest and attraction necessary to preserve the emotional tie that is the cement of the relationship" (p. 58).

The aforementioned changes reflect broader changes that were occurring in American society. American marriages were once institutional—meaning that unions were bound by religion, law, duty, and male domination—but that was followed by a shift to *companionate marriages* (Burgess & Locke, 1945). Companionate marriages were characterized by companionship, emotional bonds, friendship, and sexual gratification (Mintz & Kellogg, 1988). In marriages of this type, spouses gained satisfaction from serving in roles such as homemaker or breadwinner. This type of marriage was most prevalent in the 1950s. In the 1960s, a third shift occurred; during this time, *individualized marriages* arose (see Figure 16.1). Those are marriages characterized by both spouses working outside the home. Partners' roles were more flexible, and self-development was the focus.

According to Gadlin (1977), marriages underwent even further changes after the 1960s. For example, Gadlin suggested that in the 1970s, emotions were no longer a component of relationships. He felt that people were relying on technical skills (as seen in encounter groups, sensitivity groups, and human relations training) to cope with their relationships. If we fast-forward to the 21st century, instead of looking ahead, many researchers are looking back and asking whether the good old days—those days when spousal roles were socially proscribed along gender lines—were actually that great. Questions regarding marital happiness and marital success seem to be posed more often now, as we look back across time in an attempt to determine what happy families

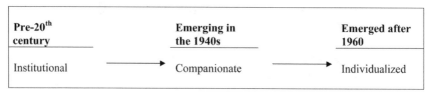

Figure 16.1 Shifts in marriage.

and marriages are like. According to the opening lines of Leo Tolstoy's *Anna Karenina* in 1877 (translated by Pevear and Volokhonsky in 2000): "Happy families are all alike; every unhappy family is unhappy in its own way" (p. 1). Stephanie Coontz (2005) disagreed with Tolstoy's statement. She explained,

> the more I study the history of marriage, the more I think the opposite is true. Most unhappy marriages in history share common patterns, leaving their tear-stained—and sometimes bloodstained—records across the ages. But each happy, successful marriage seems to be happy in its own way. (p. 20)

MARRIAGE IN THE NEW MILLENNIUM

What does all this mean for today's Americans? Today, the American family, in general, and intimate relationships, in particular, are still "ever-changing and fluid" (Bryant, Bolland, Burton, Hurt, & Bryant, 2006, p. 25). Marriage is just one of many lifestyles. Moreover, there are many forms of marriage. For example, the unions of some couples may resemble institutional marriages, whereas other unions consist of the husband serving in the homemaker role, with the wife serving in the breadwinner role. Other lifestyles include lifelong cohabiting unions or even lifelong singlehood. Some believe that these alternative lifestyles reflect the declining popularity of marriage.

Use of the term *popular* or *popularity* is interesting. It is very different from *value*. Can something that is unpopular be valued? The answer to that question is yes. Three decades ago, Americans held the belief that married people were happier than single people, and most Americans continue to hold such beliefs today (Axinn & Thornton, 2000). Thus Americans do, indeed, value marriage and family life (Thornton, 1989; Thornton & Young-DeMarco, 2001). Most Americans expect to someday marry (Lichter, Batson, & Brown, 2004; Mauldon, London, Fein, Patterson, & Bliss, 2002). Moreover, the vast majority do actually marry

(Casper & Bianchi, 2002; Goldstein & Kenney, 2001). Of the women born between 1961 and 1965, 90% have married or will do so (Goldstein & Kenney, 2001). Interestingly, boys and girls who graduated from high school between 1996 and 2000 were more likely than those who graduated earlier (i.e., between 1976 and 1980) to rate having a good family life as extremely important (Whitehead & Popenoe, 2002). Thus marriage is still a strong ideal—even among the poor (Edin, 2000).

The decreased popularity of marriage is associated not with decreased value for this particular lifestyle, but, perhaps, it is instead associated with increased expectations. Increased marital expectations may consequently lead to raising the standards (or the proverbial bar, so to speak) by which we measure not only marital happiness, but also the standards by which we measure the merits of proceeding with a marital union. Perhaps people want to know that they are ready to marry; being ready can mean anything from partners feeling as though they have saved enough money for marriage and secured good jobs to feeling as though they have adequately tested their compatibility (Edin, 2000). Given the desire to forego marriage until ready as well as the rise in cohabitation rates and the decreasing stigma associated with singlehood, we should not be taken aback by the declines in marriage. Indeed, what is most astonishing is the fact that people are still actually marrying. However, not all Americans are marrying at the same rates.

African Americans have slightly different demographics with regard to marriage. In 1940, African Americans—both men and women—married earlier than did Whites (Cherlin, 1992; Tucker & Mitchell-Kernan, 1995). The 1950s and early 1960s were distinct periods for marriage; not only was the prevalence of marriage high, but early marriage was common among Whites as well as African Americans.

Approximately 34% of African Americans, 15 years of age and older, were married in 2004; about 43% were categorized as never married at that time (U.S. Census Bureau, 2007). Of the non-Hispanic Whites, about 57% were married, and 24% were never married; thus they were more likely to be married and less likely to have never married than were African Americans (see Figure 16.2). An examination of households reveals that African Americans were less likely to live in married-couple households than were non-Hispanic Whites (U.S. Census Bureau, 2007). Moreover, while only 9% of non-Hispanic White households consisted of families headed by a woman with no husband present, about 30% of African American households consisted of families headed by a woman with no husband present (see Figure 16.3). Researchers are predicting that

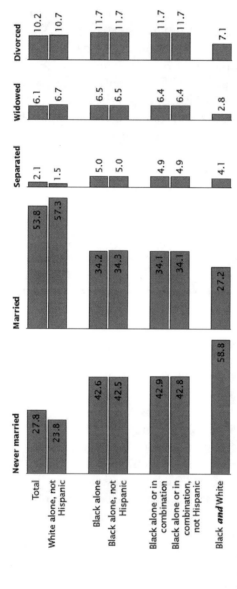

Figure 16.2 Summary of marital status (2004). Percentage distribution of population aged 15 and older. Data are based on a sample limited to the household population and exclude the population living in institutions, college dormitories, and other group quarters. Some percentages do not sum to 100.0 due to rounding. (For information on confidentiality protection, sampling error, nonsampling error, and definitions, see the U.S. Census Bureau Web site http://www.census.gov/prod/2007pubs/acs-04.pdf) Data are from the U.S. Census Bureau, 2004 American Community Survey, Selected Population Profiles, S0201.

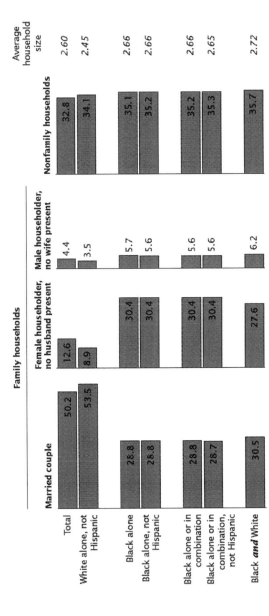

Figure 16.3 Type of household (2004). Percentage distribution. Household type is shown by the race and Hispanic origin of the householder. Data are based on a sample limited to the household population and exclude the population living in institutions, college dormitories, and other group quarters. (For information on confidentiality protection, sampling error, nonsampling error, and definitions, see the U.S. Census Bureau Web site http://www.census.gov/prod/2007pubs/acs-04.pdf) Data are from the U.S. Census Bureau, 2004 American Community Survey, Selected Population Profiles, S0201, and Detailed Tables B11001.

only about two-thirds of African American women will eventually marry (Goldstein & Kenney, 2001). About 60% of African American (compared to 20% of White) children will not grow up in a married-couple household (Bumpass & Lu, 2000). This suggests the need for a closer examination of trends involving specific populations in the United States.

As stated earlier, yes, the institution of marriage has changed. Marriage has become more voluntary and less obligatory. What may be even more noteworthy is that the social meaning of interpersonal closeness has changed, and that change may be much more profound because it has implications beyond marriage.

Statistics on divorce and domestic violence as well as numerous stories about families in crisis paint a very negative picture of marriage and family life today. However, this is not the first time in history that academics have proposed a retreat from marriage. For decades, many respected social scientists have predicted that the institutions of marriage and the family were dying:

> 1927: "In 50 years, unless there is some change, the tribal custom of marriage will no longer exist."—John B. Watson, psychologist

> 1937: "The family as a sacred union of husband and wife, of parents and children, will continue to disintegrate."—Pitirim Sorokin, Harvard sociologist

> 1947: "There is little left now, within the family itself or the moral code, to hold the family together."—Carl Zimmerman, Harvard sociologist (Bernard, 1970, as cited in Olson & DeFrain, 2006, p. 6)

It is a little difficult to determine whether their comments reflect the popularity of marriage or the value of marriage.

As suggested earlier, perhaps marriage is not dying out—it is just in a process of change. So the questions we should ask are, Is it changing for the better? Or is it changing for the worse? While some people believe that the shifts reflect the eventual disintegration of marital and familial life, others believe that the shifts are adaptations to complex stresses, social contexts, and economic circumstances. Recall that the Victorians felt that family life was fading away, as people began adapting to industrialization and urban life, just as in the later decade of the 20th century and the beginning of the 21st century, many academics, politicians, and laypersons believed that family life was fading away.

However, those observed changes also reflected adaptations: adaptations for coping with increased economic strain, as it became necessary for many families in the United States to become dual-earner households. The social, economic, and even cultural context in which families and marriages are formed and maintained must be acknowledged if we are to develop an understanding of the shifts observed in marital trends over time.

ONE NATION UNDER GOD

Social, economic, and cultural factors also influence family functions and processes. Some of the most important functions of families involve the socialization and transmission of values, norms, and culture as well as religion. Like other factors, however, there are important religious shifts that affect families. Thus the goals of this section are to provide a bit of context to religion in America, discuss strengths and limitations of the study conducted by Bengston et al., highlight emerging religious trends, and outline information that might prove instructive for similar and future studies.

Religion occupies a special place in the life of Americans. A recent poll suggested that 91% of Americans believe in God (Braiker, 2007; Meacham, 2007). A recent study of 8th, 10th, and 12th graders in the United States found that 60% of youth believed that religion was important (Wallace, Forman, Caldwell, & Willis, 2003). One of the most noted observers of American culture, Alexis de Tocqueville (1835/1948), noted, "There is no country in the world where the Christian religion retains a greater influence over the souls of men than in America" (p. 314). In fact, the late scholar Seymore Martin Lipset (1996), in his tome, *American Exceptionalism,* thoroughly outlined and described the components of American creed that distinguish it from other Western nations. With respect to social aspects, one of the defining features is America's religious character. Lipset documented that relative to other Western countries, Americans are the most churchgoing Protestants. For example, he cited comparative data which suggest that a substantially greater percentage of Americans reported attending weekly church services than did their British and West German counterparts. Also, nearly four-fifths of Americans reported religion as being important to their lives, relative to an average 45% of Europeans.

Religion is highly salient among Americans; freedom of religion is the subject of the First Amendment in the Constitution of the United States and thus the legal right of every citizen. This right also includes the right not to affiliate with a particular religion or not to subscribe to a particular religious ideology. In addition, Americans also enjoy the right to change religions or to disavow religion altogether. In keeping with this, there have been significant changes in religious affiliation over the last 30 years. Sherkat (2001) extensively examined these changes between 1973 and 1998. He found declining memberships primarily among liberal Protestants (i.e., Presbyterians, Unitarian), Episcopalians, and Catholics as well as an increasing number of persons indicating they have no religious affiliation. In light of the previously mentioned demographic and normative trends as well as the aforementioned religious trends, the study by Bengston et al., which examines the intergenerational transmission of religiosity, is timely.

The study by Bengston et al. has several important strengths. First of all, it was conducted with a large sample, which includes over 3,000 respondents between the ages of 16 and 91 within 350 multigenerational families. As such, the authors were able to test their hypotheses across four generations. Second, the study was longitudinal in nature, and the authors were able to assess religious variation over time for each cohort. The combination of the former and the latter represents a substantial contribution to social science research. Third, the study addresses nagging concerns regarding the ability of the family to continue to function as a moral agent, especially with respect to religion. The study findings suggest that families retain moral agency, which is important information for practical and policy considerations. Finally, the realities of the day suggest that grandparents are increasingly involved with their grandchildren for a variety of reasons, including longer life expectancies and the "increasing importance of relations across two generations" (Bengston, 2001, p. 2). Therefore the authors incorporate grandparents into their examination of the process of family socialization as it relates to religious transmission. Again, this represents a significant contribution to the literature.

While there are notable strengths to the study, there are also a few limitations. LSOG participants are primarily White residents of California. Thus the findings are not generalizable to Whites nationally or to other racial or ethnic groups. California has—and has had for some time—one of the most racially and ethnically diverse populations in the nation. While all researchers encounter data constraints, in this study, there is no mention of the relative lack of diversity of the sample or any discussion of religiosity among any racial or ethnic groups in California and/or the nation. As heightened attention to racial and ethnic diversity exists, it is important to note patterns relative to other groups, namely, the religious orientation of African Americans and Latinos—two groups with sizeable populations in California and who comprise the largest minority groups in the nation.

Inclusion of information about the religiosity of other racial and ethnic groups would have been useful. For example, religion and spirituality are highly salient among Black Americans (see, e.g., Paris, 1995). This salience transcends family structure. Additionally, Latino Americans also highly value religion (see, e.g., Avalos, 2004) and often have family structures that differ from White Americans (i.e., extended families). Recent studies involving large samples of Black and Latino children found high levels of religiousness among children in both groups (Smith, Lundquist-Denton, Faris, & Regnerus, 2005; Wallace et al., 2003). Additionally, grandparents play more active roles in the lives of Black and Latino children (Cherlin & Furstenberg, 1985, 1992; Fields, 2003; Hernandez & Meyers, 1993; Zambrana, 2004). Broadening the discussion of intergenerational transmission of religion (i.e., similar or dissimilar patterns) to include these two groups in particular would have made this study even more compelling.

The self-report measure used in the study might warrant further attention. There seems to be some inconsistency, namely, among males, between reports of church attendance and religiosity. It is possible that persons are inflating reports of church attendance. For example, according to a study by Hadaway and Marler (2005), the common figure often cited regarding the proportion of Americans attending church services during a given week is about 40%. The authors stated, "That more than four out of ten Americans actually worship in a church or synagogue during an average week struck many denominational leaders and some social researchers as unlikely" (p. 307). Their study concluded that it is more likely that about 21% of Americans attend weekly church services. Another study by Kohut et al. (2000) suggested that church service had actually declined since the mid-1960s—along with religious salience. Studies found that the self-reported church attendance measure is often inflated as persons do not report actual behavior (Burton & Blair, 1991; Silver, Anderson, & Abramson, 1986); rather, persons report on past or intended behavior—especially when such behavior is socially sanctioned.

Missing in the study was some measure of parent–child, grandparent–grandchild relationship quality. Relationship quality undoubtedly facilitates the transmission of religion between parents and children as well as grandparents and grandchildren. Coleman (1998), specifically as it relates to social capital, which is a by-product of religion, stated, "The social capital of the family is in the relations between children and parents (and when families include other members, relationships with them as well)" (p. S110). He went on to state,

> Social capital within the family that gives the child access to the adult's human capital depends both on the physical presence of adults in the family and on the attention given by the adults to the child. . . . Even if adults are physically present, there is a lack of social capital in the family if there are not strong relations between children and parents. (p. S111)

Including some measure of relationship quality between grandparents and grandchildren in particular would enhance the study findings.

A recent study by King and Elder (1999) parceled out grandparent religiousness into public and private dimensions when examining grandparent involvement with their grandchildren. The public dimensions included attended church services as well as the following: having led a religious service, taught Sunday school or other religious class, and attended a religious class or religious discussion group. Private dimensions of religiousness included religious orientation along with the following: having read the Bible, tuned to a religious broadcast, and prayed privately. The authors found that both types were significant predictors of grandparent involvement with grandchildren. Thus it might be particularly useful to expand the measures of grandparent religiousness to determine if the additional components of public and private religiousness specifically facilitate the intergenerational transmission of religion within families.

Bengston et al. found that grandmothers in particular significantly influenced religiosity and conservative beliefs among their grandchildren—primarily among granddaughters. The authors shed little light on this gendered effect. What is it about grandmothers that drive their influence? Why is the so-called grandmother effect particularly strong for granddaughters? A recent article by Miller and Stark (2002) provided some insight that might prove instructive in helping to address these questions. The authors reviewed the literature about the near-universal gender differences with respect to religiosity and religious commitment, with women being more religious than men. The authors summarized previous explanations for the gender differences: Women are socialized to be nurturing and submissive, and thus religious commitment is more common; the mother role encompasses aspects of religiousness (i.e., teaching morality to children); women have more time to invest in religion because they often are not in the labor force; religion falls under the rubric of family life, and the division of labor allocates family matters to women; due to differences in social power, women seek religion as a refuge; and feminine personality traits and religiousness are related. Miller and Stark investigated whether gender differences with respect to religion are due to the fact that irreligion is akin to risk taking, and men are socialized to engage in riskier behaviors, while women are socialized to be more cautious and minimize risk taking. The authors found support for several hypotheses, including the following: Gender differences will be greater when the consequences of irreligion are riskier.

The discussion of individualism by Bengston et al. was given short shrift. Individualism is a core American value and a defining feature of American culture (Lipset, 1996). Individual autonomy is now a more common driver of religious choices—as it is with marital and familial choices. With respect to religion today, there is less denominationalism and more limited connections to formal religious institutions as well as a quest for spirituality (Anderson, 2001). Persons are more selective in the spiritual marketplace, where, according to Turner (2005), "individual[s] should be free to choose any religion or combination of religion to feel good" (p. 314). Indeed, Turner suggested that a sense of "believing without belonging" (p. 309) exists. These trends are not insignificant, and they will undoubtedly continue to influence religiosity and religious practices on both the individual and family levels for years to come.

Since the LSOG began in 1970, technological advances, such as the Internet, have become integral facets of daily American life. However, in the Bengston et al. study, there is no discussion of technology, the Internet in particular, and how it might shape or influence religiousness. A Pew Research Center (2005) report indicated the following: (a) 82,000,000 Americans have used the Internet for religious or spiritual purposes; (b) in 2004, 6,000,000 persons looked for religious and spiritual information online on a typical day; (c) 73% of female respondents obtained spiritual or religious information online, compared with 56% of male respondents; and (d) 21% of respondents indicated that they belonged to an online religious organization. While the Internet may not supplant actual church attendance (Corrigan, Morgan, Silk, & Williams,

2006; Larsen, 2004), use of the Internet to engage in religious or spiritually based activity clearly complements and/or extends existing religious and/or spiritual practices. Hence future use of the Internet as well as other technological advancements may come to exert greater or more direct influence on individuals with respect to religious routines (i.e., routines may become less traditional).

Bengston et al. provide little discussion about how emerging social and religious trends might influence the religiosity and religious practices of younger cohorts. However, recent articles centering on emerging adults are instructive. Arnett (2000) suggested that emerging adulthood represents a developmental period for those aged 18–25. Arnett and Jensen (2002) characterized emergent adulthood as including the following: questioning the beliefs in which they were raised, placing greater emphasis on individual spirituality than affiliating with a religious institution, and picking and choosing certain aspects of religion. In their study, Arnett and Jensen also found no relationship between emerging adults' religious socialization in childhood and their current church attendance or current religious views. This suggests that, at least for a time, the family's influence on emerging adults' religiosity is diminished.

Hervieu-Leger (1993) suggested that religion is often viewed as a *symbolic toolbox*, where individuals select particular aspects of a religion, but not all. As persons reduce their affiliation with specific denominations, preferring instead to customize their religious beliefs and practices, today's young adults are following suit. Emergent adults' preferences are less adaptive than they might have been in childhood and suggest that they desire to adopt religious and spiritual components that best meet their needs at the time. This reality may have less to do with familial influences and more to do with developmental needs, the increased trends of individualism, and the diversity of religious and/or spiritual options available in America. Thus future patterns of religiosity for younger cohorts may be less predictable than with previous cohorts.

The study by Bengston et al. yields interesting preliminary information regarding the role of grandparents in the process of the intergenerational transmission of religious values. Future studies should include families with more racial and ethnic diversity. In addition, a broader range of family structures should be included in future analyses. Certainly, given the demographic, normative, and religious shifts occurring in America in particular, there is more to understand about the intergenerational transmission of religion across cohorts, especially younger cohorts. Additionally, the persistence of the moral agency and resiliency of the family will continue to be put to the test, as future trends and technological advancements emerge.

CONCLUSION

Three key factors link the work of Hayward and Bengston et al.: (a) the role of individualism, (b) family, and (c) context. The focus on self-development (i.e., individualism) has had a profound effect on marriage. Moreover, individualism is an inherent component of religion in our culture in that adopting any given religion is the right of every American. Marriages are shaped by sociohistorical, economic, familial, and cultural contexts—as is religiousness, to a great extent. Thus American youth coming of age today will likely experience shifts in marital trends, in addition to shifts in religious values, as a result of changes in the contexts in which they live. If the desire for individualism grows, so, too, may the desire of these youth to find their own religious paths—rather than adopting their families' beliefs. Only time will tell, as trends shift and shift again.

REFERENCES

Anderson, L. (2001). Religion and family. In J. M. Hawes (Ed.), *The family in America: An encyclopedia* (pp. 808–816). Santa Barbara, CA: ABC-Clio.

Arnett, J. J. (2000). Emerging adulthood: A theory of development from the late teens through the twenties. *American Psychologist, 55,* 469–480.

Arnett, J. J., & Jensen, L. A. (2002). A congregation of one: Individualized religious beliefs among emerging adults. *Journal of Adolescent Research, 17,* 451–467.

Avalos, H. (2004). *Introduction to the U.S. Latina and Latino religious experience.* Boston: Brill.

Axinn, W. G., & Thornton, A. (2000). The transformation in the meaning of marriage. In L. J. Waite (Ed.), *The ties that bind: Perspectives on marriage and cohabitation* (pp. 147–165). New York: Aldine de Gruyter.

Bengston, V. L. (2001). Beyond the nuclear family: The increasing importance of multigenerational bonds. *Journal of Marriage and Family, 63,* 1–16.

Bernard, J. (1970). Women, marriage, and the future. *Futurist, 4,* 41–43.

Braiker, B. (2007, March 31). Newsweek Poll: 90% believe in God. *Newsweek.* Retrieved March 10, 2008, from http://www.msnbc.msn.com/id/17879317/site/newsweek/print/0/displaymode/1098/

Bryant, C. M., Bolland, J. M., Burton, L., Hurt, T., & Bryant, B. (2006). The changing social context of relationships. In P. Nollar & J. Feeney (Eds.), *Close relationships: Functions, forms and processes* (pp. 25–47). New York: Psychology Press.

Bumpass, L. L., & Lu, H. (2000). Trends in cohabitation and implications for children's family contexts in the United States. *Population Studies, 54*, 29–41.

Burgess, E. W., & Locke, H. J. (1945). *The family: From institution to companionship.* New York: American Book Company.

Burton, S., & Blair, E. (1991). Task conditions, response formulation processes and response accuracy for behavioral frequency questions in surveys. *Public Opinion Quarterly, 55*, 50–79.

Casper, L., & Bianchi, S. M. (2002). *Continuity and change in the American family.* Thousand Oaks, CA: Sage.

Cherlin, A. (1992). *Marriage, divorce, remarriage.* Cambridge, MA: Harvard University Press.

Cherlin, A., & Furstenberg, F. (1985). Styles and strategies of grandparenting. In V. L. Bengston & J. F. Robertson (Eds.), *Grandparenthood* (pp. 97–116). Beverly Hills, CA: Sage.

Cherlin, A. J., & Furstenberg, F. F. (1992). *The new American grandparent: A place in the family, a life apart.* Cambridge, MA: Harvard University Press.

Coleman, J. S. (1998). Social capital in the creation of human capital. *American Journal of Sociology, 94*(Suppl.), S95–S120.

Coontz, S. (2005). *Marriage, a history: How love conquered marriage.* New York: Penguin Books.

Corrigan, J., Morgan, D., Silk, M., & Williams, R. H. (2006). Forum: Electronic media and the study of American religion. *Religion and American Culture: A Journal of Interpretation, 16*, 1–24.

de Tocqueville, A. (1948). *Democracy in America.* New York: Alfred A. Knopf. (Original work published 1835)

Eden, K. (2000). Few good men: Why poor mothers don't marry or remarry. *American Prospect, January 3*, 26–51.

Fields, J. (2003). *Children's living arrangements and characteristics: March 2002* (Current Population Reports No. P20-574). Washington, DC: U.S. Census Bureau.

Fukuyama, F. (1997). *The Tanner Lectures on human values.* Oxford, England: Brasenose College.

Fukuyama, F. (1999). *The great disruption.* New York: Free Press.

Gadlin, H. (1977). Private lives and public order: A critical view of the history of intimate relations in the United States. In G. Levinger & H. L. Raush (Eds.), *Close relationships: Perspectives on the meaning of intimacy* (pp. 33–72). Amherst: University of Massachusetts Press.

Goldstein, J. R., & Kenney, K. T. (2001). Marriage delayed or marriage forgone? New cohort forecasts of first marriage for U.S. women. *American Sociological Review, 66*, 506–519.

Hadaway, C. K., & Marler, P. L. (2005). How many Americans attend worship each week? An alternative approach to measurement. *Journal for the Scientific Study of Religion, 44*, 307–322.

Hernandez, D. J., & Meyers, D. E. (1993). *America's children: Resources from family, government, and the economy.* New York: Russell Sage Foundation.

Hervieu-Leger, D. (1993). Present-day emotional renewals: The end of secularization or the end of religion? In W. H. Swatos (Ed.), *A future for religion? New paradigms for social analysis* (pp. 129–148). Thousand Oaks, CA: Sage.

King, V., & Elder, G. H. (1999). Are religious grandparents more involved grandparents? *Journals of Gerontology, Ser. B, 54,* S317–S328.

Kohut, A., Green, J. C., Keeter, S., & Toth, R. (2000). *The diminishing divide: Religion's changing role in American politics.* Washington, DC: Brookings Institution Press.

Larsen, E. (2004). Deeper understanding, deeper ties: Taking faith online. In P. N. Howard & S. Jones (Eds.), *Society online* (pp. 43–56). Thousand Oaks, CA: Sage.

Layard, R. (2005). *Happiness: Lessons from a new science.* New York: Penguin Books.

Lichter, D. T., Batson, C. D., & Brown, J. B. (2004). Welfare reform and marriage promotion: The marital expectations and desires of single and cohabiting mothers. *Social Service Review, 78,* 2–24.

Lipset, S. M. (1996). *American exceptionalism.* New York: W. W. Norton.

Marler, P. L., & Hadaway, C. K. (2002). "Being religious" or "being spiritual" in America: A zero-sum proposition? *Journal for the Scientific Study of Religion, 41*(2), 289–300.

Mauldon, J. G., London, R. A., Fein, D. J., Patterson, R., & Bliss, S. (2002). *What do they think? Welfare recipients' attitudes toward marriage and childbearing.* Cambridge, MA: Abt Associates.

Meacham, J. (2007, April). Is God Real? [U.S. Edition]. *Newsweek, 149*(14), 54.

Miller, A. S., & Stark, R. (2002). Gender and religiousness: Can socialization explanations be saved? *American Journal of Sociology, 107,* 1399–1423.

Mintz, S., & Kellogg, S. (1988). *Domestic revolutions: A social history of American family life.* New York: Free Press.

Olson, D., & DeFrain, J. (2006). *Marriages and families: Intimacy, diversity, and strengths.* Boston: McGraw-Hill.

Paris, P. J. (1995). *The spirituality of African peoples.* Minneapolis, MN: Fortress Press.

Pew Research Center. (2005). *Trends 2005.* Washington, DC. Retrieved on March 7, 2008, from http://pewresearch.org/assets/files/trends2005.pdf

Sherkat, D. E. (2001). Tracking the restructuring of American religion: Religious affiliation and patterns of religious mobility, 1973–1998. *Social Forces, 79,* 1459–1493.

Silver, B., Anderson, B. A., & Abramson, P. R. (1986). Who over-reports voting? *American Political Science Review, 80,* 613–624.

Smith, C., Lundquist-Denton, M., Faris, R., & Regnerus, M. (2005). Mapping American adolescent religious participation. *Journal for the Scientific Study of Religion, 41,* 597–612.

Thornton, A. (1989). Changing attitudes toward family issues in the United States. *Journal of Marriage and Family, 51,* 873–893.

Thornton, A., & Young-DeMarco, L. (2001). Four decades of trends in attitudes toward family issues in the United States: The 1960s through the 1990s. *Journal of Marriage and Family, 63,* 1009–1037.

Tolstoy, L. (2000). *Anna Karenina.* R. Pevear & L. Volokhonsky (Trans.). London: Penguin Books. (Original work published in 1877.)

Tucker, M. B., & Mitchell-Kernan, C. (1995). Trends in African American family formation: A theoretical and statistical overview. In M. B. Tucker & C. Mitchell-Kernan (Eds.), *The decline in marriage among African Americans* (pp. 3–26). New York: Russell Sage Foundation.

Turner, B. S. (2005). Talcot Parson's sociology of religion and the expressive revolution. *Journal of Classical Sociology, 5,* 303–315.

U.S. Census Bureau. (2007, February). *The American community—Blacks: 2004.* American Community Survey Reports. Retrieved February 29, 2008, from http://www.census.gov/prod/2007pubs/acs-04.pdf

Wallace, J. M., Forman, T. A., Caldwell, C., & Willis, D. S. (2003). Religion and U.S. secondary school students: Current patterns, recent trends and sociodemographic correlates. *Youth and Society, 35,* 98–125.

Whitehead, B. D., & Popenoe, D. (2002). *Why men won't commit: Exploring young men's attitudes about sex, dating and marriage.* The State of Our Unions: The Social Health of Marriage in America, The National Marriage Project. Retrieved March 7, 2008, from http://marriage.rutgers.edu/Publications/SOOU/SOOU2002.pdf

Zambrana, R. (2004). *Understanding Latino families: Scholarship, policy, and practice.* Thousand Oaks, CA: Sage.

Subject Index

Exercise programs, recruiting older
  adults into, 51
Experience sampling paradigms, 118
Exterogestation, 5
Extraversion, 160

Factories and firms, 271
Faith-based human service
  initiatives, 93
Falls in older people, 53, 62, 64
Families
  and careers, 202
  religious socialization, 307, 308, 327
  and television, 287, 295
  traditional and nontraditional
    families, 347
  See also International family change
Family and community life, Vietnam,
  television, and the elderly, 297
Family structure and social institutional
  forces, 335–344
  changes in women's and men's labor
    market positions, 338–339
  commentary on, 346–355
  demographic shifts, 346
  first demographic transition,
    339, 341
  grandparents rearing grandchildren,
    340–341
  historical context, 346–347
  individualism and self-fulfillment, 339,
    346, 347, 361
  public policy implications, 335,
    341–343
  retreat from marriage, 336–338.
    See also Marriage
  second demographic transition,
    339–341, 343, 346
  social stratification, 340, 343
  traditional and nontraditional
    families, 347
Famines, 276
Fast-food industries, 16
Feral children, 4–5
First demographic transition,
  339, 341
Flexibility of *Homo sapiens*, 5–6, 18
Flexible life course (three-box life), 206,
  207, 208
fMRI. *See* Functional magnetic resonance
  imaging
Foraging, 258, 259, 260, 262–263

Foraging bands, 262–263, 276, 281
Foster care, 341
Functional magnetic resonance imaging
  (fMRI), 125, 161

Gatekeeping, 11
GATT agreement, 277
Gender effect, Religion and
  intergenerational transmission over
  time, 358–359
Generativity, 219, 223
Genotypes and phenotypes, changes in,
  176–177
Geographic stability, and careers, 203
George's story, 271–272, 278, 280
Gerontechnology, 168
Gerontological Society, 246
Gerontology
  emerging as a science, 233–234
  theories of change in, 255–257
  See also Cultural tansformations,
    history, and aging
"Gerontranscendance"
  (Joan Erikson), 241
Globalization, 243, 257, 282
  as cultural transformation, 276,
    277–278
  of economic activity, 173–174, 225
  of international family change
    media, 289
Goal setting, 53–54
Grandparents
  rearing grandchildren, 340–341
  religious influence and parental
    divorce, 323–325
  religious influence on grandchildren,
    309, 321, 323, 345

Haida communities, 267–268
Health behavior pathways (levels),
  98–99
  connections among, 50–60, 102,
    103
  life span perspective, 27
  physiological processes, 59–60, 99
  psychology of the aging self,
    51–55, 99
  social/cultural context, 55–58, 99
  theoretical model for, 26, 27,
    98–99
  See also Behavioral change in reduction
    of health risk

Author Index

Printed in the United States
202978BV00001BC/1/P

9 780826 124081